second edition

PHARMACOLOGY
for technicians

Don A. Ballington, M.S.
Midlands Technical College
Columbia, South Carolina

Mary M. Laughlin, Pharm.D., M.Ed.
Regional Medical Center
Memphis, Tennessee

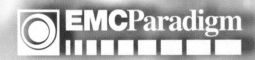

EMCParadigm

Developmental Editor	Christine Hurney
Associate Editor	Desiree Faulkner
Editorial Assistant	Susan Capecchi
Indexer	Nancy Fulton
Photo Researcher	Joan D'Onofrio
Cover and Text Designer	Michelle Lewis
Illustrator	Precision Graphics
Photos	Credits follow index

Publishing Management Team

George Provol, Publisher; Janice Johnson, Director of Product Development; Tony Galvin, Acquisitions Editor; Lori Landwer, Marketing Manager; Shelley Clubb, Electronic Design and Production Manager

---

Library of Congress Cataloging-in-Publication Data

Ballington, Don A.
   Pharmacology for technicians / Don A. Ballington, Mary M. Laughlin.-- 2nd ed.
     p. cm.
   Includes index.
   ISBN 0-7638-1527-6 (text)
    1. Pharmacology. 2. Pharmacy technicians. I. Laughlin, Mary M. II. Title.

   RM300 .B22 2003
   615'.1--dc21   2001054476

Text ISBN 0-7638-1527-6
Product Number 01563

Care has been taken to verify the accuracy of information presented in this book. The authors, editors, and publisher, however, cannot accept responsibility for errors or omissions or for consequences from application of the information in this book and make no warranty, expressed or implied, with respect to its content.

Some of the product names used in this book have been used for identification purposes only and may be trademarks or registered trademarks of their respective manufacturers.

Printed in the United States of America.

10 9 8 7 6 5 4 3 2

Contents

UNIT 4
RESPIRATORY, GI, RENAL, AND CARDIAC DRUGS......191

UNIT 5
NONNARCOTIC ANALGESICS, MUSCLE RELAXANTS, HORMONES, AND TOPICALS........................309

UNIT 6
CHEMOTHERAPY, HERBS, AND MISCELLANEOUS DRUGS 397

Chapter 17
Recombinant Drugs and Chemotherapy 399

Chapter 18
Vitamins, Nutritional Supplements, Natural Supplements, Antidotes, and CODE Blue Emergencies 429

Contents

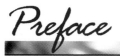
Preface

Pharmacology for Technicians, Second Edition by Don Ballington and Mary M. Laughlin is designed to support a comprehensive pharmacology course that allows students to acquire the drug knowledge and dispensing information needed for completing certification requirements and securing employment as pharmacy technicians.

The role of the pharmacy technician in today's pharmacy is both challenging and rewarding. Technicians are asked to perform many critical tasks. It is extremely important that they perform these tasks in the correct way, and they must be well versed in basic pharmaceutical concepts.

Material in this text is presented with the goal of giving students full insight into the dispensing of medications. An emphasis is placed on drug classes and the mechanisms of action in order to provide an understanding of why certain drugs are prescribed for particular disease states. This important background information will help students make intelligent decisions when dispensing drugs and will help them play an active role in avoiding errors.

This book is designed to help students develop a commitment to the pharmacy field with the hope that, as pharmacy technicians, they will be challenged by this constantly changing field and motivated to learn more about the body and the drugs that heal and make patients' lives more comfortable.

Improvements to the second edition include

- ◇ expanded treatment of generic drugs, the drug approval process, and pharmacokinetics
- ◇ Internet research exercises that introduce students to important sources of information about drugs and diseases
- ◇ warning sidebars alerting students to look-alike and sound-alike drug names
- ◇ full-color diagrams and enhanced layout to improve presentation of information

How This Text Is Organized

Pharmacology for Technicians, Second Edition is divided into six units.

- ◇ Unit 1 The Science of Pharmacology
- ◇ Unit 2 Anti-Infectives and Drugs for the Common Cold
- ◇ Unit 3 Narcotic Pain Relievers and Other Nervous System Drugs
- ◇ Unit 4 Respiratory, GI, Renal, and Cardiac Drugs
- ◇ Unit 5 Nonnarcotic Analgesics, Muscle Relaxants, Hormones, and Topicals
- ◇ Unit 6 Chemotherapy, Herbs, and Miscellaneous Drugs

The chapters within Unit 1 provide important foundation material to help students understand the specific drug information provided in the later units. Within this section, the discussion of the drug testing and approval process, pharmacokinetics, and issues related to drug actions and responses have been expanded. Later chapters apply this foundation information to the treatment of specific diseases and conditions.

How Chapters Are Organized

Each chapter begins with Learning Objectives and ends with a Chapter Summary. These pedagogical tools will help students study and remember the important points raised in each chapter.

Units 2 through 6, including a total of fifteen chapters, provide an overview of the drug group and the diseases these medications are designed to treat is provided along with tables of the most-commonly used agents in the particular group. A discussion of the major side effects and associated dispensing issues is included for key drugs in the group. Warning sidebars highlight possible dispensing errors due to look-alike and sound-alike drug names.

Chapters in these units also include a summary of the drugs presented in the chapter, and the Chapter Review section provides an opportunity for students to test their comprehension of the concepts presented in the chapter. Two new Internet research exercises have been added to each chapter to encourage students to use the Internet to expand and update chapter materials. These exercises are designed to encourage critical thinking and practice communicating using the language of pharmacology.

Resources for the Student

In addition to the end-of-chapter exercises found in the textbook, students are encouraged to use the workbook to reinforce the information taught in the text. The workbook that accompanies *Pharmacology for Technicians, Second Edition* includes additional exercises for Chapters 2 through 18. New exercises in this edition of the workbook include communication exercises that can be completed as individual writing assignments or group discussion problems. Each chapter includes a new exercise type called "Alert the Pharmacist: Prevention of Medication Errors" which asks students to deal with common prescription problems. Exercises also include items that ask students to interpret drug labels and prescriptions and provide students with the opportunity to demonstrate their understanding of generic and brand drug names.

Online quizzes and drug name practice is available on the Internet Resource Center for this title at www.emcp.com.

Resources for the Instructor

In addition to suggested course syllabus information, the Instructor's Guide that accompanies *Pharmacology for Technicians, Second Edition* includes answers for all end-of-chapter exercises and all workbook exercises. It also provides teaching hints for each chapter and ready-to use tests for chapter, unit, midterm, and final examinations.

Tests and an item testbank are available at the password-protected section of the Internet Resource Center for this title at www.emcp.com.

WebCT and Blackboard Web course management systems are available. Each comes preloaded with course information, contents, and quizzes.

In addition to *Pharmacology for Technicians, Second Edition*, Paradigm Publishing Inc. also publishes *Pharmacy Practice for Technicians, Second Edition*, and *Pharmacy Calculations for Technicians, Second Edition*. Both of these titles are supported with instructor's guides, testbank, and Web course management systems. A workbook is also available for the *Pharmacy Practice for Technicians, Second Edition* title.

About the Authors

Don A. Ballington, M.S., serves as program coordinator for the pharmacy technician training program at Midlands Technical College in Columbia, South Carolina. He has served as president of the Pharmacy Technician Educators Council and consulting editor for the *Journal of Pharmacy Technology*. Over the course of his career at Midlands Technical College, he has developed and refined a set of training materials. These materials were developed into *Pharmacology for Technicians, Pharmacy Calculations for Technicians,* and *Pharmacy Practice for Technicians*. All of these books are now available in second editions.

Mary M. Laughlin holds a Pharm.D. and an M.Ed. In addition to being co-author of *Pharmacology for Technicians,* she is co-author of *Pharmacy Calculations for Technicians*. Dr Laughlin has been an item writer for both NABPLEX and the PTCE. Currently she is assistant director of the pharmacy at the Regional Medical Center in Memphis, Tennessee and assistant professor of pharmacology and pharmacoeconomics at the College of Pharmacy, located on the campus of the University of Tennessee, Health Science Center in Memphis, Tennessee.

Acknowledgments

The authors would like to thank the editorial team at Paradigm Publishing Inc. as well as the following list of reviewers and contributors for their expert advice and opinions on how to make this an effective textbook program.

Gail B. Askew, Pharm.D., FCSHP
Santa Ana College
Santa Ana, CA

Ruben Baray
United Education Institute
Irvine, CA

Cheri Boggs, CPhT, BA
El Paso Community College
El Paso, TX

Richard Franco
Apollo College
Tucson, AZ

Gloria Gendi, RPh, BS
San Jacinto College North
Houston, TX

James R. Hickmon
Cape Fear Community College
Wilmington, NC

Beulah Hofmann, RN, MSn, BSn, CMA
Ivy Tech State College
Terre Haute, IN

Carol Lee Jarrell, MLT
Commonwealth Business College
Merrillville, IN

Cindy Johnson
Arapaho Community College
Littleton, CO

Leonard Lichtblau, PhD
EduMed, Inc.
Bloomington, MN
University of Minnesota School
   of Nursing
Minneapolis, MN

Shawn Madison
Eastern School of Technology
Virginia Beach, VA

Ann Malosh, M.Ed.
Linn-Benton Community College
Albany, OR

Doris Monroe
American Institute of Health
  Technology, Inc.
Boise, ID
Saint Luke's Regional Medical Center
Boise, ID

Kathy Moscou, RPh, BS
North Seattle Community College
Seattle, WA

Pamela L. Neu, CMA, BS
International Business College
Wolcottville, IN

David Olugbami
Richland College
Dallas, TX

Bruce Raby
San Jacinto College, South
Houston, TX

Deborah J. Randall
Children's Healthcare of Atlanta
Atlanta, GA
Professional Career Development
  Institute
Norcross, GA

Kathy Ricossa
Mission Community College
Santa Clara, CA

Sandra Simon, RPh
Foothill College
Los Altos Hills, CA

Tina Stacy, Pharm.D., BCOP
Northside Hospital
Atlanta, GA

Debbie Sturm
Gray's Harbor College
Aberdeen, WA

Gregory R. Tausz, RPh, BS
Rutgers, The State University of
  New Jersey
Morristown, NJ

Sandi Tschritter, CPhT
Spokane Community College
Spokane, WA

Valerie L. Wagner
California Paramedical and
  Technical College
Long Beach, CA
Southeast Regional Occupational
  Program
Cerritos, CA

Neal F. Walker, RPh
University Medical Center—Mesabi
Hibbing, MN
University of Minnesota College
  of Pharmacy
Minneapolis, MN

The authors and editorial staff encourage your feedback on the text and its supplements. Please reach us by clicking the "Contact Us" button at www.emcp.com.

The Science of Pharmacology

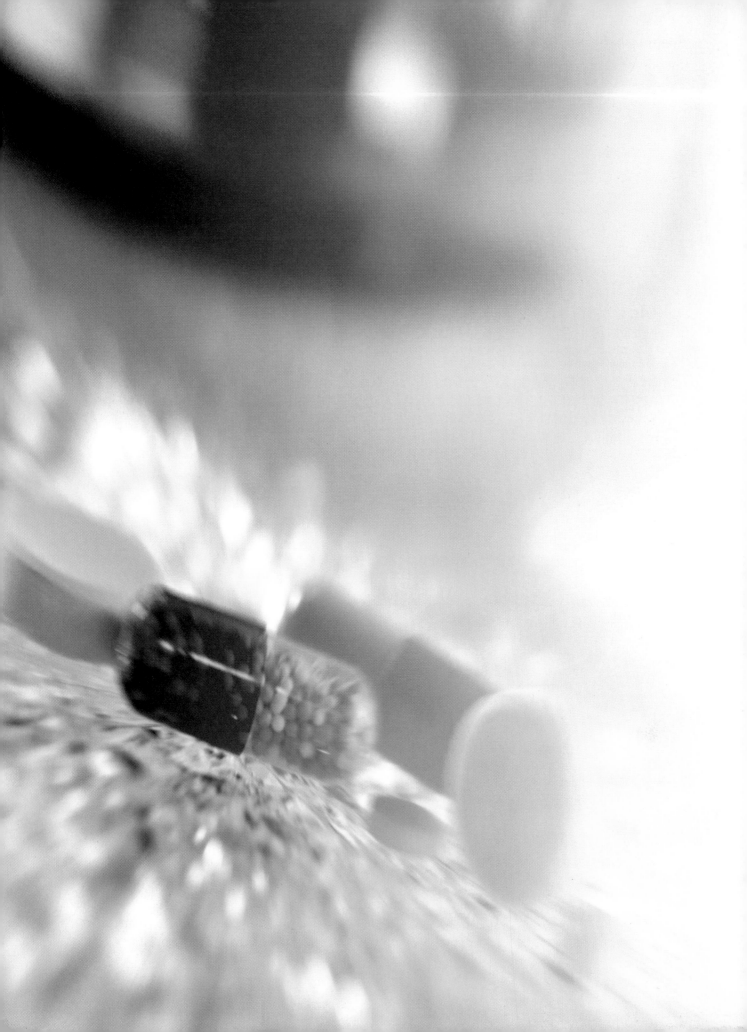

The Evolution of Medicinal Drugs

Chapter

1

Learning Objectives

◇ Recognize the important figures, events, and resources in the development of pharmacology through the ages.

◇ Know what is meant by pharmacology.

◇ Define drugs, identify their sources, and understand how they work.

◇ Be familiar with the federal laws that regulate drugs and the agencies that administer them.

◇ Be familiar with the procedure for getting a new drug to market.

The use of drugs to treat illnesses has changed dramatically since early civilizations first attempted to heal the sick. Pharmacology today is based on solid science and systematic research rather than anecdotal information and trial and error. During the twentieth century, the discovery of many new drugs has revolutionized medical care, and a rational system of laws governing drug manufacture and distribution has been developed to protect patients. Under current law, all new drugs need proof that they are effective, as well as safe, before they can be approved for marketing.

THE HISTORY OF MEDICINAL DRUGS

Ancient documents indicate that people have been treating physical and mental ailments with some type of medicine for thousands of years. Clay tablets from Babylonia, from the eighteenth century B.C., list more than 500 medicinal remedies. What has changed over the centuries is how the causes of disease are determined and which substances are used as medicine.

Early humans believed the world was controlled by good and evil spirits. The sick were considered victims of evil forces or of a god's anger. Religious leaders largely controlled medical treatment. These shamans, or priests and priestesses, guarded their healing knowledge closely. By their trial and error, folk knowledge of the healing properties of natural substances grew.

Early Remedies

Plants and naturally occurring substances were the main sources of early medicine. They were administered in some of the same ways used today: topically, orally, and rectally. The *Ebers Papyrus*, an Egyptian medical source compiled around 1550 B.C., lists more than 700 different herbal remedies used by healers. These remedies consisted of drugs drawn from the natural environment, using botanical drugs such as castor bean, garlic, and poppyseed for internal use. The most common mixtures

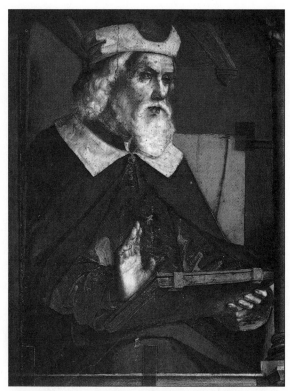

Hippocrates proposed that disease came from natural rather than supernatural causes and was the first to dissect the human body to study the functions of specific organs.

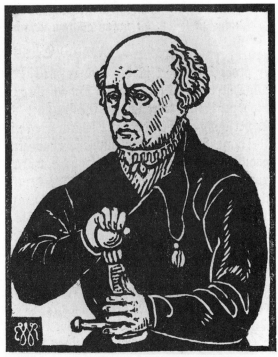

Paracelsus understood that if not dosed correctly, a medicine could easily become a poison.

were laxatives and enemas. Early Greek records include the concept of drug, or *Pharmakon*. This word means magic spell, remedy, or poison.

Hippocrates (c. 460–377 B.C.) was first to propose that disease came from natural rather than supernatural causes. Although he practiced herbal medicine, he rejected unsupported theory and superstition in favor of observation and classification, or empirical learning. Hippocrates was also first to dissect the human body to study the functions of specific organs.

Another Greek, Galen (c. A.D. 130–201), lived in Rome and built on Hippocrates' ideas of empirical learning. A follower of Aristotelian concepts, he believed disease was caused by an imbalance of one of four "humors"—blood, phlegm, black bile, and yellow bile. Illnesses were cured with an herbal compound of an opposing quality (moist, dry, cold, or warm). Galen's vast writings about these compounds, known as galenicals, influenced medical knowledge for more than 1,000 years.

The document *de Materia Medica*, compiled by Dioscrides in the first century A.D., was a major influence on European pharmaceutical knowledge until the sixteenth century. In it, Dioscrides scientifically described and classified 600 plants by substance rather than by the disease they were intended to treat.

Drugs in the Middle Ages

During the Middle Ages, as the Christian church became a stabilizing cultural force, the practice of medicine and pharmacy passed again from lay practitioners to religious leaders. Monasteries became centers of treatment and intellectual life. Monks wrote medical texts and grew herb gardens of medicinal plants.

The Swiss surgeon Paracelsus (1493–1541) was the first to challenge the teachings of Galen. He denounced the philosophy of humors in medicine and advocated use of individual drugs rather than mixtures or potions. He reasoned that treating diseases with individual drugs would make it easier to identify what agent helped, what made the patient worse, and how much of a drug was needed. These concepts are still used today.

Near the end of the Middle Ages, two of the earliest official listings of medical preparations, or pharmacopoeias, were written. The *Nuovo Receptario* was compiled by doctors in Florence,

Italy and published in 1498. In 1546, Valerius Cordis published the *Dispensatorium* in Nuremberg, Germany.

Drugs in the Modern Age

The seventeenth and eighteenth centuries were times of advancement in pharmacy and chemistry. London physicians eliminated many outlandish drug preparations when the first London pharmacopoeia was compiled in 1618. Some drug mixtures introduced at this time, such as tincture of opium, cocoa, and ipecac, are still used today.

In the nineteenth century, French physiologist Claude Bernard (1813–1878) advanced the knowledge of how drugs work on the body when he demonstrated that certain drugs have specific sites of action within the body. He is credited with starting the field of experimental pharmacology because of his use of laboratory methods to study drugs.

Claude Bernard demonstrated that certain drugs have specific sites of action within the body and used laboratory methods to study drugs.

American Pharmacology

Unlike Central and South America with their treasures to confiscate or spices to export, North America held little to attract medical personnel. As a result, early settlers were left to rely on domestic or kitchen medicine from home remedies. As the colonies grew in the eighteenth century, they attracted a broader range of immigrants, including apothecaries (early pharmacists) from England.

During this time, as in Europe, most physicians owned the dispensary or pharmacy. They prescribed, prepared, and dispensed drugs imported from Britain. The American Revolution forced American physicians, druggists, and wholesale distributors of drugs to manufacture their own chemically based drugs and make common preparations of crude drugs.

In 1820, the United States' first official listing of drugs, the *Pharmacopoeia of the United States*, was published by the Massachusetts Medical Society, with approval from a national convention of physicians. By the nineteenth century, in the United States and Europe, a division between those medical practitioners who treated patients and those primarily interested in preparing medicines had emerged. Practitioners who treated patients supported the growth of the pharmaceutical profession because it released them from compounding medicines and stocking a shop. Not until after the American Civil War (1861–1865) were boundaries between the professions clearly drawn.

William Proctor Jr. is considered to be the father of American Pharmacy. His statue resides in the rotunda of the American Pharmaceutical Association in Washington, D.C.

Twentieth Century Pharmacology

By the second half of the nineteenth century, pharmacology, the science of drugs and their interaction with the systems of living animals, had become a scientific discipline.

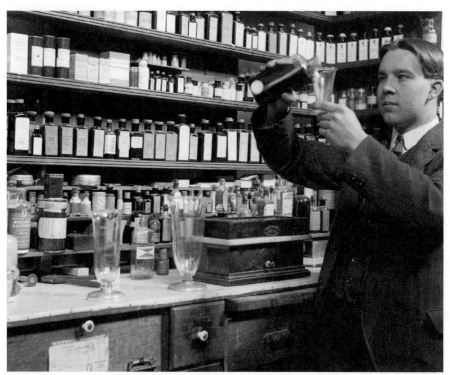

Dr. Emil King prepares medicine in his pharmacy in Fulda, MN, 1905.

Departments of pharmacology were opened in several European universities, a movement led by Oswald Schmiedeberg (1838–1921) at the University of Strasbourg in Germany.

Major breakthroughs in medical care came with the discovery of several important drugs. Ignaz Philip Semmelweis helped reduce death from puerperal fever in 1847 by requiring those entering maternity wards to first scrub their hands in chlorinated lime water. In the 1860s, Joseph Lister introduced antiseptics into surgery with his use of carbolic acid for cleansing instruments and ligatures.

Paul Ehrlich, a German bacteriologist, introduced arsphenamine, or Salvarsan, to treat syphilis in 1907. This rudimentary antibiotic was the first chemical agent used to treat a disease. In 1923, Sir Frederick Banting, a Canadian physiologist, and his assistant Charles Best successfully extracted the hormone insulin from the pancreas to create the first effective treatment for diabetes.

In 1935, the first antibiotic, the sulfa drug prontosil, was introduced by the German Gerhardt Domagk. It was followed about ten years later by the introduction of penicillin drugs after their discovery by bacteriologist Sir Alexander Fleming at St. Mary's Hospital in London.

PRESENT-DAY PHARMACOLOGY PRACTICE

Contemporary pharmacology is a science based on systematic research to determine the origin, nature, chemistry, effects, and uses of drugs. The growth of present-day pharmacologic knowledge has been greatly stimulated by the development of synthetic organic chemistry, which provided new tools and led to the development of new therapeutic agents.

As new drugs are introduced, it is essential that those who prescribe them also thoroughly understand them. Various practitioners are essential to carrying out the tasks required for appropriate and effective use of drugs in medical practice.

The Pharmacist and Pharmacy Technician

The pharmacist and pharmacy technician are important professionals on the healthcare team. The primary responsibility of the pharmacist is to see that drugs are dispensed properly and used appropriately. The technician assists the pharmacist in this endeavor.

It has become increasingly important for pharmacists to focus their expertise and judgment on direct patient care and counseling. Accordingly, responsibilities related to dispensing have shifted to the pharmacy technician.

A pharmacy technician is defined as an individual working in a pharmacy who, under the supervision of a licensed pharmacist, assists in activities not requiring the professional judgment of a pharmacist. The rules and regulations that set limits on the roles and responsibilities vary from state to state. Technicians are involved in all facets of drug distribution. A few of their responsibilities include

- receiving written prescriptions or requests for prescription refills from patients or their caregivers
- verifying that the information on the prescription is complete and accurate
- counting, weighing, measuring, and mixing the medication
- preparing prescription labels and selecting the container
- establishing and maintaining patient profiles
- ordering and stocking prescription and over-the-counter medications
- assisting with drug studies
- taking prescriptions over the telephone
- transferring prescriptions
- tracking and reporting errors
- "tech check tech" in preparation of medicine carts

Four organizations—the American Pharmaceutical Association (APhA), the American Society of Health System Pharmacists (ASHP), the Illinois Council of Health-System Pharmacists (ICHP), and the Michigan Pharmacists Association (MPA)—have joined together to form the Pharmacy Technician Certification Board (PTCB) and to create a national certification program. The PTCB fosters standards and acts as the nationally recognized credentialing agency. It also administers the National Pharmacy Technician Certification Examination. Certified technicians must be recertified every two years. Pharmacy technicians with higher qualifications bring greater value to the pharmacy, enabling the healthcare team to bring an increased quality of care to the patient.

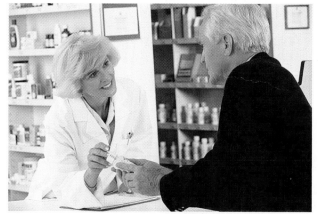

The pharmacist plays an important role in dispensing medications as well as instructing patients about side effects of medications, food and drug interactions, and dosing schedules.

Medicinal Drugs

Drugs (medications) are medicinal substances or remedies used to change the way a living organism functions. Drug actions on a living system are known as pharmacologic effects. Drugs are often classified according to their use. Therapeutic drugs relieve symptoms of a disease while prophylactic drugs are used to prevent or decrease the severity of disease.

[handwritten: to prevent the disease]

Drug Origins and Sources

The study and identification of natural sources for drugs is called pharmacognosy. Drugs come from a variety of sources: plant parts or products, animals, minerals, chemicals, and recombinant deoxyribonucleic acid (DNA).

Various parts of many plants can be used to make drugs. Examples of drugs that come from plants are ergotamine from rye fungi, digoxin from foxglove, and morphine from the opium poppy. Drugs from animal products include thyroid and insulin, which are obtained from domestic animal sources. Drugs from minerals include vitamins and silver nitrate.

Chemical substances are made into drugs synthetically. Drugs made synthetically include sulfonamides, aspirin, sodium bicarbonate, and many others. Bioengineered drugs are produced by recombinant DNA technology and are some of the most expensive drugs available. Current examples are Betaseron (interferon beta-1b), Avonex (interferon beta-1a), and Epogen (erythropoietin). Table 1.1 provides specific examples of drug sources along with corresponding drug names and therapeutic effect.

Drug Names and Classifications

Every drug has three names: a chemical name, a generic name, and a brand name. The chemical name describes the drug's chemical make-up. It is usually long and difficult to pronounce. The generic name is the name the manufacturer gives a drug. It often is a shortened version of the chemical name. The brand name, also called the trade name, is the name under which the manufacturer has patented the drug. It is copyrighted and used exclusively by that company.

The generic name for a commonly used drug begins with a lowercase letter—for example, erythromycin—whereas the trade name begins with a capital letter—such as E-Mycin. Both terms refer to the same drug. One generic drug can be manufactured by a variety of companies.

DRUG LEGISLATION AND REGULATION

The manufacture, sale, and use of drugs is regulated by our legal system. Federal laws govern the development, prescribing, and dispensing of drugs, providing a

Table 1.1	Drug Sources, Drug Names, and Their Therapeutic Effect	
Drug Source	**Drug Name**	**Therapeutic Effect**
plant: Foxglove	digitalis	cardiotonic
animal: stomach of hog and cow	pepsin	digestive enzyme
mineral: silver	silver nitrate	anti-infective
synthetic: omeprazole	Prilosec	gastric acid inhibitor
bioengineering: erythropoietin	Epogen	RBC stimulant

rational system of checks and balances to ensure everyone's safety. These laws have been developed and refined over the past century.

The Food and Drug Administration (FDA)

In 1906, the Federal Food and Drug Act, often referred to as the Pure Food and Drug Act, was passed as the first attempt by the United States government to regulate the sale of drugs or substances that affect the body.

In 1927, the Food, Drug, and Insecticide Administration was formed. In 1930, its name was changed to the Food and Drug Administration (FDA). This branch of the federal government is responsible for ensuring that any drug or food product approved for marketing is safe when used as directed on the label.

When the Food, Drug, and Cosmetic Act of 1938 passed, it required all new drugs to be proven safe before being marketed, initiating a system of drug regulation in the United States. The FDA controls adulteration or purity, labeling accuracy, and product safety. The basic definition of "safe" under this act was "nontoxic" when used in accordance with the conditions set forth on the label. This act also required that every new drug has been the subject of an approved New Drug Application (NDA) before United States commercialization. The NDA is the vehicle through which drug sponsors formally propose that the FDA approve a new pharmaceutical for sale and marketing in the United States. The NDA will be discussed further in the Drug Testing and Approval subsection of this chapter.

In 1951, the Durham-Humphrey Amendment established two classes of drugs. Legend drugs are sold only by prescription and are labeled, "Caution: Federal (U.S.A.) law prohibits dispensing without prescription." or "Rx only." Over-the-counter (OTC) drugs are sold without a prescription.

The FDA has the responsibility of regulating both legend and OTC drugs as well as medical and radiological devices, food, cosmetics, biologics, and veterinary drugs. The FDA does not test drugs itself, although it does conduct limited research in the areas of drug quality, safety, and effectiveness. (It is the responsibility of the company seeking to market a drug to test it and submit evidence that it is safe and effective.)

Controlled Substances Act

The Controlled Substances Act, Title II of the Comprehensive Drug Abuse Prevention and Control Act of 1970, was designed to combat escalating drug abuse. It promoted drug education and research into the prevention and treatment of drug dependence; strengthened enforcement authority; and designated schedules, or categories, for controlled substances according to their probability of abuse.

The Drug Enforcement Administration (DEA) was established in 1973 as a branch of the U.S. Justice Department. The DEA is responsible for regulating the sale and use of specified drugs. It works at the national, state, and local levels. Individuals and institutions which handle or prescribe any controlled substances must be registered by the DEA. The prescriber's DEA registry number must be associated with the prescription when it is filled.

There are five categories, or "schedules," of controlled substances. These schedules set the restrictions on the prescription of such substances. For example, schedule I drugs have the highest potential for abuse and have no accepted medical use. They may be used solely for research purposes. Table 1.2 overviews the five controlled substances schedules and includes the corresponding abuse potential, accepted medicinal uses, and example drugs for each category.

Table 1.2   **Schedules for Controlled Substances**

Schedule	Manufacturer's Label	Abuse Potential	Accepted Medical Use	Examples
schedule I	C-I	highest potential for abuse	For research only. Must have license to obtain. No accepted medical use in the United States.	heroin, lysergic acid diethyl-amide (LSD)
schedule II	C-II	high possibility of abuse, which can lead to severe psychological or physical dependence	Dispensing is severely restricted. Cannot be prescribed by phone except in an emergency. No refills on prescriptions.	morphine, oxycodone, meperidine, hydromor-phone, fentanyl
schedule III	C-III	less potential for abuse and addiction	Prescriptions can be refilled up to five times within six months if authorized by a physician.	codeine with aspirin, codeine with acetamino-phen, anabolic steroids
schedule IV	C-IV	low abuse potential; associated with limited physical or psychological dependence	Same as for schedule III.	benzodiazepines, meprobamate, phenobarbital
schedule V	C-V	lowest abuse potential	Some sold without a prescription depending on state law, purchaser must be over 18 and is required to sign a log and show a driver's license.	liquid codeine preparations

DRUG TESTING AND APPROVAL

The FDA requires that the manufacturer of any new drug provide evidence of its safety and effectiveness. Before a drug enters the United State's market, it must be proven safe through an intensive testing process. This process is undertaken by a drug sponsor—usually a pharmaceutical company. Drug sponsors are responsible for testing the drug's efficacy and safety on animals and, later, on human subjects through controlled clinical trials.

Before the clinical testing begins, researchers analyze the drug's main physical and chemical properties in the laboratory and study its pharmacologic and toxic effects in laboratory animals. A drug sponsor must request permission from the FDA to test any new drugs. Any hospital, physician, or researcher involved in experimental drug testing must also get FDA approval.

It is the responsibility of the company seeking to market a drug to test it and submit evidence that it is safe and effective. All test results are made available to the FDA through the New Drug Application (NDA), which also specifies the proposed labeling for the new drug.

The NDA details the entire history of the drug's development and testing. It documents the results of the animal studies and clinical trials; describes the drug's components and composition; explains how the drug behaves in the body; and provides the details of manufacturing, processing, and packaging, with a special emphasis on quality control. The FDA also requires that the NDA include samples of the drug and its labels. A team of FDA physicians, statisticians, chemists, pharmacologists, and other scientists then review the contents of the NDA. If proven safe and effective, the FDA will approve a drug.

Clinical Trials

If initial laboratory and animal model research on a particular drug is sufficiently promising, the developer will submit an application to the FDA requesting permission to begin testing the drug on humans. Human testing, referred to as a clinical trial, is used to determine whether new drugs or treatments are both safe and effective. Protocols for testing are typically developed by researchers and are subject to the approval of an FDA review board. These protocols describe what type of people may participate in the trial, the schedule of tests and procedures, medications and their dosages, and the length of the study. Throughout the trial phases, participants are monitored to determine the safety and efficacy of the drug. Only about twenty percent of the drugs that enter clinical trials are ultimately approved for marketing.

During clinical trials patients are typically separated into two groups. The experimental group receives the drug to be tested, while the control group receives either a standard treatment for the illness or a placebo. A placebo is an inactive substance that has no treatment value. In general, neither trial participants nor the study staff know whether a particular participant is in the experimental or control group. This practice, which allows for greater objectivity on the part of the investigators, is referred to as double-blinding.

Clinical trials of new drugs proceed through four phases.

- ◇ **Phase I** The drug is administered to a small group of people (20–100) to evaluate its safety, determine a safe dosage range, and identify side effects. Phase I studies assess the most common acute adverse effects and clarify what happens to a drug in the human body.
- ◇ **Phase II** The drug is studied in patients who have the condition it is intended to treat. It is determined at this point whether the drug has a favorable effect on the disease state. Short-term, placebo-to-drug comparisons are made in double-blind trials to determine the range and response of various doses.
- ◇ **Phase III** The drug treatment is compared to commonly used treatments. During this phase, investigators collect information that will allow the drug to be used safely. This phase continues the double-blind, placebo-to-drug comparisons begun in phase II. Dose escalations are used to determine the efficacy of the drug in treating the target disease.
- ◇ **Phase IV** Once the drug has been approved for marketing, phase IV studies continue testing it to collect information about its effects in various populations and to identify any side effects associated with long-term use.

The FDA Approval Process

In the past, the entire FDA approval process took from seven to ten years. However, the FDA has taken steps to make urgently needed drugs available sooner. The Prescription Drug User Fee Act of 1992 instituted reforms which shortened the review process for new drugs. This act required that drug companies pay fees upon the submission of NDAs and thereby created the funds to hire an adequate number of reviewers. The standard application for new drugs must now be acted on within ten months, and priority applications for drugs used to treat serious diseases must be acted on within six months.

The order in which applications are reviewed is determined with the aid of a classification system. Priority is given to drugs with the greatest potential benefit. Drugs that offer a significant medical advantage over existing therapies for any given disease state are assigned "priority status." Drugs for life-threatening diseases are considered first.

It is important to remember that no drug is absolutely safe. The FDA's approval is based on a judgment about whether a new drug's benefits to users will outweigh its risks. The FDA will allow a product to present more of a risk when its potential benefit is great—especially for products used to treat serious, life-threatening conditions.

Post-marketing Surveillance

The consumer's well-being is the FDA's most important concern. Public health cannot be safeguarded without procedures to monitor the quality of drugs once they are marketed. The FDA has a branch, the Office of Compliance, which oversees the drug manufacturing process, ensuring that manufacturers follow good manufacturing practices (GMPs) as spelled out in FDA regulations.

Some adverse reactions do not become apparent until after a drug has been approved and has been used by a significant number of people. Therefore, post-marketing surveillance to ensure that drugs that pose serious safety threats are promptly removed from the market is critical. MedWatch, the FDA Medical Products Reporting Program, is a system through which professionals and consumers can report serious adverse reactions. The purpose of this program is to improve the post-marketing surveillance of medical products and to ensure that new safety information pertaining to drug use is rapidly communicated to the medical community, thereby improving patient care. If a drug poses a health risk, the FDA will remove it from the market even though it has already been approved.

Generic Drugs

At some point in the drug development process, a drug sponsor will apply for patent protection. The patent protects the investment in the drug's development by granting the sponsor the sole right to manufacture the drug while the patent is in effect. Under patent protection, the drug's generic and brand names both belong to the sponsor. The manufacturer's proprietary right to the drug expires as soon as the patent expires, leaving other companies free to produce this drug as a nonpropri-etary, or generic, drug—either under their own brand name or under the generic name. When this occurs, the price differential between the brand name drug and the generic preparation is frequently substantial.

The substitution of generic drugs for more expensive brands is an important means of reducing healthcare costs and many insurance companies often require the use of generics if they are to reimburse patients for drug costs. Some insurance companies actually provide a list of brand name drugs whose cost they will cover.

Drug companies must submit an Abbreviated New Drug Application (ANDA) for approval to market a generic product. In approving a generic drug, the FDA requires many rigorous tests and procedures to assure that the drug is interchangeable with the innovator drug under all approved indications and conditions of use. The generic drug must meet the following requirements. It must

◇ contain the same active ingredients as the original brand name drug
◇ be identical in strength, dosage form, and route of administration

◇ have the same use indications
◇ meet the same batch requirements for identity, strength, purity, and quality
◇ yield similar blood absorption and urinary excretion curves for the active ingredient

When the above criteria are met, the generic drug will elicit similar pharmacologic effects to the innovator drug.

The FDA has devised an A/B rating system to establish the therapeutic equivalence of generic drugs. The rating indicates whether a drug has been judged by the agency to be therapeutically equivalent to the innovator drug by meeting the criteria of pharmaceutical equivalence, bioequivalence, labeling, and good manufacturing practices. The FDA has also identified generics that are not therapeutically equivalent. Although few drugs fall in this category, be aware that such drugs do exist.

Part of the responsibility of the healthcare practitioner is to decrease costs. Healthcare costs have risen at an alarming rate in this country, but pharmaceutical costs have not increased at the same rate—primarily because of generic drugs. According to the Congressional Budget Office, generic drugs save consumers an estimated $8 to $10 billion a year at retail pharmacies. Even more billions are saved when hospitals use generics.

FDA FOOD HEALTH CLAIMS

Weighing risks against benefits is the primary objective of the FDA. By ensuring that products and producers meet certain standards, the FDA protects consumers and enables them to know what they are receiving.

In July of 1999, the FDA authorized a new health claim that allowed food companies to promote disease-fighting and cancer-fighting benefits of whole grains in various breakfast cereals. Manufacturers of whole grain foods that contain 51% or more of whole grain ingredients by weight can now make the following claim: "Diets rich in whole grain foods and other plant foods and low in total fat, saturated fat, and cholesterol may reduce the risk of heart disease and certain cancers." In October of 1999, the FDA authorized the use of health claims about the role of soy protein in reducing the risk of coronary heart disease on the labels of foods. Consumers must realize that these products are not to be substituted for prescribed medications but are to be used in conjunction with drug therapy.

Chapter Summary

The History of Medicinal Drugs
- ◇ The very concept of influencing bodily function via an outside force must be considered one of humanity's greatest advances.
- ◇ Drugs have been used to gain increased control over our lives to make them better and longer. Throughout history, drugs have held a special fascination for humans.
- ◇ The twentieth century brought major breakthroughs in medical care. The first antibiotic, sulfa, was soon followed by penicillin.

Present-Day Pharmacology Practice
- ◇ Interactions between potent chemicals and living systems contribute to our knowledge of biologic processes and provide effective methods for diagnosing, treating, and preventing many diseases. Compounds used for these purposes are called drugs.
- ◇ Pharmacology is a broad term that includes the study of drugs and their actions on the body.
- ◇ Sources of drugs are plants, animals, minerals, synthetic materials, and bioengineering advances.

Drug Legislation and Regulation
- ◇ Laws govern the drug industry and protect patients' rights.
- ◇ Federal law divides controlled substances into five schedules according to their potential for abuse and clinical usefulness.

Drug Testing and Approval
- ◇ The FDA requires that all new drugs be proved effective and safe before they can be approved for marketing.
- ◇ Controlled clinical trials, in which results observed in patients getting the drugs are compared to the results in similar patients receiving a different treatment, are the best way to determine what a new drug really does.
- ◇ It is when the benefits outweigh the risks that the FDA considers a drug safe enough to be approved.
- ◇ Generic drugs must be equivalent to the brand name drugs and the FDA has devised an A/B rating system to establish this.

FDA Food Health Claims
- ◇ The FDA sets food labeling standards to ensure that consumers know what is in the food they are buying.

Chapter Review

Understanding Pharmacology

Select the best answer from the choices given.

1. The word *Pharmakon* means
   a. dosing methods.
   b. remedy.
   c. pharmacist in Greek.
   d. None of the above

2. Pharmacognosy is
   a. a broad term that includes the study of drugs and their actions on the body.
   b. the study and identification of natural sources of drugs.
   c. the treatment of disease.
   d. the combined effect of two drugs.

3. Claude Bernard
   a. was a French physiologist who demonstrated that certain drugs have specific sites of action within the body.
   b. grew herbs of medicinal value.
   c. is the father of American pharmacology.
   d. discovered penicillin.

4. Pharmacology is
   a. a broad term that includes the study of drugs and their actions on the body.
   b. the study and identification of natural sources of drugs.
   c. the treatment of disease.
   d. an unusual or unexpected response to a drug.

5. A pharmacy technician should never
   a. take prescriptions over the telephone.
   b. advise patients about the use of their medicine.
   c. mix IV solutions.
   d. maintain patient profiles.

6. The FDA is required to
   a. ensure that a drug is safe and effective.
   b. monitor drug safety after a drug has been approved for sale.
   c. approve drugs in a timely manner.
   d. All of the above

7. Which of the following drug schedules has no accepted medical use in the U.S.?
   a. Schedule I
   b. Schedule II
   c. Schedule III
   d. Schedule IV

8. Which of the following federal laws was designed to prevent drug abuse?
   a. Federal Food and Drug Act
   b. Durham-Humphrey Amendment
   c. Controlled Substances Act
   d. Prescription Drug User Fee Act

9. MedWatch is
   a. a program to shorten the review process for new drugs.
   b. an organization that sets standards for clinical trials.
   c. an initiative to encourage healthcare professionals to monitor for and report adverse drug events.
   d. an organization that registers pharmacists.

10. The FDA's approval of a new drug is based on
    a. the completion of the first three phases of clinical trials.
    b. evidence that a drug is effective in treating the condition for which it was intended.
    c. a judgment that a new drug's benefits to users will outweigh its risks.
    d. All of the above

The following statements are true or false. If the answer is false, rewrite the statement so it is true.

_F_ 1. Hippocrates introduced antiseptics to prevent infection.

_F_ 2. Dioscrides first dissected the human body to study the function of specific organs.

_T_ 3. Paracelsus advocated the use of individual drugs rather than mixtures or potions.

_F_ 4. Lister wrote *de Materia Medica.*

_T_ 5. The FDA requires that the manufacturer of any new drug provide evidence of its safety and effectiveness.

_T_ 6. The A/B rating system is a system for assessing generic drug equivalence.

_F_ 7. Controlled substances are divided into seven schedules.

_T_ 8. The DEA is a branch of the U.S. Justice Department that regulates manufacturing, distributing, and dispensing controlled substances.

_T_ 9. If two preparations are generically equivalent and their administration yields similar blood absorption and urinary excretion curves for the active ingredient, they are assumed to be therapeutically equivalent and to elicit similar pharmacological effects.

_____ 10. Once a patent expires, the drug may be produced in the generic form. The price differential is considerable when this occurs.

Pharmacology at Work

1. What are the requirements for dispensing schedule II and III prescriptions? Name some examples of each.
2. Describe the four phases in getting a drug to market. What would be the ramifications if the fourth stage were dropped?
3. Explain which requirements must be met before a generic drug is considered to be therapeutically equivalent to the brand. Would you or your family use generics?

Internet Research

Use the Internet to complete the following assignments.

1. Research the career options for trained pharmacy technicians. Write a short (two to three paragraphs) report outlining the qualifications sought by potential employers and explaining how this course will help you succeed in the job market. List at least two Internet sources.
2. Go to the FDA's Web site. Describe two pages within that site which you believe will be of interest to you in your career as a pharmacy technician. How does/will the information contained in those pages impact the marketing of drugs in the United States? List the complete URLs for the pages you selected.

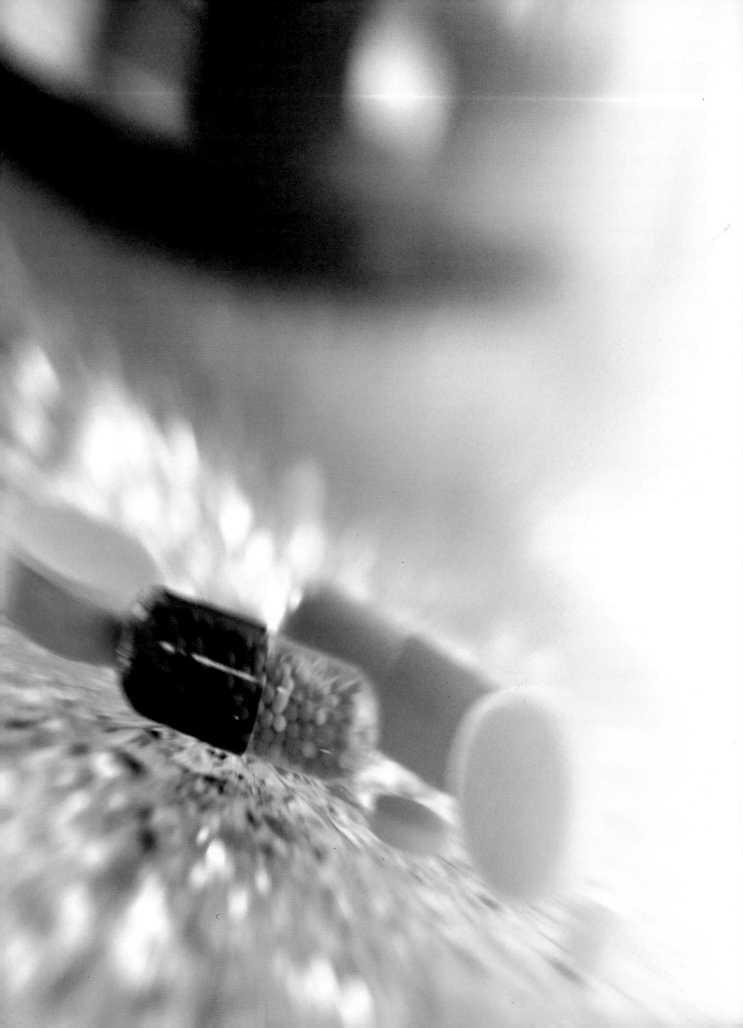

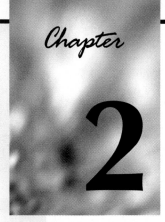

Introduction to Pharmacology

Learning Objectives

- ◇ Understand receptors and their function in mechanisms of drug actions.
- ◇ Be aware of the pharmacokinetics involved in developing and testing drugs.
- ◇ Understand that some drug effects are beneficial while others can be harmful.
- ◇ Be familiar with the common terms used to describe drug interactions.
- ◇ Understand the immunization process.

The goal of drug therapy is to produce a response in the body that results in the cure or control of a specific disease or condition. Drugs work via a series of processes, which can be described in the terms of pharmacokinetics. Pharmacokinetic studies reveal how drugs work in the body and provide critical insight for predicting the effects of each specific drug. An understanding of these processes enables the development of safe and effective treatments for various diseases.

RECEPTORS

To maintain homeostasis within a body, it is essential that the body's cells have the ability to communicate with each other. One of the ways that cells communicate is through the action of chemical messengers. These messengers, produced by cells, are sent out into the extra-cellular fluids of the body. Histamine, prostaglandin, and bradykinin are some important endogenous (i.e., originating from within the body) chemical messengers. These will be discussed in detail in Chapter 3.

Once the messenger has been released it can diffuse throughout the extra-cellular fluid to reach its "target cell." The target cell is recognized and communicated with via specific protein molecules present on the surface of or within the cell. These molecules are called receptors. A receptor is a molecule on the surface of or within a cell that recognizes and binds with specific molecules, producing some effect in the cell.

The various cell types within the body differ with regard to the types of receptors they contain, and only certain cell types possess the receptor required for combination with a particular chemical messenger. To bind with a specific cell type, the messenger must have a chemical structure which is complementary to the structure of that cell's receptors. This property of a receptor site is known as specificity. For example, the cells involved in immune responses have receptors that are highly specific to bacteria, viruses, and some cancer cells. Receptors mediate many important bodily functions such as blood clotting and smooth muscle contraction, and play an important role in the body's protection against injury and infection.

The strength by which a particular messenger binds to its receptor site is referred to as its affinity for the site. Affinity is an important concept for understanding how drugs work in the body.

MECHANISMS OF DRUG ACTION

Drugs often act like the chemical messengers described above to exert powerful and specific actions in the body. Some drugs bind to a particular receptor and trigger the cell's response in a similar way to the body's own chemical messenger. These drugs are termed agonists.

Other drugs work via a competitive mechanism to block the action of the endogenous messenger. These drugs have a similar structure to the endogenous messenger and so may have a high affinity for the receptor site. When the drug binds to the receptor site, it blocks the action of the endogenous messenger. However, unlike the endogenous chemical, these drugs do not trigger the cell's response. These drugs are termed antagonists.

When two drugs have an affinity for a particular receptor, they will compete for available receptor sites. The relative number of receptors occupied by each drug will depend on the relative concentrations of each drug as well as the relative affinities of the receptor site for each drug. When two drugs try to bind to the same receptor, site antagonism occurs.

Some drugs produce their effects by interacting with chemically nonspecific membrane lipids. Their effectiveness is related to lipid solubility and does not depend on receptor sites. Examples of drugs that work this way are the volatile anesthetic agents.

Drugs can also combine with other proteins—such as enzymes, transport proteins, and with nucleic acids—rather than receptors. Some antidepressants work this way by blocking the uptake of serotonin by nerve terminals.

Other drugs act without any direct interaction with the cell. For example, drugs can work through an osmotic effect. Mannitol is such a drug. It interferes osmotically with water reabsorption by the kidneys.

PHARMACOKINETICS

Medications are given to produce a response that results in cure, control, or prevention of a specific disease. The study of pharmacokinetics enables researchers to understand how a drug works within the body to affect both normal physiology and disease. Pharmacokinetics describes the action of drugs in the body over a period of time. As such, it can be conceived of as a series of processes which produce specific effects.

Pharmacokinetic Processes

Each drug's pharmacokinetics can be described in terms of four processes of interaction with the body. These processes are absorption, distribution, metabolism, and elimination. An understanding of these processes provides an important framework for researchers who are responsible for the development of drugs. Figure 2.1 presents a schematic model of these processes.

Figure 2.1

The Pharmaco-kinetic Process
The main phases of drug/body interactions are absorption, distribution, metabolism, and elimination (ADME).

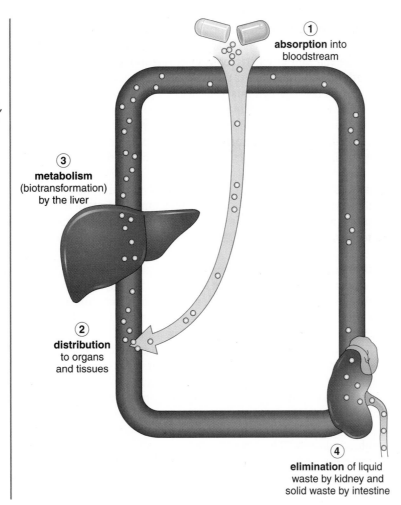

① **absorption** into bloodstream

③ **metabolism** (biotransformation) by the liver

② **distribution** to organs and tissues

④ **elimination** of liquid waste by kidney and solid waste by intestine

ABSORPTION Absorption describes the process whereby a drug enters the circulatory system. The absorption of a drug depends on its route of administration, solubility, and other physical properties. The solubility of the drug refers to its ability to dissolve in body fluids (e.g., blood). The form of the drug is an important factor in controlling its solubility. For example, drugs in liquid solution are already dissolved so they are absorbed more readily than those in capsule form.

The most common route of administration is the oral route. Other routes include intramuscular, subcutaneous, rectal, sublingual, transdermal, inhalation, and epicutaneous (topical) routes. Intravenous and intra-arterial administration (directly into systemic blood circulation) do not require absorption, as the drug is immediately available.

When an oral medication is not given as a solution, its rate of absorption is slowed by the time necessary for the tablet or capsule to release the drug (dissolution) and for the drug to dissolve in the gastrointestinal (GI) tract. Disintegration and dissolution depend on the physical properties of the drug and its dosage form. Factors affecting dissolution include the chemistry of the drug, the surface area of its particulates, as well as manufacturing variables. Some drugs interact with certain gastric contents, such as food. This effect subsequently reduces the amount of drug available for absorption.

The small intestine is the primary site of absorption because of its large surface area. When drugs are given orally, the degree of GI motility also affects absorption. The faster the rate of gastric emptying, the more rapid the absorption rate.

In the small intestine, the drug must cross the cell membrane of the epithelial cells. Membranes are composed of lipids, proteins, and carbohydrates. Pores are small openings or empty spaces in this membrane through which low-weight molecules pass freely. Lipid-soluble molecules, small hydrophilic molecules, and ions readily pass through this barrier. Some drugs may be metabolized by enzyme action within the epithelial cell before they reach systemic blood.

DISTRIBUTION Distribution is the process by which a drug moves from the blood-stream into other body fluids and tissues and ultimately to its sites of action, the receptors. Blood flow is the rate-limiting factor for distribution of a drug. Three additional factors also affect the rate and degree of distribution.

⬦ **Binding to Plasma Proteins** The biological activity of a drug is related to the concentration of "free" drug in circulation. The protein-bound portion of the drug is restricted from reaching its site of action and is essentially inactive. Once saturation binding occurs, the unbound drug increases and is available to be distributed to its site of action. This competition increases the plasma concentration of the free drug, which remains unbound and active. Disease states can also affect protein binding. Renal failure, for example, may result in a loss of plasma proteins (with less available for binding) or in the accumulation of metabolic wastes that could potentially displace some bound drugs. Liver disease may also result in fewer plasma proteins to transport drugs.

⬦ **Binding to Cellular Constituents** Drugs can also bind to other tissues besides blood plasma. This type of binding usually occurs when the drug has an affinity for some cellular constituent.

⬦ **Blood-Brain Barrier** The capillaries in the central nervous system (CNS) are enveloped by glial cells, which present a barrier to many water-soluble compounds though they are permeable to lipid-soluble substances. This barrier prevents many substances from entering the cerebrospinal fluid from the blood. Therefore, many drugs cannot get to the CNS because they are unable to pass through the blood-brain barrier. However, pathologic states such as inflammation will reduce this resistance and the barrier becomes more permeable. For example, while general anesthetics penetrate this barrier with ease, penicillin cannot penetrate the CNS unless the meninges are swollen.

METABOLISM Metabolism is a process by which drugs are converted to compounds and then excreted through metabolic pathways. These pathways are the routes for a number of processes. Through oxidation, electrons are lost and oxygen is added to a molecule. In the reduction pathway, electrons are gained and oxygen is lost. In conjugation, drug molecules combine with a highly water-soluble compound. In hydrolysis, adding water cleaves a compound, the hydroxyl group being incorporated into one portion and the hydrogen atom into another.

In general, metabolism converts drugs to more water-soluble (less lipid-soluble) forms. Once in a more water-soluble state, drug metabolites may be more easily excreted by the liver and kidney.

Many factors can alter metabolism and elimination. If given together, two drugs may decrease or enhance the metabolism of each other. Some drugs decrease the metabolism of other drugs by competitive or complete inhibition of a particular drug-metabolizing enzyme. Other drugs enhance drug metabolism by induction of these same enzyme systems. Disease states, age, and genetic predisposition all affect the way the body metabolizes drugs.

Enzymes in the cell's endoplasmic reticular membrane convert drugs from fat-soluble to water-soluble. These enzymes exist and play a major role in metabolism of endogenous substances (i.e., steroids, fat-soluble vitamins, and fatty acids). They are responsible for the metabolism of most drugs as well as toxins such as those in tobacco smoke, charcoal-broiled meat, polychlorinated biphenyls (PCBs), herbicides, and general combustion by-products. The enzymes convert lipophilic substances into more readily excreted water-soluble metabolites. Enzyme levels may be hyperstimulated, resulting in excessively rapid metabolism of drugs, or hypostimulated, increasing a compound's toxicity.

Two processes, induction and inhibition can control specific enzymes.

- ◇ **Induction** The concentration of a particular enzyme can be affected by some drugs, foods, and smoking. Drugs that increase these enzymes can decrease the pharmacologic response to other agents (e.g., phenobarbital increases the metabolism of warfarin) or to themselves (e.g., some barbiturates stimulate self-metabolism).
- ◇ **Inhibition** Some agents can slow or block enzyme activity, which impairs the metabolism of drugs and may increase their concentration and toxic or pharmacological effects. An example is Tagamet (cimetidine).

ELIMINATION Elimination occurs primarily in the kidney and the bowel, but other routes exist. Drugs may be exhaled by the lungs or excreted in perspiration, saliva, and breast milk. The elimination rate of a drug from a specific volume of blood per unit of time is referred to as its clearance.

Important Pharmacokinetic Parameters

An understanding of the pharmacokinetic processes enables researchers to make determinations regarding how a particular drug should be administered to the patient to obtain a specific response. Safe and effective drug therapy requires that drugs be delivered to their target sites in concentrations within a range that will treat the disease state for which it is intended without toxicity.

A dose is the quantity of a drug administered at one time. As greater doses of a drug are given, a greater response will be noted until a point is reached when no improved clinical response occurs with increased dosage. This is called the ceiling effect. Figure 2.2 illustrates the typical dose-response curve. Increased dosing beyond the ceiling effect may result in side effects, toxicity, or even death.

Dosages are fairly universal from patient to patient. In some cases, however, dosage must be individualized to the patient because of variables such as age, size, weight, sex, race, nutritional state, pregnancy, as well as other drugs the patient may be taking. A determination of individual patient dose and dosing intervals can be made, if necessary, based on the testing of drug concentrations in body fluids such as blood, plasma, and urine. Testing of these fluids over specified time intervals provides an indication of how the patient is metabolizing the drug.

Typically, only a portion of the dose administered becomes biologically active in the body. The fraction of the administered dose that is available to the target tissue is an expression of the drug's bioavailability. Drugs taken orally must pass through the intestinal wall and traverse the liver before reaching systemic sites. This process is referred to as the first-pass effect. If a drug which is absorbed from the GI tract is metabolized by the liver to a great extent before it reaches the systemic circulation (first-pass effect), oral bioavailability will be decreased. Some drugs have such a substantial first-pass effect that their use is essentially limited to the parenteral route (i.e., injection).

Figure 2.2

Dose-Response Curve
The ceiling effect is when greater doses of a drug are given and a greater response is noted until a point is reached when no increased response occurs with increased dosing.

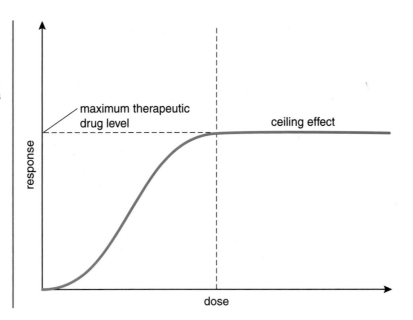

The therapeutic window of serum concentrations for a particular drug should provide the optimum probability of achieving the desired response with the least probability of toxicity. Figure 2.3 illustrates this concept. A defined therapeutic range provides the best chance for successful therapy. Some patients may require concentrations of drug below or above the therapeutic range.

Doses and dosing intervals are determined by clinical trials but may need to be adjusted on an individual basis. This is done based on a blood sample and is particularly beneficial for attaining the desired concentration for a drug with a narrow therapeutic range. When the amount of drug in a patient's blood gives the desired response, it is said to be at the therapeutic level. The length of time a drug is at this level is referred to as its duration of action. This concept is illustrated by the curve in Figure 2.4.

The time required to achieve therapeutic levels of a drug can be shortened by the administration of a loading dose—an amount of drug that will bring the blood concentration rapidly to a therapeutic level. Loading of the drug may be accomplished by the administration of a single loading dose. Alternatively, if a large single dose poses a risk of toxicity, loading can be accomplished by the administration of the

Figure 2.3

Therapeutic Range
Optimum dosage yields a range of therapeutic effects while underdosing has little effect and overdosing can lead to toxicity and death.

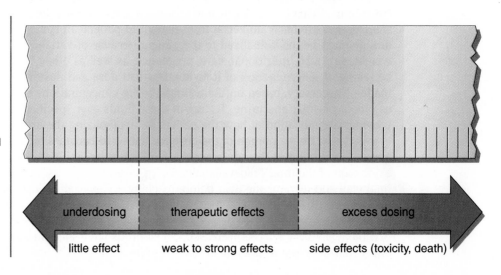

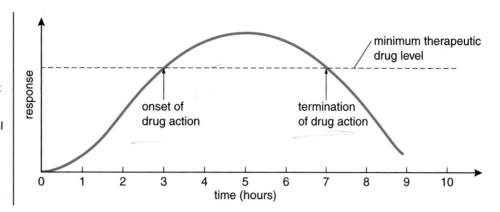

Figure 2.4

Duration of Action

Plasma drug concentration must reach a minimum therapeutic level before physiological activity is noted.

loading amount in a series of doses. Maintenance doses are then given to keep the drug at a therapeutic level. The volume of distribution, which describes the relationship between the blood concentration attained and the dose of drug given, is important for prescribing the loading dose; whereas clearance, the removal of a drug from a specific volume of blood per unit of time, is important for calculating the maintenance dose.

The time necessary for the body to eliminate half of the drug in circulation at any time is the half-life, written $T_{1/2}$. The longer the half-life, the longer the drug action. It takes about five to seven half-lives to consider the drug "removed" from the body—meaning that less than 3% remains. If the $T_{1/2}$ of a drug is two hours, then the drug would be gone in ten to fourteen hours. If the $T_{1/2}$ is thirty hours, then it would take 150 to 210 hours, or six to nine days, to eliminate the drug. A drug with a long half-life may produce effects for days or even weeks after being discontinued.

Pharmacokinetic Modeling

Studies on drug absorption, distribution, metabolism, and elimination have advanced the concept that the body may be considered as consisting of different compartments. In the simplest form, a drug passes from one compartment to another in direct proportion to its concentration gradient.

Pharmacokinetic modeling is a method of describing the process of absorption, distribution, metabolism, and elimination of a drug within the body. For some drugs, elimination is a zero-order process; that is, a fixed quantity of drug is eliminated per unit of time. The best example is alcohol. For the majority of drugs, elimination is said to be "first order." That is, a constant fraction of remaining drug is eliminated per unit of time. Two pharmacokinetic models, based on the compartment theory, have been developed. In the one-compartment model, the drug is distributed into blood volume. This model assumes an instantaneous and homogenous distribution of drugs throughout the body. In the two-compartment model, the drug is distributed into blood volume and then into body tissue. This more complex model better describes the distribution of many drugs.

DRUG EFFECTS

The pharmacokinetic models described above provide critical insight for predicting the effects of each specific drug. Some effects are beneficial, while others can be detrimental or dangerous. Just as each person is different, each person's reaction to a drug may be different. Thus, each patient must be monitored closely to ensure that his response to the drug he is taking is appropriate.

Beneficial Responses

The desired action of a drug in the treatment of a particular disease state or symptom is referred to as a therapeutic effect. The therapeutic effect is the action for which the drug is prescribed. Drugs can act locally or they can act on the body as a whole. A local effect is confined to a specific part of the body. A systemic effect, on the other hand, has a generalized, all-inclusive effect on the entire body.

Sometimes drugs are prescribed to prevent the occurrence of an infection or disease. In this case, the drug effect is referred to as prophylaxis. Patients who will be undergoing surgery will, in some cases, be administered prophylactic drugs, which will work to prevent the occurrence of infections.

In selecting a drug for an individual patient, the healthcare practitioner considers its approved uses and situations in which it should or should not be given. The indications for a drug are the diseases, symptoms, and conditions for which the drug is known to be of benefit. The contraindications are the diseases, symptoms, and conditions in which the drug will not be beneficial and may indeed do harm.

Side effects are secondary responses to a drug other than the primary therapeutic effect for which the drug was intended. Drugs can on occasion be prescribed for their side effects.

Harmful Responses

ALLERGIC RESPONSES An allergic reaction is a local or general immune response. In essence, an allergy is an instance of the immune system overreacting to an otherwise harmless substance. The first exposure to an allergen generally gives little or no observable response. Rather, what is critical about the initial exposure is the resulting "memory storage" which characterizes active immunity. Thus, upon re-exposure, the body recognizes ("remembers") the antigen and responds with a more potent antibody response. This response can elicit a range of reactions from uncomfortable to life threatening. Some responses start within minutes of exposure; others may be delayed. Exposure to the allergen may cause mild, moderate, or in some cases, severe inflammation. Some common allergic reactions to drugs include hives, nasal secretions, swelling, wheezing, an excessively rapid heart rate, and, in rare cases, even death.

Anaphylactic reactions are severe allergic responses resulting in immediate life-threatening respiratory distress, usually followed by vascular collapse and shock and accompanied by hives. Idiosyncratic reactions are unusual or unexpected responses to a drug, unrelated to the dose given.

DRUG DEPENDENCE, ADDICTION, ABUSE, AND TOLERANCE Drug dependence describes a state in which a person's body has adapted physiologically and psychologically to a drug and cannot function without it. Dependence should not be confused with addiction, which is a dependence characterized by perceived need to take a drug to attain the psychological and physical effects of mood-altering substances. One sign of addiction is a decrease in psychological well-being and social or vocational functioning. Patients who are being treated for various disease states may become dependent on medications, without exhibiting the signs of addiction.

Drug abuse is the use of a drug for purposes other than those prescribed and/or in amounts that were not directed. It is generally thought of as experimental or recreational use of a substance that may have adverse effects. Abusive use of drugs can be, but is not always, linked to addiction.

After a patient has been taking a drug over a significant period of time, he or she may begin to develop a decreased response to the drug. This decrease in response to the effects of a drug due to its continued administration is referred to as tolerance. As tolerance develops, there may be a need to increase the dosage of the drug in order to maintain a constant response.

Drug Interactions

Another reaction to drugs involves that of interaction. In this case, one drug alters the action of another. Foods, alcohol, and nicotine can also interact with drugs. A system of enzymes tagged as cytochrome P-450 has been identified as the factor that contributes to many drug interactions. Cytochrome P-450 plays a key role in the oxidative biotransformation of drugs.

It is important that the physician and pharmacist have a complete list of all drugs—prescription and over-the-counter—that a patient is taking so that potential interactions can be recognized and appropriately handled. The pharmacy technician should routinely ask the patient for this information.

Table 2.1 describes a number of common drug relationships.

Table 2.1	Common Drug Relationships
Drug Relationship	**Description**
addition	The combined effect of two drugs. It is equal to the sum of the effects of each drug taken alone.
antagonism	The action of one drug negates the action of a second drug.
potentiation	An effect that occurs when a drug increases or prolongs the action of another drug, and the total effect is greater than the sum of the effects of each drug used alone. If one drug prescribed alone cannot get the desired effect, another drug can be prescribed to increase the first drug's potency. This term is used when a drug has little or no action when given alone and the second drug increases the potency of the first drug.
synergism	The joint action of drugs in which their combined effect is more intense or longer in duration than the sum of their individual effects. Drugs that work synergistically are usually prescribed together.

Chapter Summary

Receptors

- A receptor is a molecule on the surface of or within a cell that recognizes and binds with specific molecules producing some effect in the cell.
- Drugs bind to receptors on or within body cells.
- One drug can compete with another drug for its intended receptor.

Mechanisms of Drug Action

- Drugs can mimic or block the action of chemical messengers to exert powerful and specific actions in the body.

Pharmacokinetics

- Pharmacokinetics is the study of the time course of absorption, distribution, metabolism, and excretion of drugs and their metabolites in relation to the time they are present in the body.
- Testing body fluids over time demonstrates how the body handles the drug. Before certain drugs are dispensed, the pharmacy technician may be responsible for making sure the laboratory reports have been received and that the pharmacist has reviewed them.
- The volume of distribution is important for loading dose, clearance for maintenance dose, and half-life for determining the dosing interval.
- The primary sites of elimination are the kidney and the liver. Drugs may also be exhaled by the lungs or excreted in perspiration.

Drug Effects

- Drugs can interact with other drugs, food, and the patient's own body.
- Drug effects include therapeutic effects, adverse reactions, and side effects.
- Two drugs may be prescribed together because the combination has fewer or more tolerable side effects than a high dose of either.

Chapter Review

Understanding Pharmacology

Select the best answer from the choices given.

1. Responses other than the intended therapeutic one are
   a. side effects.
   b. synergism.
   c. potentiation.
   d. additive.

2. Which term refers to the treatment of disease?
   a. Side effects
   b. Synergism
   c. Therapeutics
   d. Addiction

3. Increasing resistance to the usual effects of an established dosage of a drug as a result of continued use is
   a. an idiosyncratic reaction.
   b. an anaphylactic reaction.
   c. tolerance.
   d. dependence.

4. A response that is unusual, unexpected, or opposite from the expected response to a drug is
   a. an idiosyncratic reaction. — *unusual*
   b. an anaphylactic reaction. → *severe allergic effect*
   c. tolerance.
   d. dependence.

5. Severe allergic life-threatening response with breathing difficulty, vascular collapse, and shock, accompanied by urticaria, pruritus, and angioedema is
   a. an idiosyncratic reaction. *hives   itchy   swallowing*
   b. an anaphylactic reaction.   *around the mouth.*
   c. tolerance.
   d. dependence.

6. Complete removal of a drug from a specific volume of blood per unit of time is
   a. pharmacokinetics.
   b. bioavailability.
   c. volume of distribution.
   d. clearance.

7. What describes the relationship between the dosage of drug given and the blood concentration attained?
   a. Pharmacokinetics
   b. Bioavailability
   c. Volume of distribution
   d. Clearance

8. The degree to which a drug becomes available to the target tissue is
    a. pharmacokinetics.
    b. bioavailability.
    c. volume of distribution.
    d. clearance.

9. A study to understand drug behavior in the human body is
    a. pharmacokinetics.
    b. bioavailability.
    c. volume of distribution.
    d. clearance.

A M
D E
Absorption   Metabolize
Distribution.   Excretion.

10. A method of describing the process of absorption, distribution, and elimination of a drug within the body is
    a. drug interactions.
    b. disintegration and dissolution.
    c. routes of administration.
    d. pharmacokinetic modeling.

The following statements are true or false. If the answer is false, rewrite the statement so it is true.

___T___ 1. Side effects are secondary responses to a drug other than the therapeutic effect.

___F___ 2. Potentiation is when the combined effect of two drugs is equal to the sum of the effect of each drug taken alone. Addition.

___F___ 3. Addition is an effect that occurs when a drug increases or prolongs the action of another drug, the total effect being greater than the sum of the two parts. Potentiation

___F___ 4. Half-life is the time required for the drug to eliminate 75% of the drug in circulation at any given time. 50%

___F___ 5. GI motility does not affect absorption.

___T___ 6. Blood flow is the rate-limiting factor for distribution of a drug.

___T___ 7. Pharmacokinetics is the study of the time course of absorption, distribution, metabolism, and elimination of drugs over a period of time.

___T___ 8. Only a portion of the dose administered becomes biologically active in the body.

___F___ 9. Drugs can pass through the blood-brain barrier quite easily. lipid soluble

___T___ 10. When two drugs try to bind to the same receptor, this is called site antagonism.

Pharmacology at Work

1. Explain the statement "Pharmacists must consider the effect the body has on the drug as well as the effect the drug has on the body."
2. Explain the concepts receptor, agonist, and antagonist.
3. Define half-life. If a drug's half-life is six hours, how long would it take to remove the drug from the body?
4. Define ceiling effect and its importance in dosing medication.

Internet Research

Use the Internet to complete the following assignments.

1. Go to the National Library of Medicine's PubMed Web site at www.ncbi.nlm.nih.gov. This site provides a comprehensive index of medical journal articles. Find two journal article abstracts that describe pharmacokinetic studies of new drugs and, for each, list the full citation of the article along with the name(s) of the drug(s) included in the study. Note the abstracts' use of the terms introduced in this chapter (e.g., clearance, half-life, bioavailability) and record an example of one sentence containing such terminology within each of the abstracts. Describe your search strategy.
2. Research flu vaccines. Who should get a flu vaccine, and when should they get it? What is the vaccine composed of? Why must the vaccine be given every year? Locate and list at least three sites. Which site(s) were most helpful to you in answering the questions listed above? Which site(s) would be most useful to an individual concerned about contracting the flu? Which site(s), if any, would be most useful to a scientist studying infectious diseases?

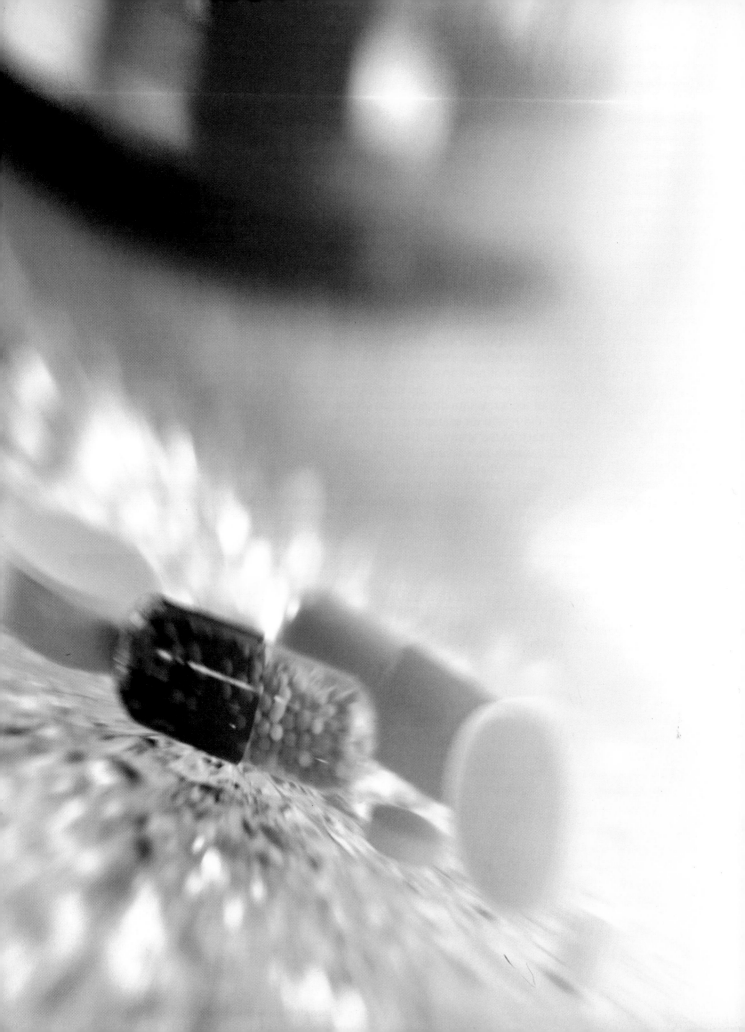

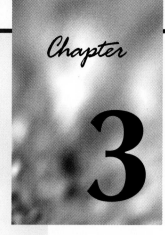
Administration of Pharmacologic Agents

Learning Objectives

- Know the components of the prescription, including the accepted standard abbreviations.
- Understand the five rights of correct drug administration.
- Recognize common dosage forms.
- Know the routes of administration.
- Recognize factors that influence the effects of drugs, particularly in the elderly and pediatric populations.
- Know the affects natural chemicals have on drug action and response.

Pharmacy technicians play a key role in the dispensing of pharmacologic agents. This role requires a thorough understanding of the components of the drug prescription and the responsibilities of pharmaceutical personnel. The prescription includes all the information necessary for the pharmacist to fill the prescription with the correct dosing form and for the patient to take the medication correctly. Two age groups of patients, elderly and pediatric, have special needs to be considered in dispensing drugs.

THE DRUG PRESCRIPTION

A prescription is an order written by a physician to be filled by a pharmacist indicating the medication the patient needs. The prescription should contain

- the patient's name
- the date the prescription was written
- the inscription, which states the name of the drug, dose, and quantities of the ingredients
- the *signa,* often referred to as the sig, which gives directions to be included on the label for the patient to follow in taking the medication
- an indication of the number of refills allowed, or "no refills" if that is the case
- the signature (handwritten, not stamped) and address of the prescribing physician
- indication whether generic substitution is permitted

The DEA number of the prescribing physician must be on the prescription if it is for the dispensing of a controlled substance. Figure 3.1 is an example of a prescription with the essential elements labeled. Pharmacy technicians should always double-check a prescription for accuracy and to ensure that all of the legal requirements have been met. The label on the medication container given to the patient must include the patient's name, date written, inscription, signa, number of refills, expiration date, the physician's name, and the phone number and address of the pharmacy.

Figure 3.1

The Essential Elements of a Prescription
The pharmacy technician should always check the first six elements.

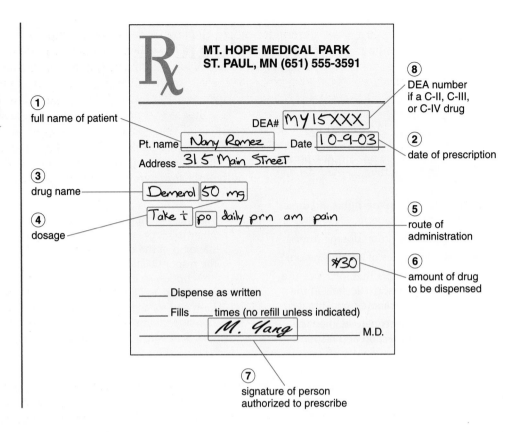

① full name of patient

③ drug name

④ dosage

MT. HOPE MEDICAL PARK
ST. PAUL, MN (651) 555-3591

DEA# MY15XXX

Pt. name _Nancy Ramez_ Date _10-9-03_
Address _315 Main Street_

Demerol _50 mg_
Take ī _po_ _daily prn am pain_

_*30_

_____ Dispense as written

_____ Fills_____ times (no refill unless indicated)
M. Yang _____ M.D.

⑧ DEA number if a C-II, C-III, or C-IV drug

② date of prescription

⑤ route of administration

⑥ amount of drug to be dispensed

⑦ signature of person authorized to prescribe

Table 3.1 **Abbreviations Used in Writing Prescriptions**

Abbreviation	Translation	Abbreviation	Translation
ac	before meals	NKA	no known allergy
AD	right ear	npo	nothing by mouth
AS	left ear	OD	right eye
AU	both ears	OS	left eye
bid	twice a day	OU	both eyes
c̄	with	pc	after meals
cap	capsule	po	by mouth
cc	cubic centimeter (milliliter)	prn	as needed
		q	every
DAW	dispense as written	qd	every day
D/C	discontinue	qh	every hour
g	gram*	q2h	every 2 hours
gr	grain	qid	four times a day
gtt	drop	qs	a sufficient quantity
hs	at bedtime	SC	subcutaneous
ID	intradermal	sig	write on label
IM	intramuscular	ss	one half
IV	intravenously	stat	immediately
L	liter	syr	syrup
mcg	microgram	tab	tablet
mEq	milliequivalent	tid	three times daily
min	minute	ud	as directed
mL	milliliter	wk	week

* Gram is sometimes abbreviated as gm.

Note: Some prescribers may write abbreviations using capital letters or periods.

To fill the prescription safely, the pharmacy technician should be familiar with common abbreviations used in prescriptions, listed in Table 3.1. While these abbreviations are standard usage for physicians, pharmacists, and their technicians, the instructions to the patient are spelled out in full and as simply as possible to ensure proper use of the medication. Most pharmacies provide the patient an information sheet with additional details regarding the proper way to take the medication (especially in regard to food intake), possible side effects, and situations in which the prescribing physician should be consulted. Limiting the number of refills allowed without another physician consultation is a way to prevent the patient from encountering severe side effects or addiction from overuse of the medication.

FIVE "RIGHTS" FOR CORRECT DRUG ADMINISTRATION

There are five "rights" of medication administration that offer useful guidelines when filling prescriptions for patient medications. These concepts have been widely used to avoid medication errors. A drug misadventure occurs whenever these are not followed correctly. Figure 3.2 illustrates the concepts, and the five rights are overviewed below.

- **Right Patient** Always verify the patient's name before dispensing medication.
- **Right Drug** Always check the medication against the original prescription and the patient's disease state. The medication label contains important information about the drug that will be dispensed to the patient.
- **Right Strength** Check the original prescription for this information and pay attention to the age of the patient. Pediatric or elderly patients can easily get the wrong dose.
- **Right Route** Check that the physician's order agrees with the drug's specified route of administration. Many medications can be given by a variety of routes and the route of administration can affect the medication's absorption.
- **Right Time** Check the prescription to determine the appropriate time for the medication to be administered. Some medications must be taken on an empty

Figure 3.2

Five "Rights" for Correct Drug Administration

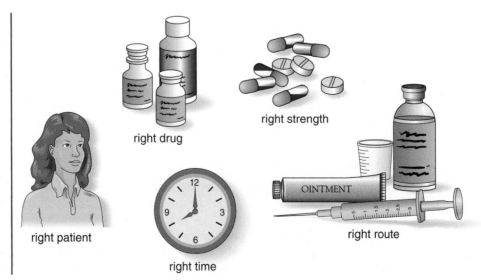

right drug

right strength

right patient

right time

right route

Figure 3.3

Medication Label on a Dispensing Container
Important information, such as the drug name, dosage form, dosage strength, precautions, and usual dosage and frequency of administration will be provided on the medication dispensing container.

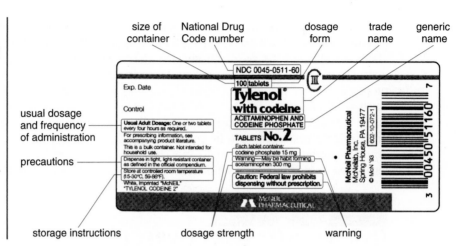

size of container · National Drug Code number · dosage form · trade name · generic name

usual dosage and frequency of administration

precautions

storage instructions · dosage strength · warning

stomach (one hour before or two hours after a meal) while others should be taken with food. Sometimes, a certain time span is needed between doses to maintain a therapeutically effective blood level.

DOSAGE FORMS AND ROUTES OF ADMINISTRATION

There are many different forms into which a medicinal agent may be placed for the convenient and efficacious treatment of disease. The route and dosage form are determined by many factors. Among these are the disease being treated, the area of the body which the drug needs to reach, and the chemical composition of the drug itself. Each drug has its own characteristics related to absorption, distribution, metabolism, and elimination. Drugs are prepared for administration by every conceivable route. There are three routes of administration: oral, parenteral, and topical. Table 3.2 lists a few examples of these.

Medications are available in a variety of forms, and frequently a single drug will be available in a number of different forms. Examples of the common drug forms associated with the three administration routes are overviewed in Table 3.3.

The age and condition of the patient often determine the dosage form that will be used. Pediatric and geriatric populations frequently have special needs. These two groups often need liquid dosage forms. Convenience may also play a role in the selection of the appropriate dosage form. It has also been found that drugs with distinctive sizes, shapes, and colors are inherently easier to identify. Dosage forms that reduce the frequency of administration without sacrifice of efficacy are often advantageous and facilitate patient compliance.

Oral Routes

The oral route is the most economical and most convenient way to give medications. The term oral means that the medication is given by mouth in either solid form, as a tablet or capsule, or in liquid form, as a solution or syrup. Once the medication enters the mouth, it must be swallowed to reach the stomach. Then it must pass to the point of absorption, most commonly the small intestine, although some medications are absorbed in the stomach.

This process takes time and is affected by several factors including the presence of food (which slows the process) or digestive disorders. It is important to refer to a reliable drug reference guide to determine if the medication should be

Table 3.2   **Dosage Routes**

Route	Example
oral (by mouth)	swallowed sublingual (under the tongue) buccal (dissolves in the cheek)
parenteral (injection through veins, etc. for rapid entry of the drug into the circulatory system)	IV (vein) intrarterial (artery) intracardiac (heart) intraspinal/intrathecal (spinal fluid) intrasynovial (joint-fluid area) subcutaneous (beneath the skin) intramuscular (muscle)
topical (applied to surface of skin or mucous membranes)	transdermal (skin surface) conjunctival (conjunctiva) intraocular (eye) intranasal (nose) aural (ear) intrarespiratory (lung) rectal (rectum) vaginal (vagina) urethral (urethra)

Table 3.3   **Common Dosage Forms**

Route	Primary Dosage Forms
oral	tablets capsules solutions syrups elixirs suspensions magmas gels powders trouches/lozenges
parenteral	solutions suspensions
topical	ointments creams pastes powders aerosols lotions transdermal patches sprays inhalants suppositories enemas emulsions sponges

given with or without food and whether any specific assessments should be done before dispensing it.

Sublingual (under the tongue) and buccal (between the cheek and gum) routes of administration are used when a rapid action is desired, or when a drug is specifically designed to be easily absorbed into blood vessels. The medication enters the bloodstream directly from the richly vascularized mucous membrane of the mouth and produces its effects more quickly than drugs that are swallowed. This dosage form cannot obtain the same effect if swallowed.

When taking medication by the sublingual route, the patient should hold the tablet under the tongue until it is completely absorbed. For buccal administration, the patient should place the tablet between the cheek and gums, close the mouth, and hold the tablet there until it is absorbed. It is important to remind the patient not to drink water or swallow excessively until the tablet is completely absorbed.

Parenteral Routes

Medications that are injected directly into the tissues of the body do not pass through the liver before entering the bloodstream. Avoiding this "first pass effect" prevents medications from being inactivated in the liver. Drugs may be injected into

- ◇ a muscle: intramuscular
- ◇ a vein: intravenous
- ◇ the skin: intradermal
- ◇ the tissue beneath the skin: subcutaneous
- ◇ the spinal column

Drugs such as insulin are inactivated in digestive juices, so swallowing them would be ineffective.

Parenteral routes also offer the potential for quick absorption of injected medication into the bloodstream and a rapid effect (especially for the intravenous route). Disadvantages include pain during administration and the possibility of infection since the skin is punctured. Also, once the medication is injected, there is no way to retrieve it if an error has been made.

Topical Routes

Topical medications are applied to the surface of the skin or mucous membranes. The desired effect can be local or systemic. Other topical routes are inhalation, ophthalmic, otic, nasal, and rectal.

The inhalation route delivers medications to the respiratory system. These medications are intended to produce one or more of the following effects. They are intended to alter the condition of the mucous membranes, alter the character of the secretions in the respiratory system, and treat diseases and infections of the respiratory tract.

Administration of medications via the ophthalmic route includes the instillation of a cream or ointment or placing of drops of a liquid preparation into the conjunctival sac of the eye.

A drug preparation for the otic route is a drug that is used locally to treat inflammation or infection of the external ear canal or to remove excess cerumen (wax) or foreign objects from the canal. Eardrops come in solutions and suspensions. If the patient has a tube in the ear, a suspension rather than a solution should be used.

Medications can be administered into the nose by instillation or spray.

Medications that are administered by the rectal route are most commonly in suppository form and enemas. Suppositories are rounded, soft pieces of easily melted glycerin. They dissolve at body temperature and release the medication to be absorbed through the walls of the large intestine.

The prominent advantage to rectal administration is that the medication does not depend on the digestive system to be absorbed into the bloodstream. Therefore, it is frequently used to treat nausea and vomiting. Suppositories also can be used for local effect to treat constipation. Additionally, the rectal route is ideal for treating fever in infants and young children.

Medications given by the vaginal route can be used to treat local infections caused by either bacteria or fungi.

FACTORS THAT INFLUENCE DRUG EFFECTS

A variety of factors can influence the effects of drugs and may require dosage adjustment. Pediatric patients and the elderly may require less of a drug because of their smaller size or inability of the liver to metabolize the medication adequately. In these instances, if the dosage is not decreased, it may have toxic effects on the patient. The physician can use a variety of formulas when prescribing medications for elderly and pediatric patients.

Gender also needs to be considered when prescribing some medications, especially hormonal preparations, since men and women have different amounts of hormones.

Patients with specific diseases may be unable to absorb, metabolize, or excrete various medications. Impaired gastrointestinal function may affect absorption, impaired liver function may affect metabolism, and impaired kidney function may affect elimination. Inadequate nutritional intake may also adversely affect the metabolism of drugs. Therefore, the patient's disease condition must be evaluated before prescribing medications.

Other factors physicians consider when prescribing medications include psychological and genetic factors. The mental state of a patient can influence the body's ability to release chemical substances needed to appropriately absorb or metabolize a drug. Genes can also control the release of chemicals and how the body absorbs or metabolizes various medications. Unfortunately, these factors are less predictable than age, gender, and disease condition. However, if the patient does not seem to be responding to a medication, these factors should be considered.

Immune responses should also be evaluated for all patients before medications are prescribed. Allergic responses to medications should be documented in the medical record, and each time a new medication is dispensed, the pharmacy technician should ask whether the patient has had any additional allergic responses in order to keep the records up to date.

Special Considerations in Elderly Patients

The elderly tend to have more chronic disease than the young. They use more drugs—both prescription and nonprescription. For some elderly patients, medication is often the difference between an independent ambulatory lifestyle and confinement in a long-term care facility. Many elderly individuals take three to four medications, three to four times daily; and four out of five in this age group have at least one chronic disease. As a result, geriatric medicine has emerged as a new and important medical specialty of the healthcare system. A listing of the drugs most often used by elderly patients is given in Table 3.4. Pharmacy technicians should be familiar with both the brand and generic names of these drugs.

CHANGES IN PHYSIOLOGIC FUNCTION   The concept of aging has traditionally been linked to declining mental function; however, physiologic changes do not occur equally or predictably in an individual patient. Successful aging is characterized by nonpathologic losses in physiologic function. Usual aging is characterized by minimal physiologic loss when compared with that of average persons in the same age group. Impaired aging represents pathologic physiologic changes.

These changes occur slowly or with increasing rapidity in a wide range of body systems.

⋄ **Optic Changes** As the lenses become less elastic, more dense, and yellow, visual acuity is compromised; this is often correctable with eyeglasses. Macular degeneration and cataracts become a problem, often necessitating surgery.
⋄ **Auditory Changes** Hearing loss occurs in all frequencies, but especially in the high ranges. Impairment of sound localization and loudness perception is a

Table 3.4	Most-Commonly Used Agents for Elderly Patients		
Generic Name and Class		**Brand Name**	**Dosage Form**
Nonsteroidal Anti-Inflammatory Drugs			
acetaminophen		Tylenol	tablet, caplet, liquid, chewable, suppository
aspirin		Bayer	tablet, caplet, chewable
ibuprofen		Advil	tablet, caplet, gel caplet, oral suspension
		Motrin	tablet, caplet, gel cap
naproxen		Aleve	tablet, caplet
Antidepressants			
fluoxetine		Prozac	capsule, liquid, tablet
paroxetine		Paxil	capsule, oral solution, suspension, tablet
sertraline		Zoloft	tablet, liquid
Miscellaneous			
albuterol		Proventil	tablet, aerosol, solution, syrup
celecoxib		Celebrex	capsule
clonidine		Catapres	tablet, transdermal
conjugated estrogen		Premarin	tablet, IM, IV, cream
digoxin (glycoside)		Lanoxin	tablet, elixir, capsule, IV, IM
furosemide		Lasix	tablet, solution, IM, IV
levothyroxin		Synthroid	tablet, IV
lisinopril		Zestril	tablet
loratidine		Claritin	tablet, syrup
triamterene/HCTZ (diuretics)		Dyazide, Maxzide	capsule, tablet
warfarin		Coumadin	tablet
zolpidiem		Ambien	tablet

problem for many elderly patients. A delay in central processing of auditory messages results in an increase in the time it takes for the person to respond to a question.

◇ **Gastrointestinal Changes** These changes create many problems, among them decreases in saliva production, esophageal motility, hydrochloric acid secretion, absorptive surface, and a reduction in the rate of gastric emptying. Constipation is a daily complaint; the elderly are often preoccupied with this physiologic function. Overuse of stimulant laxatives is a significant problem for some elderly patients.

◇ **Pulmonary Changes** Many elderly patients have chronic obstructive pulmonary disease (COPD). Aging brings on increased rigidity of the chest wall, decreased vital capacity (maximum intake and exhalation), decreased response to hypoxia (reduced oxygen in the blood), and hypercapnia (increased carbon dioxide in the blood). If an elderly patient also has cardiac disease, these conditions are further compromised.

◇ **Cardiovascular Changes** Hypertension and coronary artery disease are major issues to address. Healthy persons at rest have little age-related loss of cardiac output; during exercise, however, cardiac responses needed to meet the increased oxygen demand are diminished. To compenste, the sympathetic nervous system releases more norepinephrine and epinephrine. As a result, a compensatory increase in stroke volume occurs, and cardiac output is maintained. In elderly patients with cardiac disease, these compensatory mechanisms are impaired, resulting in decreased output.

◇ **Urinary Changes** These changes can result from a decrease in the number of functioning nephrons and in renal blood flow. The elderly have a higher incidence of renal insufficiency (reduced capacity to perform). Incontinence (inability to retain urine in the bladder) is often a problem, and diapers become a necessity. Instability of bladder muscle, overflow, and sphincter weakness are the causes. Diuretics, often necessary medications to treat an existing illness, may aggravate this condition. Urinary retention may be the result of prostatic hypertrophy, malignant states, stones, anticholinergic drug intake, and urinary tract infections.

◇ **Hormonal Changes** Functional changes are a natural consequence of aging.

◇ **Compositional Body Changes** The proportion of total body weight composed of fat increases with age, while lean body mass and total body mass decrease. Albumin production decreases with aging, possibly as the result of poor nutrition, hepatic disorders, or other disease states. Loss in bone density (osteoporosis) causes some loss of height. Arthritis also takes its toll on the skeletal system.

ALTERED DRUG RESPONSES Age-related changes in organ function and body composition can alter the response to medication. These factors play an important part in selecting a drug and its dosage.

◇ **Absorption Changes** Changes in GI function with aging may affect dissolution, enzymatic breakdown, and drug ionization. Reduction in the rate of gastric emptying may delay absorption of some drugs. For most, the rate and extent of absorption are determined by passive diffusion during contact with the surface area of the gut. Reduction in absorptive surface reduces absorption. GI fluids and GI motility also decrease.

◇ **Distribution Changes** Alterations in body composition, such as protein binding (less protein, more free drug in plasma), affect distribution of drugs. If the drug is highly protein-bound, it may have enhanced pharmacologic or toxic effects in elderly patients. Other factors that affect distribution are decreases in total body water, lean body mass, and cardiac output.

- ◇ **Elimination Changes** Metabolism occurs in the liver, and the kidneys are responsible for elimination. Both processes may be altered with aging, with serious effects on blood levels of a drug. Varying degrees of renal and hepatic dysfunction may be present, depending on the patient's disease states, the drugs used, and the degree of successful aging.
- ◇ **Metabolism Changes** During metabolism, a drug is transformed biochemically to a more water-soluble compound. Elderly patients may have impaired metabolism, therefore decreasing clearance and allowing the drug to accumulate, sometimes reaching toxic levels. Normally, blood flow per minute decreases about 1% per year as an individual ages, beginning at about age 35 (40% from ages 35 to 75).

Older patients are more likely to have chronic diseases requiring long-term treatment. Many take from three to twelve medications, and they tend to have a disproportionate number of adverse drug reactions (ADRs). Maintaining medication profiles is important in these cases.

Polypharmacy is the term used for excessive use of unnecessary medication. ADRs are often the result of overprescribing. Owing to slowing of drug metabolism with aging, the elderly can often obtain the desired pharmacologic effect with a much lower dose than normally prescribed. When many drugs are prescribed for a patient, especially when the patient sees more than one physician, the potential for drug interactions or other problems is high.

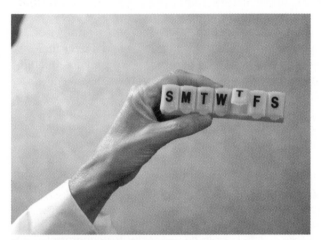

Using tools such as this pillbox will help patients who must take medications daily to remember to take them. The pharmacy technician can help inform patients about such medication management strategies.

Aging can also affect cognitive abilities. An inadequate understanding of the need for the medication and dosage directions for the medication (e.g., taken with or without food) can lead to failure to take the drug, unintentional overdosing, taking the medication for the wrong reason, or taking drugs prescribed for another person. This failure to adhere to the appropriate drug regimen is referred to as noncompliance and is especially prevalent among the elderly. Pharmacy technicians can provide invaluable services in this area. They can make sure the patient gets written information and provide aids to dosing and ways to remember to take medication. Some adverse reactions more common in the elderly are listed in Table 3.5.

Table 3.5	**Common Adverse Reactions in the Elderly**	
◇ central nervous system (CNS) changes (often misdiagnosed as disease manifestations)	◇ GI upset
◇ constipation	◇ incontinence
◇ dermatitis	◇ insomnia
◇ diarrhea	◇ rheumatoid symptoms
◇ drowsiness	◇ sexual dysfunction
◇ falls	◇ urinary retention
	◇ xerostomia (dry mouth)

Special Considerations in Pediatric Patients

Providing drug therapy to children presents a unique set of challenges. As they grow, children undergo profound physiologic changes that affect drug absorption, distribution, metabolism, and elimination. Failure to understand these changes and their effects can lead to underestimating or overestimating drug dosage, with the resultant potential for failure of therapy, severe adverse reactions, or perhaps fatal toxicity.

Age may be the least reliable guide to drug administration in children because of the wide variation in the relationship between age and degree of organ-system development. Height better correlates with lean body mass than does weight. Body surface area may be the best measure because it correlates with all body parameters; however, it is not easily determined. Body weight is most commonly used because of its ease of calculation. Children who are small for their age should receive conservative doses, but larger children may require a dose recommended for the next higher age bracket.

Dosing pediatric patients can be a challenge. Pediatricians often prescribe an over-the-counter medication for a child without telling the parent how to dose the drug, or they forget, thinking the dosing instructions will be on the package. A caretaker may purchase the medication only to find the drug is intended for use in an older child and appropriate dosage information for a smaller child is not provided with the medication. The pharmacist may have to determine the child's dose for the caretaker. The pharmacy technician should always refer these questions to the pharmacist. Many factors need to be considered before recommending a drug dosage that goes beyond the printed instructions on the box.

The following considerations are important when dosing children.

◇ Reevaluate all dosages at regular intervals.
◇ Be sure the dosage is appropriate for the child's age. A dose appropriate for a neonate may not be so for a premature infant or a toddler.
◇ Always double-check all computations.

Immunization

Immunization is a process whereby the immune system is stimulated to acquire immunity to a specific disease. This is generally achieved via the use of a vaccine, which is a suspension of microorganisms or fraction thereof administered to induce immunity.

There are two types of immunity, active and passive. Active immunity results from coming into contact with an infectious agent or an inactivated part of an infectious agent through a vaccine. As a result, the body develops antibodies which protect the body from the disease. Passive immunity is the result of receiving antibodies that were formed by another person or animal who had developed them in response to being infected.

Some early vaccines made from live or attenuated organisms caused serious reactions, and their efficacy was questionable. The recent development of recombinant deoxyribonucleic acid (DNA) technology and the success of peptide sequencing and synthesis have helped in developing new and safer vaccines. Synthetic vaccines use chemically synthesized antigens (usually peptides) as the immunizing agent. The success of these vaccines depends on the ability of an antibody elicited in response to a small, defined peptide to recognize and bind to that peptide sequence. Synthetic vaccines have two advantages. First, they are quite safe because they do not rely on live or attenuated viruses. Second, the antigenic peptides can be synthesized on a large scale.

Immunotherapy is an important part of pediatric medicine. Development of safe, effective vaccines to prevent infectious diseases has been responsible for the substantial decline in morbidity and mortality associated with smallpox, rabies, diphtheria, pertussis, tetanus, yellow fever, poliomyelitis, measles, mumps, and rubella.

TEACHING PATIENTS TO MANAGE THEIR MEDICATIONS

The pharmacy technician can play an important role in helping patients learn how to manage medications. Compliance refers to the patient's adherence to the dose schedule and other particular requirements of their specific drug regimen. A patient's failure to follow the drug regimen is often the result of a lack of understanding or lack of motivation. If the drug does not enter the body or enters it incorrectly, it will not work as desired. The pharmacy technician can positively affect patient compliance by providing clearly written instructions and aids to implement the process.

Information about prescription drugs must be provided to the patient by the pharmicist filling the prescription. Federal law requires that patient history regarding drugs prescribed as well as side effects and adverse reactions experienced by the patient is collected. The pharmacy technician can positively affect patient drug therapy by accurately collecting and recording the patient's medication history in the patient's profile. It is also required that the patient be given information about the drugs ordered and their proper administration. The pharmacist can help the patient understand administration instructions, as well as precautions. Specific instructions to emphasize include

- ◇ methods for administering the drug
- ◇ how to make swallowing easier
- ◇ times and time intervals for administration
- ◇ whether a medication can or should be taken with or without food
- ◇ possible side effects and which ones should be reported to the physician
- ◇ how long the medication should be taken

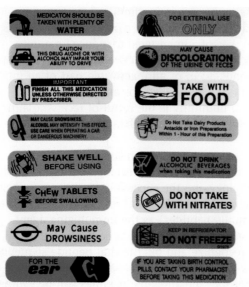

When a patient receives a prescription, it will sometimes include labels that provide instructions for how to properly self-administer the medication. These labels use color and logos to communicate their message.

In some states, technicians can ensure that patients understand how to read medication labels. Important items to look for include the trade name and/or generic name, the dosage strength, frequency and route of administration, precautions and warnings, and potential interactions. It is important to remember, however, that technicians cannot—by law—counsel patients! Figure 3.4 provides an example of a doctor's prescription and the corresponding medication label that should be affixed to the drug container. The label provides directions that the patient needs to understand and follow.

Over-the-counter (OTC) drugs that patients take often help relieve many common, uncomplicated symptoms. However, they can interfere with the desired effects of prescription drugs ordered by the physician. That is why it is so important to obtain information about the patient's OTC drug use as well as information about prescription medications.

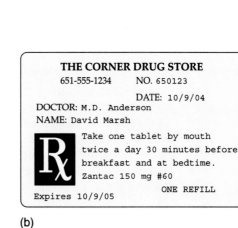

Figure 3.4

Medication Label Information
The information on a prescription as shown in (a) is translated for the patient as instructions on the medication label, as shown in (b). This label also includes the MD's name and the date the prescription was written, the drug name, the number of refills, and the pharmacy's address and phone number.

Many drugs now available over-the-counter once required a prescription. This change occurred because they were found to help with common problems and carry a relatively lower risk of adverse efffects. However, it is important that patients read the information provided with these drugs to understand their action, interactions, cautions, and possible side effects.

NATURAL CHEMICALS THAT AFFECT DRUG ACTION AND RESPONSE

The body naturally produces several chemicals that invariably affect the metabolism of drugs. Some important chemicals are histamine, prostaglandins, and bradykinin.

Histamine

Histamine is a decarboxylation product formed from the amino acid histidine. Stress and infections can increase histidine decarboxylase activity in some tissues. Histamine is widely distributed in body fluid and almost all organs. The highest concentration is in the lungs, but significant amounts are also found in the gut, liver, skin, and peripheral nerve trunks. Histamine is bound in the mast cells, where it is stored in large cytoplasmic granules.

When an antigen (a foreign substance) enters the body, it evokes a tissue response in the form of an antibody, which is synthesized specifically to combat the particular antigen. The complex reactions that follow are believed to trigger the release of histamine. It is this body chemical that evokes the symptoms more commonly known as the allergic reaction: red watery eyes, sneezing, urticaria (hives), rash, and bronchiolar constriction. Gastric mucosal cells (particularly the acid-secreting parietal cells) also stimulate the secretion of histamine. Histamine may be released from the mast cells by the action of competing compounds (binding sites), the process of exocytosis, and leakage due to damage to the mast cells. The aggregation of migrating leukocytes in the affected tissue is part of the inflammatory response resulting from cell degeneration. The release of histamine is the body's mobilization of a protective mechanism. Various physical and chemical stimuli, including certain chemical compounds and drugs and antigen-antibody reactions, can trigger this release. Histamine release is definitely involved in anaphylactic shock. It is a major mediator of allergic reactions like hay fever.

Histamine acts on two separate and distinct receptors, termed H_1 and H_2. Contraction of smooth muscle of the bronchi and intestine is mediated by H_1 receptors and is antagonized by a drug class identified as antihistamines. There are basically two types of drugs that block the histamine receptors. The antihistamines block the H_1 receptors in the upper respiratory system. The H_2 blockers affect the cells in the gastrointestinal tract. These drugs are discussed in Chapter 6. H_2 receptors mediate the action of histamine on gastric secretion and cardiac acceleration. The antagonists of this histamine are Tagamet (cimetidine), Zantac (ranitidine), Pepcid (famotidine), and Axid (nizatidine). These are thought of as H_2 blockers rather than antihistamines. Both are antihistamines that block histamine receptors. The H_2 blockers are discussed in Chapter 11.

THE ALLERGIC RESPONSE Allergy is a state of heightened sensitivity as a result of exposure to a particular substance. In the United States, 8% to 10% of the population responds to normally harmless substances with immune responses. A side effect of immunity is an abnormal immune reaction. Common allergens include pollens, mold, house dust, animal dander, feathers, wool, dyes, industrial chemicals, insect stings, foods, and medicines. Most allergens are moderately large molecules of protein that resist degradation by heat or acid.

The first exposure to an allergen generally gives little or no observable response; the second and subsequent exposures, however, can elicit a range of reactions from uncomfortable to life threatening. Some responses start within minutes of exposure; others may be delayed. The allergen may cause mild, moderate, or in some cases, severe inflammation. At the first exposure, the allergic individual produces and secretes immunoglobulin G (IgG) that binds to mast cells. When the immunoglobulin E (IgE) on mast cell membranes binds with antigen, the mast cells secrete histamine, prostaglandins (PGs), leukotrienes, and other substances that cause the inflammatory response.

Nasal entrances into the body are protected by cells capable of recognizing and destroying foreign substances before they injure cells. Macrophages, neutrophils, and eosinophils (found in tissues and blood) ingest and digest foreign particles. Mediator cells include mast cells, basophils, platelets, neutrophils, and enterochromaffin cells. When properly stimulated, these cells release chemical mediators.

The body responds with dilation of blood vessels, edema, constriction of smooth muscles, and recruitment of other cells to the immune response site. The resulting inflammatory response is an effective means of countering the invasion of foreign particles. In some persons, the response is too easily triggered or persists too long.

The cell types involved in these reactions are mast cells and basophils. Mast cells are found in the skin, nasal area, conjunctival mucosa, respiratory tissue, and the gut. Basophils, found normally in circulation, migrate into tissues during certain immune reactions. Both types of cells have receptors on their membranes with a high affinity for IgE. IgE binds to allergens and sends the chemical signal. Basophils contain preformed mediators that are released on the signal that IgE has bound to the antigen. Granules or pockets of mediators then open and release the chemicals, resulting in an immediate allergic reaction.

As allergens enter the bloodstream, lymphocytes produce antibodies that react with them to induce allergic inflammation and irritation in sensitive body areas, such as the eyes, nose, lungs, and digestive system. Itching and nasal symptoms (sneezing, rhinorrhea, and congestion) result from IgE activation of mast cells, which in turn release reactive mediators. Individuals disposed to reaction to allergens produce IgE on the mast cell membranes. IgE binds with the allergen causing mast cell degranulation and the release of mediators, which in turn cause inflammation. The effects of mediators are vasodilation (causing nasal blockage and stuffiness) and increased permeability of nasal vessels and glandular secretion (causing rhinorrhea). Nerve stimulation produces itching and sneezing.

Many mediators are chemotactic in that they attract various white cells (e.g., eosinophils, neutrophils, and T cells), setting off another release of mediators that further enhance the inflammatory process. The development of nasal hypersensitivity is an important result of the inflammation. Thus, the patient has an increased susceptibility to lower levels of allergens that otherwise would not cause a problem.

The mediator chemicals are primarily histamine and various enzymes (tryptase, chymase, and acid hydrolase). Other substances produced by mediator cells on IgE activation are leukotrienes, PGs, platelet-activating factor, and adenosine. Leukotrienes and PGs are of special concern in bronchoconstriction, as well as being potent chemotactic factors, causing additional movement of inflammatory cells into the site.

When histamine is released, the body reacts rapidly to its intense pharmacologic actions. Blood vessels dilate, causing a fall in peripheral resistance and increased capillary filling. The drop in blood pressure may be offset by the release of catecholamines. Capillary permeability increases, and bronchial and GI muscles constrict, causing difficulty in breathing. Stomach acid secretion increases, causing the gastric contents to become highly acidic. Local edema, pain, and itching occur, often leading to a phenomenon known as the triple response of flush, wheal, and flare. A flush is a reddening of the skin caused by increased blood flow into dilated vessels. A wheal is an elevated, smooth area on the skin surface, noticeably redder or paler than the surrounding skin, caused by leakage of fluids and some small proteins into the tissue, along with in-migration of white or other protective cells, or both. A flare is itching, pain, or a burning sensation caused by stimulation of nerve endings.

The significance of the triple response is the mobilization of the body's protective mechanism at the site of injury, including the increased passage of plasma proteins and white blood cells into tissue spaces because of traumatic tissue injury. Such injury may be the result of mechanical, thermal, or chemical means; ultraviolet radiation (sunburn); histamine-releasing drugs; animal venoms and toxins; plant poisons; bacterial toxins; or allergic reactions.

Anaphylaxis is an acute reaction to an antigen introduced into the bloodstream of a person with a level of antibodies against it. The results are local cellular damage at the entry site and the release of mediator chemicals, of which histamine and leukotrienes are thought to cause the most damage. Histamine causes severe peripheral vasodilation, loss of fluids through the capillary membranes, and bronchiolar spasm. The most unusual result is severe circulatory collapse with perhaps some respiratory difficulty, and the person is likely to die within the next few minutes if the reaction is severe enough.

As much as twenty percent of the population of the United States suffers from some degree of allergic rhinitis. The number with food allergy is not known; however, with milk, sensitivity is as high as 7.5%.

ALLERGIC DISEASES Allergic diseases have a wide range of causes and may involve any body system. Hay fever is caused by an allergic reaction of the nasal mucosa to the pollen of trees, grasses, weeds, and molds. It may occur in spring, summer, or fall and may last until frost. It is characterized by attacks of inflammation of the mucosa of the upper respiratory tract and conjunctiva, with excessive secretion from the nasal mucosa (rhinitis) and the tear ducts (watery eyes). The patient has spells of sneezing, itching and weeping eyes, running nose, and burning in the palate and throat. Asthma may sometimes be a complication. Inhibition of histamine release contributes to relief.

Allergic rhinitis causes nasal congestion, sneezing, and a runny nose due to allergies, often seasonal. Symptoms may, however, last year-round if caused by such allergens as house dust, animal dander, and foods.

Allergic dermatitis, or eczema, is a noncontagious, itchy rash that often occurs in the creases of the arms, legs, and neck, although it can cover the entire body. It is often associated with allergies.

Contact dermatitis comes from direct skin contact with an irritant; common irritants are animals, plants, chemicals, and minerals. Poison ivy is the most common causative agent of this condition.

Urticaria (hives) is an outbreak of itchy welts of varying size. They may develop on the face, lips, tongue, or throat; in the eyes or ears; or internally. Allergies to food or drugs, particularly penicillin and aspirin, are well-known causes.

DRUG THERAPY FOR ALLERGIES Treating allergies involves clearing the environment of allergens (if possible). If a particular food is a problem, it must be avoided. The most frequently used agents for symptomatic treatment are antihistamines (discussed in Chapter 6) and corticosteroids (discussed in Chapter 15).

Short-term relief of symptoms is often gained through antihistamines; long-term desensitization programs may be of benefit. First, the patient undergoes skin tests to identify the causative allergens. Gradual administration of larger and larger doses of the antigen stimulates the patient's body to make IgG instead of IgE. With each dose, the body makes more circulating IgG antibodies and IgG memory cells. IgG antibodies bind with the allergens blocking attachment of IgE to mast cells, thus blocking inflammation.

Medications and/or immunizing injections must be administered at the proper time. Remember that antihistamines work better at preventing the allergic symptoms than stopping it.

Prostaglandins

Prostaglandins (PGs) are mediators of several physiologic processes and are synthesized from arachidonic acid, a fatty acid. They are formed by intact tissues and cells and by extracts. They produce diverse, complex pharmacologic actions in several body systems and metabolic pathways.

ENDOCRINE SYSTEM ACTIONS In the endocrine system, PGF causes intense uterine contraction, while PGE, PGA, and PGB cause uterine relaxation. They are involved in the transport of semen in male and female tracts and assist nutrition of sperm by vasodilation of genital mucosal membranes. Sufficient PGs are absorbed from semen through vaginal mucosa to affect their motility through the fallopian tubes and thus facilitate the transport of spermatozoa to the ovum. PGs promote strong contractions in uterine smooth muscle, and their release at the appropriate time initiates parturition. They may be responsible for uterine spasms and other smooth-muscle activity during menstruation.

CARDIOVASCULAR SYSTEM ACTIONS In the cardiovascular system, PGs reduce blood pressure and increase heart rate and cardiac output (perfusion to tissues, liver, and kidneys). Reduced peripheral resistance is due to relaxation of arterial smooth muscle. Through renal action they promote the loss of water and sodium ions. Increased blood flow into the kidney cortex increases filtration and decreases reabsorption. PGs may act as natural antihypertensives by causing vasodilation or by promoting diuresis with sodium and water loss, or both. Elevation of free fatty acids by catecholamines and hormones is antagonized, causing lipolysis. Inhibition of adenylate cyclase in adipose tissue then prevents formation of cyclic adenosine monophosphate (cAMP), resulting in lower blood lipids.

GASTROINTESTINAL SYSTEM ACTIONS PGE and PGA stimulate gastrointestinal mucosal secretion. Aspirin and other nonsteroidal anti-inflammatory drugs (NSAIDs) inhibit PG formation and release. Gastric irritation and ulcers may then form, owing to loss of effect on gastric secretions, which protect gastric mucosa from acid and proteolytic enzymes.

PULMONARY SYSTEM ACTIONS Lungs remove PGs from the blood. PGs stored in the lung parenchyma and bronchial walls can produce bronchodilation to oppose constrictor activity of histamine, serotonin, and other constrictors.

INFLAMMATORY ACTIONS Endotoxins (complexes in bacterial cell walls that are pyrogenic and increase capillary permeability) stimulate the synthesis and release of prostaglandins, which act on the temperature center to produce fever. Antipyretic drugs inhibit PG synthesis. PG lowers the stimulatory threshold of sensory receptors, thereby allowing substances like bradykinin to stimulate receptors, causing pain. PG release is thought to cause the pain and inflammation of arthritis.

Bradykinin

Bradykinin is a polypeptide first discovered in urine. Researchers found that with IV administration, it would lower blood pressure. Bradykinin is formed from plasma alpha globulin and causes contraction of intestinal, uterine, and bronchial smooth muscle. Aspirin and some NSAIDs can block this reaction. It causes arterial dilation that is offset by the pressor action of increased heart rate, increased permeability (edema), and increased lymph production. It stimulates autonomic ganglion cells in contact with sensory nerve endings, which causes pain. Aspirin and other anti-inflammatory drugs antagonize this action by inhibiting synthesis of PGs, which potentiates the pain-producing action of bradykinin.

Chapter Summary

The Drug Prescription

◇ A prescription is an order written by a physician to be dispensed by a pharmacist and indicating the medication the patient needs.

Five "Rights" for Correct Drug Administration

◇ The five rights for correct drug administration are the right patient, the right drug, the right strength, the right route, and the right time.

Dosage Forms and Routes of Administration

◇ The three routes of administration are: oral, parenteral, and topical. The pharmacy technician must be familiar with each dosage form. The most common are:

oral	parenteral	topical
tablets	intravenous	ointments
capsules	injections	creams
syrups		gels
		suppositories
		patches
		lotions
		inhalants

Factors that Influence Drug Effects

◇ Altered drug responses in the elderly are due to age-related changes in organ function and body composition. These physiologic changes include visual, auditory, gastrointestinal, pulmonary, cardiovascular, renal, hormonal, and compositional alterations.

◇ Some special problems of the elderly are poor nutrition, adverse drug reactions, poor compliance with drug regimens, and the need for caregivers.

◇ Body surface area is the best method to determine a dosage for children; however, owing to the difficulty of ascertaining this measurement, weight is most frequently used.

◇ Immunization is the process whereby the immune system is stimulated to acquire immunity to a specific disease.

◇ Development of safe, effective vaccines to prevent infectious diseases has been responsible for the substantial decline morbidity and mortality associated with those diseases.

Teaching Patients to Manage Their Medications

◇ Patient compliance to dose schedule and to specific requirements of a drug regimen are important.

◇ A pharmacy technician can positively influence patient drug therapy by accurately collecting and recording patient medication history in the patient profile.

- Pharmacy technicians can help patients understand how to read medication labels.
- Patients should read the information provided with OTC drugs to understand their action, interactions, cautions, and possible side effects.

Natural Chemicals that Affect Drug Action and Response

- The body produces several chemicals naturally that invariably affect the metabolism of drugs. The important chemicals discussed in this chapter are histamine, prostaglandins (PGs), and bradykinin.
- Histamine is a chemical widely distributed in tissues and cells. The highest concentrations in humans are in the lungs, skin, and stomach. Histamine is released from the mast cells by compounds competing for receptor sites, by exocytosis, and by leakage from damaged mast cells.
- There are two types of histamine receptors. Antihistamines block the H_1 receptors. A class of drugs referred to as H_2 blockers blocks the H_2 receptors.
- Histamine release is clearly involved in anaphylactic shock, hay fever, and various other allergies and reactions.
- The classic allergic reaction is the phenomenon known as the triple response: flush, wheal, and flare.

Chapter Review

Understanding Pharmacology

Select the best answer from the choices given.

1. Which factor does not need to be considered when dosing a child?
   a. Clothes
   b. Age
   c. Height
   d. Weight

2. A prescription must contain the following parts, except the
   a. patient's name.
   b. drug and dose.
   c. *signa*.
   d. patient's age.

3. All the listed factors influence dosing, except the patient's
   a. age.
   b. disease state.
   c. body size.
   d. hair color.

4. Which route of medication administration is the most economical and convenient?
   a. Oral
   b. Topical
   c. Parenteral
   d. None of the above

5. Immunization has been found to
   a. cure some disease states.
   b. decrease morbidity and mortality associated with specific disease states.
   c. increase morbidity and mortality associated with specific disease states.
   d. None of the above

6. Federal law requires that pharmacists collect
   a. donations for hospitals.
   b. a patient history regarding the drug prescribed.
   c. pharmacokinetic data on animal models.
   d. a list of all the physicians in their state.

7. Which of the following drug forms are administered via the oral route?
   a. Tablets
   b. Syrups
   c. Capsules
   d. All of the above

8. Factors that determine the best route of administration include all of the following, except the
   a. patient's condition.
   b. type of container to be used.
   c. site of desired action.
   d. rapidity of the desired response.

9. A prescription label must have
   a. the patient's and physician's names.
   b. the dosage and how to take the drug.
   c. the address of the pharmacy and original date of fill.
   d. All of the above

10. Parenteral forms
    a. do not pass through the liver before entering the bloodstream.
    b. are inactivated in digestive juices.
    c. are the most common drug forms.
    d. are the most painless way to administer medications.

The following statements are true or false. If the answer is false, rewrite the statement so it is true.

___F___ 1. Pharmacists do not need to consider the natural chemicals of the body when dispensing drugs.

___T___ 2. The pharmacist must fill and interpret prescriptions. A part of this process includes determining the appropriateness and cost of the drug.

___F___ 3. In most states, physicians may stamp their name on the prescription.

___F___ 4. Elderly people do not spend much money on drugs and are, therefore, unconcerned about the cost.

___F___ 5. Constipation is never a problem for the elderly.

___F___ 6. It is easy to dose pediatric patients.

___F___ 7. Weight is the best method to dose children; however, body surface area is the most used.

___T___ 8. The physician's DEA must be on the prescription if it is a C-II, C-III, or C-IV drug.

___T___ 9. Many drugs now available OTC once required a prescription.

___F___ 10. A drug prepared for the otic route may be used in the eye.

Match the following prescription abbreviations with their correct meaning.

1.	qid	_____	a.	four times daily
2.	hs	_____	b.	after meals
3.	OS	_____	c.	at bedtime
4.	pc	_____	d.	left eye
5.	prn	_____	e.	intravenously
6.	IV	_____	f.	subcutaneously
7.	IM	_____	g.	as needed
8.	SC	_____	h.	intramuscularly
9.	gtt	_____	i.	right eye
10.	OD	_____	j.	drop
11.	OU	_____	k.	both eyes
12.	po	_____	l.	by mouth
13.	mcg	_____	m.	microgram
14.	g	_____	n.	cubic centimeter
15.	gr	_____	o.	grain
16.	cc	_____	p.	gram
17.	bid	_____	q.	daily
18.	tid	_____	r.	immediately
19.	stat	_____	s.	three times daily
20.	qd	_____	t.	twice daily

Pharmacology at Work

1. List the components of a prescription label.

2. List the components of a medication label on a container given to a patient.

3. List causes for and discuss altered drug response in the elderly.

4. List and explain three things to keep in mind when dosing a child.

Internet Research

Use the Internet to complete the following assignments.

1. Determine the immunization schedule for a twelve-month-old child. What immunizations should a child have within the first twelve months? List your Internet source(s).
2. Many elderly patients take more than one medication. Find information on the Internet that might be useful to these patients in managing their medications. What is the best way for an elderly patient to prevent drug interactions? Did any of your Internet sources address this question? Compare at least three sites. Which site was the most reliable source and why?

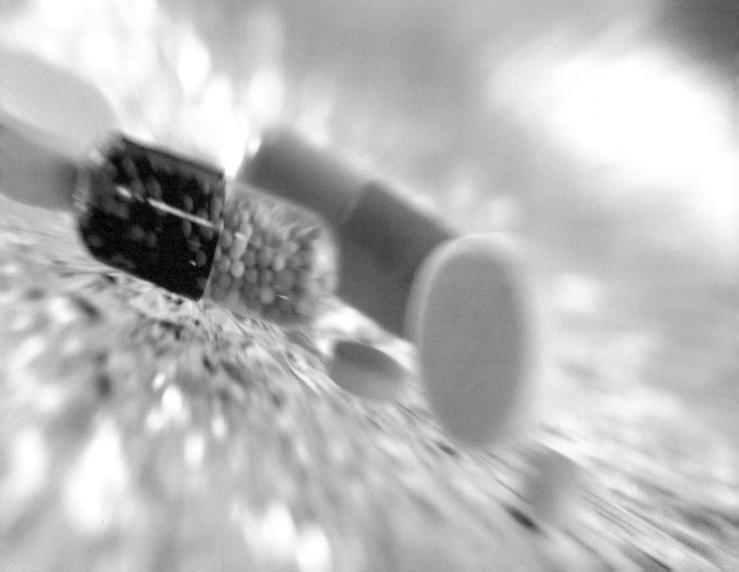

Anti-Infectives and Drugs for the Common Cold

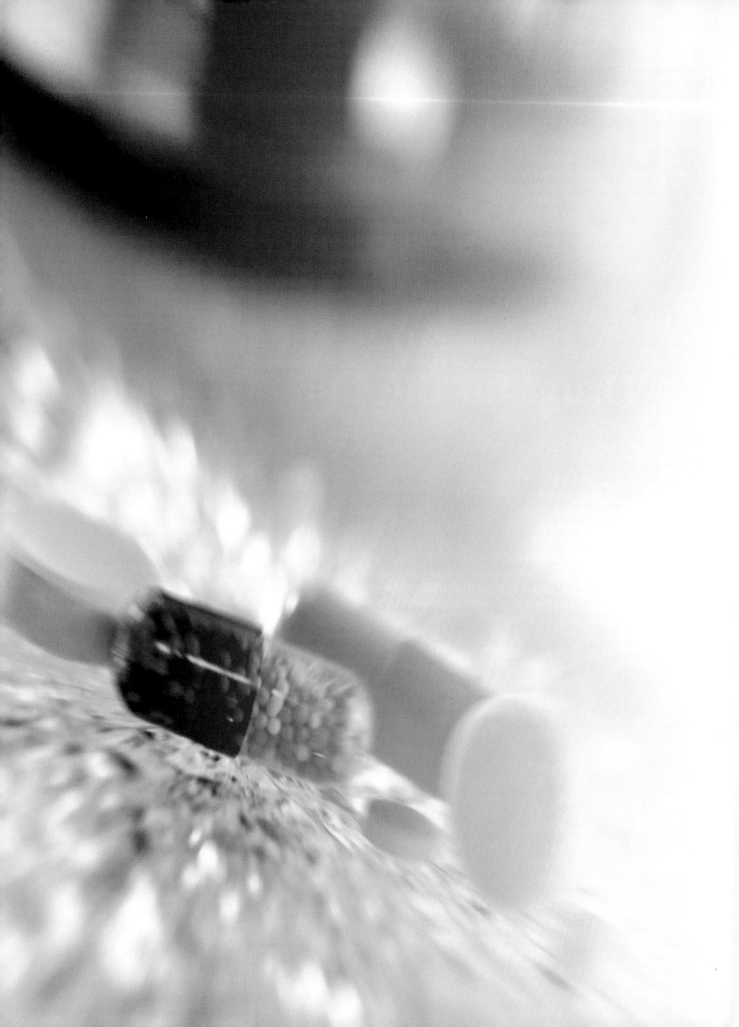

Antibiotics

4

Learning Objectives

- ◇ Identify the major types of antibiotics by drug class.
- ◇ Know indications for the major antibiotics.
- ◇ Define therapeutic effects, side effects, and administration routes of major antibiotics.
- ◇ Use antibiotic and general drug terminology correctly in written and oral communication.

Antibiotics are a major class of natural and synthetic pharmaceutical agents that kill or inhibit the growth of infection-causing microorganisms (bacteria). Antibiotics are frequently dispensed for community-acquired infections, which account for more outpatient visits to physicians than any other medical condition.

FIGHTING BACTERIAL INFECTIONS

Bacteria are single-celled organisms found almost everywhere. When bacteria penetrate body tissues, they establish an infection where their toxins can cause tissue damage. The body's immune system fights back to destroy the bacteria, usually resulting in fever and inflammation. The body can overcome many simple infections, but more serious infections often require the assistance of antibiotics to kill the invaders.

Although infectious diseases have existed for thousands of years, it was not until the nineteenth century that the cause—bacteria—was identified through the work of Louis Pasteur and other scientists. By the early twentieth century, the organisms that cause cholera, syphilis, bubonic plague, gonorrhea, leprosy, and other illnesses had been isolated and identified.

In 1907, German physician Paul Ehrlich patented the drug arsphenamine as a treatment for syphilis. Although this drug marked a breakthrough in eradicating a major infectious disease, it was not until 1936 that the first true antibiotic, sulfonamide, was discovered. When penicillin became widely available in the 1940s, physicians finally had a powerful weapon to use against several common infections, including strep throat, pneumonia, and venereal disease. Today a wide variety of antibiotics are used to combat bacteria-caused infections. Each drug is effective against specific kinds of bacteria.

Types of Bacteria

Bacteria are classified in several ways. Broadly, they are grouped into two types based on their need for oxygen. If the bacterium (singular form of bacteria) needs oxygen to survive, it is called aerobic; if it can survive in the absence of oxygen, it is called anaerobic. Aerobic bacteria cause most infections. Anaerobic bacteria are often found in nosocomial infections, infections acquired by patients while they are in the hospital.

Determining the appropriate antibiotic to use against a specific bacterium requires laboratory culture testing. A sample of material from the infected area is stained, observed under the microscope, and classified according to two characteristics which help determine the drug to prescribe. The first characteristic is the bacteria's shape and size. Bacteria cells may be round, rod-shaped, curved, or spiral (see Figure 4.1) and range in size from 0.5 micron (one-millionth of a meter) to 5 microns. The second characteristic is the bacteria's staining properties. Depending on their chemical makeup, bacteria turn certain colors during the testing technique called Gram's staining. If the stain they absorb is crystal violet (blue), the bacteria are gram-positive. If the stain is safranin (red), the bacteria are gram-negative. Figure 4.2 provides an example of the Gram's stain colors. Table 4.1 lists examples of these two bacteria characteristics and provides an example of a disease for each characteristic.

Symptoms of Bacterial Infections

The general signs that an infection may be of bacterial origin are a fever of 101°F or greater and an increased number of white blood cells (> 12,000). The onset of fever alone, however, is not diagnostic of a bacterial infection. A fever also may be caused by a self-limiting viral illness, or some types of malignancy and autoimmune disorders. In many situations, localizing symptoms or physical findings are necessary to explain the fever.

Figure 4.1

Characteristic Bacteria Shapes
(a) Round cocci
(b) Rod-like bacilli
(c) Spiral-shaped spirochetes

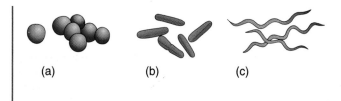

(a)　　　　(b)　　　　(c)

Figure 4.2

Gram's Stain
(a) Gram-positive bacteria turn a purple color.
(b) Gram-negative bacteria appear red.

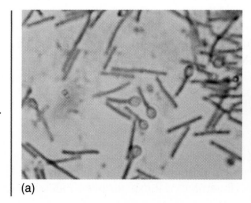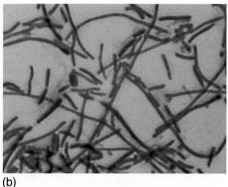

(a)　　　　(b)

Table 4.1	Examples of Bacteria Shapes, Gram's Stain Results, and Related Diseases

Shape	Gram's Stain	Bacteria	Related Diseases
rods	gram-positive	*Corynebacteria*	endocarditis
	gram-negative	*E. coli*	urinary tract infections (UTIs)
spheres	gram-positive	*Staphylococcus*	toxic shock syndrome (associated with tampon use)
	gram-negative	*Neisseria*	gonorrhea
curved or spiral rods	gram-negative	*Campylobacter*	septicemia
spirochetes	gram-negative	*Treponema palladium*	syphilis

Antibiotic Treatment and Action

Antibiotic treatment can be started after or before culturing the bacteria. The outcome of antibiotic treatment can be evaluated in two ways: (1) the clinical response, meaning the signs and symptoms disappear, or (2) the microbiological response, meaning the organism is completely eradicated.

When a patient has a serious or life-threatening infection, antibiotic treatment begins immediately. The patient is given a broad-spectrum antibiotic, which covers multiple organisms. The physician is not aware of the causative organism and probably does not have time to culture and get a definitive diagnosis until after the treatment has started. This is referred to as empirical treatment.

Antibiotics work by gaining access to the inside of the bacterial cell, where they interfere with bacterial life processes. Antibiotics work in one of five ways. They

- ◇ block protein formation: macrolides, tetracycline, aminoglycosides
- ◇ disrupt cell membrane: polymyxins
- ◇ inhibit cell wall formation: penicillins, cephalosporins
- ◇ interfere with DNA formation: nalidixic acid
- ◇ prevent folic acid synthesis: sulfonamides

An infection is an invasion of the body by pathogens resulting in tissue response to organisms and toxins. Antibiotics to treat these infections are bactericidal agents or bacteriostatic agents. The bactericidal agent kills the invading organisms and the bacteriostatic agent inhibits the growth or multiplication of bacteria.

Antibiotic Side Effects and Dispensing Issues

The parenteral forms of antibiotics should be mixed exactly as directed by the manufacturers. If mixed inappropriately, the drugs can cause tissue or vein irritation, be ineffective, or cause renal failure or even death. When dispensing oral forms of these drugs, it is important to swab the counting tray with alcohol between drugs to prevent cross-contamination. For example, if a tray was used to dispense sulfa and was not wiped down before another drug was placed on the tray, sulfa particles could stick to the new drug. This would contaminate the new drug, and when given to the patient, who is allergic to sulfa, could result in an adverse reaction. The patient could then think that the new drug caused the adverse reaction.

As a general guideline, most antibiotics should be taken on an empty stomach to attain faster absorption. There are exceptions to this rule; for example, **Macrodantin (nitrofurantoin)** and **Ceftin (cefuroxime)**. There are also antibiotics that can cause extreme GI upset. The prudent technician will be aware of this and put a "Take with Food" auxiliary label on these drugs (e.g., doxycycline, Augmentin).

The maintenance of consistent drug serum levels would require that the antibiotics be administered around the clock. An IV administration route can facilitate around-the-clock dosing for very ill patients. Otherwise, spacing the dosage evenly throughout the day will suffice to maintain a relatively constant drug serum level.

Antimicrobial Resistance

By the early twenty-first century, many patients are being infected with diseases once controlled by antibiotics, including pneumonia, tuberculosis, and meningitis. New infections are surfacing because many existing drugs no longer work. Resistance to antibiotics is developing largely because of overuse and misuse. Broad-spectrum antibiotics are often prescribed without a specific diagnosis of bacterial infection. Patients, for their part, often do not finish an antibiotic treatment once they begin to feel better. This enables the remaining bacteria to develop a resistant species. If the infection recurs, it is more difficult to treat. If the mutant species is passed on to another individual, it is equally difficult to treat. As a result, patients must take more and stronger drugs.

The pharmacy technician's role in preventing overuse of antibiotics is to ensure that all antibiotic prescriptions display an auxiliary label on the bottle advising the patient to take all the medication.

A superinfection, a new infection complicating the course of therapy of an existing infection, may occur. This occurs because bacteria or fungi resistant to the drugs in use ivade the body.

Drug destruction by bacterial enzymes in resistant organisms is the most frequent form of antibiotic resistance. Beta-lactamase producing bacteria change antibiotics such as penicillins and cephalosporins into inactive compounds. One bacterium, *Staphylococcus aureus*, can secrete protective enzymes into its surrounding environment to inactivate antibiotics before they reach the cell.

Other bacteria, e.g., klebsiella, enterobacteria, and proteus, have a space between an outer and inner membrane into which an enzyme is injected to destroy the antibiotic before it crosses the inner membrane and enters the cell. Staphylococcus, some gram-positive, and some gram-negative organisms have developed multiple aminoglycoside enzymes that bind to the drug so it cannot attach to binding sites on the bacteria.

Another way that bacteria inactivate antibiotics is by changing the composition of the bacterial membranes or by reducing the number and size of proteins in the membrane. This prevents the antibiotics from entering the cell.

Some bacteria have developed pumps that flush antibiotics out of and away from the cell membrane. Other organisms may enzymatically inactivate the antibiotic. The target or binding site may be changed by the bacteria. There is also a form of DNA mutation of which the bacteria is capable. These mechanisms used by bacteria to develop antimicrobial resistance are referred to as (1) mutation, (2) transduction, (3) transformation, and (4) conjugation.

CLASSES OF ANTIBIOTICS

Before 1935, systemic bacterial infections could not be effectively treated with drugs. Antiseptics and disinfectants could eradicate infections when applied topically, but their systemic use was ruled out because they were not safe enough. With the discovery of sulfonamides, a new era began. Each new class of antibiotics has some similar molecular structures for all drugs of the class.

Sulfonamides

Sulfonamides, or sulfa drugs, are bacteriostatic and are effective against a broad range of microorganisms because they block a specific step in the biosynthetic pathway of folic acid. Bacteria cannot absorb folic acid; therefore, they must make it from precursors. The sulfas interfere with PABA (para-aminobenzoic acid) and folic acid formation, thereby destroying the bacteria. Table 4.2 lists the most-commonly used sulfonamides.

In addition to sulfa, several antibacterial agents are used almost exclusively to treat urinary tract infections. One is a **nitrofurantoin (Macrodantin, Macrobid)**. Its mechanism of action is unknown, but it has a wide antibacterial spectrum. It works better when taken with food. Nausea is the primary side effect, so this is another reason it is important to take this drug with food. This drug may also turn urine brown. The technician will always need to place an auxiliary label on these sulfonamides and related drugs reminding the patient to drink lots of water or other fluids.

THERAPEUTIC USES OF SULFONAMIDES Sulfonamides are among the drugs of choice for the following illnesses.

- ◇ urinary tract infections (UTIs)
- ◇ otitis media (especially in children)
- ◇ ulcerative colitis
- ◇ lower respiratory infections
- ◇ general infections
- ◇ *Escherichia coli*
- ◇ *Streptococcus pneumoniae*
- ◇ prophylaxis in neutropenic patients versus *Pneumocystis carinii*

SULFONAMIDES' SIDE EFFECTS AND DISPENSING ISSUES Sulfa drugs in use today have fewer allergic reactions than the older drugs. The most common side effect is a rash. Other side effects include nausea, drug fever (often confused with a recurrent fever from the infection), vomiting, jaundice, blood complications (acute hemolytic anemia, agranulocytosis, and aplastic anemia), and kidney damage. Stevens-Johnson syndrome—a variant form of erythema multiforme, which can be fatal—can occur from use of sulfas. Patients taking sulfa drugs should be warned to avoid the sun, which can cause severe skin rashes. Sulfonamides can crystallize in the urine and

Table 4.2	**Most-Commonly Used Sulfonamides**	
Generic Name	**Brand Name**	**Dosage Form**
sulfamethoxazole	Gantanol	tablet, oral suspension
sulfamethoxazole-trimethoprim	Bactrim, Septra	oral suspension, tablet, IV
sulfasalazine	Azulfidine	tablet, enteric-coated tablet, oral suspension
sulfisoxazole	Gantrisin	tablet, oral suspension, ointment, ophthalmic
sulfisoxazole-phenazopyridine	Azo Gantrisin	tablet

deposit in the kidneys, resulting in a painful, dangerous condition. To reduce this risk, it is important that a patient taking sulfa drugs maintain an adequate fluid intake of at least six to eight glasses a day.

Penicillins

Penicillin is a highly effective antibiotic with extremely low toxicity. Manipulating the basic molecular structure of the drug has led to many effective derivatives. It is obtained from the mold *Penicillium chrysogenum*. Penicillin kills bacteria by preventing them from forming the rigid cell wall needed for survival. The weakened cell wall allows an excessive amount of water to enter the bacterium through osmosis. The cell increases in size and lyses as the cell membrane cannot contain the cell contents. Human cells do not have cell walls; therefore, they are not affected by penicillin.

Table 4.3 lists the most-commonly used penicillins by generic and brand names and provides the dosage forms for each.

THERAPEUTIC USES OF PENICILLINS Penicillin is most active against growing and reproducing bacteria, generally gram-positive aerobes, and anaerobes. Penicillins are among the drugs of choice for the following illnesses.

- abscesses
- beta hemolytic streptococcus
- meningitis
- otitis media
- pneumonia
- respiratory infections
- tooth and gum infections
- venereal diseases (syphilis and gonorrhea)

Penicillin and other antibiotics have been shown to reduce risk of disease or death for patients with subacute bacterial endocarditis, an inflammation of the lining of the heart and its valves. These patients are at risk any time a body cavity is invaded.

Preventative dosing, or prophylaxis, is also recommended whenever patients with a heart prosthesis, idiopathic hypertrophic subaortic stenosis, congenital heart disease, mitral valve prolapse, a heart murmur, or a history of rheumatic heart disease undergo any kind of surgical procedure. The American Medical Association recommends the patient be medicated thirty to sixty minutes before the procedure and for six to ten days following it. How this is done is determined by the procedure to be performed. The most common regimen is dental prophylaxis. The American

Table 4.3	Most-Commonly Used Penicillins		
Generic Name	**Brand Name**		**Dosage Form**
amoxicillin	Amoxil, Polymox		capsule, oral suspension
ampicillin	Omnipen, Principen		capsule, oral suspension
penicillin G	various brand names, also different salts, i.e., potassium, sodium		IM, IV
penicillin V	Veetids		tablet, oral suspension

Dental Association (ADA) released new guidelines for prophylactic therapy in 1997. These guidelines recommend that a single 2 g dose of amoxicillin be administered before dental procedures. For penicillin-allergic patients 600 mg of Cleocin (clindamycin) or 500 mg of Zithromax (azithromycin) is recommended.

PENICILLINS' SIDE EFFECTS AND DISPENSING ISSUES Many penicillins should be taken on an empty stomach with water because food slows absorption, and the acids in fruit juices or colas could deactivate the drug. The most common side effect of these drugs is diarrhea. Penicillin allergy affects 7% to 10% of the population. The allergy may vary from an itchy, very red mild rash to wheezing and anaphylaxis, which can be fatal.

Some organisms are resistant to penicillin owing to the beta-lactamase enzymes. Penicillins are ineffective against staphylococcal penicillinases.

◇ **Penicillin G** is the prototype, but absorption from the gastrointestinal tract is incomplete; therefore, it is used in the injectable form.

◇ **Penicillin V** is available as a potassium salt, which exhibits greatly enhanced resistance to hydrolysis by gastric acid, so it is the preferred oral form. It is the drug of choice for strep throat.

◇ **Ampicillin** has a broader antimicrobial spectrum than penicillin G. It will cause skin rash with a 100% frequency in patients with mononucleosis and in the past was used to identify and diagnose this infection.

◇ **Amoxicillin** is dosed three times a day versus ampicillin's four times a day dosage. Amoxicillin reaches higher concentrations on a milligram per milligram basis.

Warning
Amoxicillin is dosed three times daily and ampicillin is dosed four times daily.

RESISTANT PENICILLINS Because some organisms are resistant to penicillin, three types of drugs have been developed to accommodate the ineffectiveness of penicillin in specific circumstances: (1) penicillinase-resistant penicillins, (2) extended-spectrum penicillins, and (3) penicillin combinations (see Table 4.4).

Penicillinase-resistant penicillin drugs work against most gram-positive and gram-negative aerobes and a few gram-positive and gram-negative anaerobic bacteria.

Extended-spectrum penicillins are more active than natural penicillins. They are more resistant to inactivation by gram-negative bacteria, or they are more readily absorbed into the membrane of the organism.

Penicillin is sometimes combined with other drugs to improve its effect. Certain beta-lactamase inhibitors, such as clavulanate, have been combined with amoxicillin and ticarcillin with therapeutic benefit. **Unasyn (ampicillin-sulbactam)** works on ampicillin-resistant organisms due to sulbactam inhibiting the beta-lactamase enzyme. Diarrhea and nausea are common side effects of **Augmentin (amoxicillin-clavulanate)**. **Timentin (ticarcillin-clavulanate)** has only an IV dosage form.

Cephalosporins

Cephalosporins have the same mechanism of action as penicillins, but differ in their antibacterial spectrum, resistance to beta-lactamase, and pharmacokinetics. A person allergic to penicillin has around a ten percent chance to also be allergic to cephalosporins. Most computerized drug profile systems place them in the same category; therefore, if someone has an allergy to either, the computer system will indicate that the patient is allergic to both. Most cephalosporins are divided into first-, second-, third-, and fourth-generation agents (see Table 4.5).

The first-generation cephalosporins are similar to the penicillinase-resistant penicillins with slightly greater gram-negative coverage. They are used for community-

Table 4.4 **Most-Commonly Used Resistant Penicillins**

Generic Name	Brand Name	Dosage Form
Penicillinase-Resistant Penicillins		
dicloxacillin	Dynapen	capsule, oral solution
mezlocillin	Mezlin	IM, IV
nafcillin	Unipen	capsule, tablet, IM, IV
oxacillin	Bactocill, Prostaphlin	capsule, oral solution, IM, IV
Extended-Spectrum Penicillins		
carbenicillin	Geocillin	tablet
piperacillin	Pipracil	IM, IV
ticarcillin	Ticar	IV
Penicillin Combinations		
amoxicillin-clavulanate	Augmentin	oral suspension, tablet, chewable
ampicillin-sulbactam	Unasyn	IM, IV
piperacillin-tazobactam	Zosyn	IV
ticarcillin-clavulanate	Timentin	IV

Table 4.5 **Most-Commonly Used Cephalosporins**

Generic Name	Brand Name	Dosage Form
First-Generation Cephalosporins		
cefadroxil	Duricef	capsule, oral suspension, tablet
cefazolin	Ancef, Kefzol	IM, IV
cephalexin	Keflex	capsule, oral suspension, tablet
cephalothin	Ceporacin	IM, IV
cephapirin	Cefadyl	IM, IV
cephradine	Velosef	capsule, oral suspension, IM, IV
Second-Generation Cephalosporins		
cefaclor	Ceclor	capsule, oral suspension, extended-release tablet
cefamandole	Mandol	IM, IV
cefonicid	Monocid	IM, IV
cefotetan	Cefotan	IM, IV
cefoxitin	Mefoxin	IM, IV
cefuroxime	Zinacef, Ceftin	IM, IV, oral suspension, tablet
Third-Generation Cephalosporins		
cefdinir	Omnicef	oral suspension, capsule
cefixime	Suprax	oral suspension, tablet
cefoperazone	Cefobid	IM, IV
cefotaxime	Claforan	IM, IV
cefpodoxime	Proxetil	tablet
	Vantin	oral suspension
ceftazidime	Fortaz	IM, IV
ceftibuten	Cedax	oral suspension, capsule
ceftizoxime	Cefizox	IM, IV
ceftriaxone	Rocephin	IM, IV
Fourth-Generation Cephalosporins		
cefepime	Maxipime	IM, IV

acquired infections in ambulatory patients and mild to moderate infections in institutionalized patients.

The second-generation cephalosporins have increased activity, especially against *H. influenza*, an important pathogen in the pediatric group. Second-generation cephalosporins are used for otitis media in children and for respiratory and urinary tract infections in hospitalized patients.

The most recently developed third-generation cephalosporins are active against a wide spectrum of gram-negative organisms. They are used in hospital-acquired infections. Because of their long half-life, the agents are also used in ambulatory patients, especially children, with dosing done before and after school. Orally active third-generation cephalosporins include **Suprax (cefixime)**, **Cedax (ceftibuten)**, **Omnicef (cefdinir)**, and **Vantin (cefpodoxime)**.

Maxipime (cefepime) is an injectable fourth-generation cephalosporin considered to have broad-spectrum coverage. It is approved for treating pneumonia, urinary tract infections, and skin infections. Maxipime (cefepime) is considered as effective as **Fortaz (ceftazidime)**, but it is more cost-effective because it is given twice daily versus three times daily for ceftazidime.

THERAPEUTIC USES OF CEPHALOSPORINS Cephalosporins are among the drugs of choice for the following conditions.

- deep-seated infections
- dentistry work, oral infections
- heart and pacemaker procedures
- neurosurgical operations
- OB/GYN procedures and surgery
- orthopedic surgery
- pneumonia
- upper-respiratory and sinus infections

CEPHALOSPORINS' SIDE EFFECTS AND DISPENSING ISSUES Cephalosporins share the same side effects as penicillin; however, a few have been known to initiate unique toxic reactions. These drugs are commonly used in many clinical situations, since they are associated with a lower frequency of toxicity than many other antibiotics. Use of the specific drugs should be gauged by sensitivity testing of the microorganism isolated from the patient.

Diabetic patients who are prescribed **Omnicef (cefdinir)** in oral suspension form must be informed of its high sugar content (2.86 g per teaspoonful). **Cefpodoxime** as an oral suspension is **Vantin**, and it is a tablet as **Proxetil**. Prescriptions written for the brand name will be easily distinguished, but if the physician writes for the generic, the pharmacist or pharmacy technician may need a physician verification since the dosage strengths are the same. With the exception of Suprax and Omnicef, which may be stored at room temperature, oral suspensions of cephalosporins must be refrigerated following reconstitution.

STRUCTURALLY RELATED DRUGS Several new beta-lactam drugs, differing slightly from penicillin and the cephalosporins, have been introduced. One is **Primaxin (imipenem-cilastatin)**, classified as a carbapenem with excellent in vitro and in vivo activity for gram-positive and gram-negative bacteria. Side effects are similar to other beta-lactams except seizures seem to occur more frequently. A new carbapenem, **Merrem (meropenem)**, has similar coverage, but Merrem is less likely to cause seizures. It is approved for bacterial meningitis and intra-abdominal infections.

A monobactam, **Azactam (aztreonam)**, is also being used to treat serious infections, particularly of the urinary tract, with good success and low toxicity. Aztreonam is active only against gram-negative bacilli. The advantage of this drug is an unlikely cross-allergenicity with other beta-lactams. It is used against aerobic gram-negative infections. It should be administered by intravenous push over three to five minutes or by intermittent infusion over twenty to sixty minutes. Aztreonam should be mixed not to exceed 20 mg/mL. It should be administered around the clock rather than three times a day to promote less variation in peak and trough serum levels. Patients should notify their physician immediately if skin rash, redness, or itching develops.

Another related drug is **Lorabid (loracarbef)**, which is in the carbacephem class. It is similar to a beta-lactam antibiotic and lyses the bacteria. It is most frequently given to children because the suspension is stable for fourteen days at room temperature. The drug should be taken on an empty stomach.

Tetracyclines

Tetracyclines are produced by soil organisms. They are broad-spectrum bacteriostatic antibiotics that inhibit protein synthesis in bacteria by binding to ribosomes. They suppress the infection and require phagocytes to complete eradication of bacteria. Table 4.6 lists the most-commonly used tetracyclines.

THERAPEUTIC USES OF TETRACYCLINES Tetracyclines are among the drugs of choice for the following illnesses.

- acne
- chronic bronchitis
- intra-abdominal infections
- Lyme disease
- *Mycoplasma pneumoniae* infection (walking pneumonia)
- *Rickettsia* infection (Rocky Mountain spotted fever)
- skin, soft tissue infections
- some venereal diseases, such as Chlamydia infection
- traveler's diarrhea (used as prophylaxis)

Warning

Doxycycline, an antibiotic, can be mistaken for doxepin, an antidepressant.

TETRACYCLINES' SIDE EFFECTS AND DISPENSING ISSUES The primary side effects seem to be gastrointestinal upset with nausea and vomiting. Antacids containing aluminum, calcium, or magnesium and laxatives containing magnesium, iron, and sodium bicarbonate should be separated by several hours from the tetracyclines when taking any of these drugs in the same regimen.

Patients should be warned to avoid the sun due to photosensitization. They should also be warned to avoid dairy products with most tetracyclines, with the

Table 4.6	**Most-Commonly Used Tetracyclines**	
Generic Name	**Brand Name**	**Dosage Form**
demeclocycline	Declomycin	capsule, tablet
doxycyline	Vibramycin	capsule, IV, oral suspension, tablet
minocycline	Minocin	capsule, IV, oral suspension
tetracycline	Achromycin, Sumycin	capsule, oral suspension, topical, tablet

exception of doxycycline. The tetracyclines should be avoided in pregnant women and in young children up to nine years old because of tooth discoloration and the effects on bone growth. The drug should be taken on an empty stomach to avoid chelation with minerals.

Always watch the expiration date on these drugs. It can be very dangerous to dispense an out-of-date tetracycline since an expired drug can be toxic. It is important to tell patients to take all of the drug, but if any is left it should be disposed of.

Macrolides

Macrolide antibiotics are bacteriostatic agents used primarily to treat pulmonary infections caused by *Legionella* and gram-positive organisms. Erythromycin inhibits protein synthesis by combining with ribosomes. Biaxin (clarithromycin), Zithromax (azithromycin), and Dynabac (dirithromycin) cause less gastrointestinal upset. Table 4.7 lists the most-commonly used macrolides.

THERAPEUTIC USES OF MACROLIDES Macrolides are among the drugs of choice for the following illnesses.

◇ *Chlamydia*
◇ enterococcus
◇ group A beta hemolytic strep
◇ *H. influenza*
◇ Legionnaire's disease
◇ *M. pneumoniae*
◇ *Neisseria*
◇ *S. pneumoniae*

Legionnaire's disease.

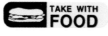 **TAKE WITH FOOD**

MACROLIDES' SIDE EFFECTS AND DISPENSING ISSUES Most antibiotics should be taken on an empty stomach to attain faster absorption; however, erythromycins usually cause such severe gastrointestinal distress that a "Take with food" sticker is placed on the prescription bottle.

Table 4.7	**Most-Commonly Used Macrolides**	
Generic Name	**Brand Name**	**Dosage Form**
azithromycin	Zithromax	capsule, oral suspension
clarithromycin	Biaxin	granules for oral suspension, film-coated tablet
dirithromycin	Dynabac	enteric-coated tablet
erythromycin	A/T/S, EryDerm, T-Stat	various topicals
erthyromycin base	Eryc, E-mycin, Ery-Tab	capsule, tablet, enteric-coated tablet, film-coated tablet
erythromycin estolate	Ilosone	capsule, oral suspension, tablet
erythromycin ethylsuccinate	E.E.S., EryPed	oral suspension, tablet, chewable, topical
erythromycin gluceptate	Ilotycin	IM, IV
erythromycin stearate	Erythrocin	film-coated tablet, IM, IV
erythromycin-sulfisoxazole	Pediazole	suspension

Some of the newer macrolides can be taken with less regard to meals. **Biaxin (clarithromycin)** may be taken without regard to meals. It is given twice daily. Biaxin XL, the extended-release form of clarithromycin, is taken only once a day and is associated with even fewer side effects. It should be taken with food. **Zithromax (azithromycin)** is dispensed in a dose pack. On the first day, the patient takes a loading dose of 500 mg. Maintenance doses of 250 mg once daily are then taken on days two through five, although this regimen can vary depending on the type of infection. **Dynabac (dirithromycin)** requires once-daily dosing and should be taken with food.

If taken over a long period, **Ilosone (erythromycin estolate)**, has a high incidence of cholestatic jaundice (patient turns yellow), especially in pregnant women. Macrolides will also inhibit the metabolism of theophylline, warfarin, carbamazepine, and cyclosporine.

Quinolones

The quinolones have strong, rapid bactericidal action against most gram-negative and many gram-positive bacteria. They antagonize the enzyme responsible for coiling and replicating DNA (for growth), causing DNA breakage and cell death. Humans do not have this enzyme, so their cells are unaffected. All quinolones cross the central nervous system. Table 4.8 lists the most-commonly used quinolones.

THERAPEUTIC USES OF QUINOLONES Quinolones are among the drugs of choice for the following conditions.

- ◇ bone and joint infections
- ◇ dental work and gum or tooth infections
- ◇ infectious diarrhea
- ◇ ophthalmic infections
- ◇ some sexually transmitted diseases
- ◇ upper respiratory infections
- ◇ urinary tract infections (UTIs)

Table 4.8	**Most-Commonly Used Quinolones**	
Generic Name	**Brand Name**	**Dosage Form**
cinoxacin	Cinobac	capsule
ciprofloxacin	Cipro, Ciloxin	tablet, oral suspension, ophthalmic, IM, IV, otic
enoxacin	Penetrex	tablet
gatifloxacin	Tequin	tablet, IM, IV
levofloxacin	Levaquin	IV
lomefloxacin	Maxaquin	tablet
moxifloxacin	Avelox	tablet
nalidixic acid	NegGram	oral suspension, tablet
norfloxacin	Noroxin	tablet
ofloxacin	Floxin	tablet, IV, otic
	Ocuflox	ophthalmic
sparfloxacin	Zagam	tablet
trovafloxacin	Trovan	IV, tablet

Trovan (trovafloxacin) has the broadest spectrum of all the quinolones and can be used as a single agent in the treatment of infections that would otherwise require a combination regimen. It should be restricted to patients with potentially life-threatening infections. Deaths have been reported due to liver toxicity induced by this drug. Therefore it is not used as an initial therapy but rather reserved for the treatment of otherwise resistant infections. It crosses the central nervous system so it is recommended that this drug be taken at bedtime or with food to reduce dizziness. Dairy products should not be taken concurrently with this drug. It is also phototoxic so patients should be advised to avoid sunlight. Because it is so potent, trovafloxacin is frequently used as a standard against which other antibiotics are measured.

QUINOLONES' SIDE EFFECTS AND DISPENSING ISSUES The side effects are primarily gastrointestinal, with nausea and vomiting. There also can be some joint swelling, dizziness, and an unpleasant taste. Antacids will interfere with their absorption. Quinolones should not be given with theophylline because of the increased risk of theophylline toxicity. These drugs are phototoxic, so patients taking these drugs should be warned to avoid exposure to the sun. Quinolones can cause joint problems and malformations. Patients on quinolones have a tendency to injure tendons. They should not be used by persons under eighteen years of age or by pregnant women.

Streptogrammins

Streptogrammins inhibit protein synthesis within the bacterial ribosomes. Quinupristin and dalfopristin are two streptogrammin antibiotics. Streptogrammins are useful in the treatment of vancomycin- and methicillin-resistant infections. Streptogrammins were granted accelerated approval under FDA because of the drug's ability to treat these life-threatening conditions.

Synercid (quinupristin-dalfopristin), a drug which combines the streptogrammins quinupristin and dalfopristin at a ratio of 30 parts quinupristin to 70 parts dalfopristin, is used primarily to treat life-threatening infections associated with vancomycin-resistant *enterococcus facium*. This class of antibiotics is an important addition to antimicrobial drug therapy since it is the alternative to vancomycin.

Streptogrammins are used for gram-positive infections, *enterococcus facium*, and vancomycin-resistant infections.

The side effects of streptogrammins are similar to those associated with the quinolones and include nausea, vomiting, joint swelling and dizziness. Synercid is administered intravenously and most patients experience an adverse reaction at the infusion site. Prior to administration, IV lines must be flushed with D_5W (5% dextrose) to ensure that the drug does not come into contact with saline or any other medications. Synercid inhibits cytochrome P-450 3A4; as a result, there are some potentially serious drug interactions. Synercid must be stored in a refrigerator.

Aminoglycosides

Aminoglycosides are commonly used to treat serious infections. Their bactericidal action inhibits bacterial protein synthesis by binding to ribosomal subunits. After the first dose, the dosage should be adjusted according to plasma concentrations of the drug in the individual patient. Table 4.9 lists the most-commonly used aminoglycosides.

Aminoglycosides are among the drugs of choice for treating life-threatening infections, sepsis (blood-borne infections), immunocompromised patients, and peritonitis.

Table 4.9	Most-Commonly Used Aminoglycosides	
Generic Name	**Brand Name**	**Dosage Form**
amikacin	Amikin	IM, IV
gentamicin	Garamycin	cream, IM, IV, ophthalmic
neomycin	Mycifradin	tablet, solution, IM, cream, ointment
netilmicin	Netromycin	IM, IV
streptomycin	(none)	IM, IV
tobramycin	Nebcin	IM, IV, ophthalmic

The major side effects of these drugs are nephrotoxicity and ototoxicity. Neuromuscular blockade can also be a problem. They may cause dose-related changes in vestibular and auditory function, ranging from equilibrium problems and hearing problems such as tinnitus to permanent deafness.

New evidence suggests that these drugs can be dosed once a day instead of two to three times daily. Bacterial growth remains suppressed for a while, even after serum levels have declined. Less frequent dosing may help to reduce their toxicity, as less drug may accumulate in the kidney and ear when there is a brief, high peak rather than steady concentrations. Once-daily dosing also reduces costs and simplifies drug monitoring. When dosing once daily, there is usually no need to measure peak drug levels; however, trough levels should be checked before the second dose to make sure the patient is eliminating the drug quickly enough.

MISCELLANEOUS ANTIBIOTICS

The following antibiotics are independent of other classes and each other due to structural differences.

Vancocin (Vancomycin)

Vancocin (vancomycin) is a bacteriocidal drug that interferes with bacterial wall synthesis. It is especially useful for methicillin-resistant *S. aureus*, pseudomembranous enterocolitis, and *C. difficile*. However, because vancomycin has been overused, bacterial resistance to this drug is increasing rapidly.

Vancomycin is among the drugs of choice for the following conditions.

◇ dialysis patients
◇ endocarditis
◇ staph infections (methicillin-resistant *Staphylococcus aureus*, MRSA)

The Centers for Disease Control (CDC) has strict guidelines for this drug due to its overuse.

Vancomycin is ototoxic and nephrotoxic. Neutropenia can be a problem. After the first dose, this drug should be dosed based on the individual patient's plasma concentrations.

When dispensed intravenously, vancomycin is usually mixed with at least 250 mL of fluid. This hydrates the patient and prevents nephrotoxicity. Even though the drug diluent ratio is 1 g per 200 mL, it is always best to mix this drug in a larger amount of fluid than the minimum required. This tactic will also prevent the drug from being infused too quickly and prevent the patient from experiencing Red Man's syndrome. The rate of infusion should not exceed 10 mg per minute or the IV solution should be infused over one hour—whichever is slower. It can also be given orally for *C. difficile*, an infection of the gastrointestinal tract. Metronidazole is also used for this purpose.

Chloromycetin (Chloramphenicol)

Chloromycetin (chloramphenicol) is a bacteriostatic antibiotic with a broad antibacterial spectrum. It was the drug of choice for typhoid fever, but because of its toxicities it is rarely given anymore. It inhibits protein synthesis by binding the ribosomal subunit. It is ineffective intramuscularly, but it can be given by mouth and intravenously. Chloromycetin (chloramphenicol) is among the drugs of choice for bacterial meningitis and salmonella with septicemia (infecting organisms present in circulating blood). Chloramphenicol use has been severely restricted because of its tendency to produce abnormalities in the blood.

Cleocin (Clindamycin)

A derivative of lincomycin, **Cleocin (clindamycin)** is a broad-spectrum antibiotic that inhibits protein synthesis. It is used for serious gram-negative infections and as a prophylaxis preceding abdominal surgery. It is also frequently dispensed in a topical form for the treatment of acne. It is effective against *Bacteroides fragilis*.

Clindamycin is among the drugs of choice for the following conditions.

◇ acne
◇ alternative in dental prophylaxis for patients allergic to penicillin
◇ anaerobic pneumonia
◇ bone infections (high concentrations in bone)
◇ bowel infections
◇ female genital infections
◇ intra-abdominal infections

Clindamycin's most serious side effect is pseudomembranous colitis (bloody diarrhea caused when toxin forms in the gut and the top layer of the colon is sloughed off). If the patient develops diarrhea, the drug must be discontinued.

Flagyl (Metronidazole)

Flagyl (metronidazole) is used primarily to treat trichomonas infections of the vaginal canal and cervix and of the male urethra. It is also used to treat amebic dysentery, giardia infections of the intestine, and serious infections caused by certain strains of anaerobic bacteria. It destroys components of the bacterium's DNA nucleus.

Metronidazole is among the drugs of choice for the following conditions.

◇ amebic dysentery
◇ *C. difficile*
◇ intestinal infections
◇ venereal diseases

Some side effects include a metallic taste, diarrhea, intolerance to alcohol, and rash. It may also discolor the urine. It may be taken with food to decrease gastrointestinal upset.

Efficacious treatment of venereal diseases requires that all sexual partners be treated at the same time and avoid sexual contact for three to four days; otherwise reinfection will occur, becoming a vicious cycle. Patients must be told to not drink alcohol with this drug.

Pentam and NebuPent (Pentamidine)

Pentam and **NebuPent (pentamidine)** are used as second line agents for *P. carinii pneumonia*. Its mechanism of action is unknown. It can be administered IV or IM once daily and by inhalation once every 4 weeks. The patient may develop sudden hypotension (low blood pressure). Thus, it is important to have emergency drugs and equipment on hand when administering this drug IV or IM.

To administer by inhalation the dose should be diluted in 6 mL of sterile water and delivered at 6 mL per minute by a jet nebulizer. Patients who develop wheezing or coughing during therapy may benefit by pretreatment (five minutes before) with a bronchodilator.

Chapter Summary

Fighting Bacterial Infections

◇ Bacteria are single-celled organisms found almost everywhere. They can penetrate body tissues and set up areas of infection.

◇ Anaerobic bacteria are often found in hospital-acquired (nosocomial) infections. Gram-negative bacteria predominate in the hospital environment.

◇ Gram-positive bacteria are most commonly isolated in community-acquired infections.

◇ General signs of infection that suggest a bacterial origin are fever (101–102°F) and an increased number (> 12,000) of white blood cells. The onset of fever alone is not diagnostic of bacterial infection.

◇ The outcome of antibiotic treatment is measured in two ways: (1) the clinical response, meaning the signs and symptoms disappear, or (2) the microbiologic response, meaning the organism is completely eradicated.

◇ Antibiotics work in one of five ways: (1) inhibit cell wall formation, (2) block protein formation, (3) disrupt cell membrane, (4) interfere with DNA formation, (5) prevent folic acid synthesis.

◇ An infection is an invasion of the body by pathogens, resulting in tissue response to organisms and toxins.

◇ A bactericidal agent kills organisms.

◇ A bacteriostatic agent inhibits growth or multiplication of bacteria.

◇ A superinfection is a new infection complicating the course of therapy of an existing infection. It is due to invasion by bacteria or fungi resistant to the drugs in use.

Classes of Antibiotics

Sulfonamides

◇ The sulfa drugs are the oldest antibiotics on the market, so the technician needs to know both the brand names and generic names of these drugs.

◇ If a patient is allergic to sulfa, the alternative drug is usually nitrofurantoin (Macrodantin, Macrobid). *It is very important that this drug be taken with food to improve absorption.* Ingestion with food also helps to avoid the GI upset that accompanies this drug. Nitrofurantoin can color the urine brown. It is also important to drink lots of water with this drug and to avoid alcohol.

◇ Sulfas are used in the treatment of UTIs, otitis media, GI infections, lower respiratory infections, and general infections.

◇ Patients taking sulfonamides should be told to drink six to eight glasses of water a day to keep the urine dilute and avoid crystallization of the drug in the urine. They should be told to avoid exposure to sunlight and to notify the physician if a rash appears (the most common side effect of the sulfas).

Penicillins

◇ Penicillin has many therapeutic uses. Ampicillin and amoxicillin have broader antimicrobial spectrums than penicillin G and V. Amoxicillin is used more often because it is dosed only three times a day; ampicillin should be dosed four times a day. Many prescribers are unaware of this difference, so to get better coverage for the patient, they should be called when the drug is dosed inappropriately.

◇ Penicillin is the drug of choice for streptococcal infections. It is used in gram-positive infections.

- The newer penicillins are penicillinase-resistant and more active against gram-negative bacilli. They are more resistant to inactivation by beta-lactamases produced by gram-negative bacteria.
- Penicillin is bactericidal in that it kills bacteria by preventing them from forming the rigid wall needed for survival. Human cells do not have cell walls and are, therefore, uninjured by penicillin.
- Penicillin should be taken on an empty stomach with water because food slows its absorption. The acids in fruit juices or colas could deactivate the drug. The most common side effect of the penicillins is diarrhea.
- Prophylaxis is recommended for patients with a heart prosthesis, congenital heart disease, idiopathic hypertrophic subaortic stenosis, murmur, mitral valve prolapse, or a history of rheumatic heart disease.
- Patients should be medicated thirty to sixty minutes before a surgical procedure, and then a dose or doses should be given afterward. This varies with the procedure. A typical regimen would be dental prophylaxis, which requires 3 g of amoxicillin thirty minutes before and 1.5 g six hours later. A new regimen recommends a single 2 g dose before dental procedures.
- A patient allergic to penicillin has a 10% possibility that an allergy to cephalosporins exists also, and vice versa. The pharmacy technician will find both allergies in the computer because most systems enter the drugs under penicillin-cephalosporin allergy.

Cephalosporins
- Cephalosporins have the same mechanism of action as penicillins but a broader spectrum of coverage.
- The first-generation cephalosporins are similar to the penicillinase-resistant penicillins, with modest gram-negative coverage. The second-generation ones have broader coverage especially against *Haemophilus influenzae*. The third-generation is active against a wide spectrum of gram-negative organisms. The new fourth-generation cephalosporin is considered "broad spectrum" with both gram-negative and somewhat less gram-positive coverage.
- Cephalosporins are probably the most-commonly used antibiotics because they cover a very wide range of organisms and have lower toxicity than other antibiotics with the same coverage.
- Primaxin has broad coverage, but patients need to be monitored for seizures. It is available only as an IV injection.

Tetracyclines
- Tetracyclines are bacteriostatic. They are the drugs of choice for Rocky Mountain spotted fever and Lyme disease, which are related.
- Tetracycline is used for prophylaxis of traveler's diarrhea. There is some discussion now about treating this phenomenon before any symptoms are exhibited.
- Patients taking tetracycline should be warned to avoid the sun, dairy products, and antacids and to take the drug on an empty stomach. The exception to these effects is doxycycline, which accounts for its popularity. Children and pregnant women should not take tetracyclines.
- Always watch the expiration date on tetracyclines. It can be very dangerous to dispense one of these drugs if it is out of date. When most drugs reach their expiration date, they simply lose effectiveness. That is not true with tetracyclines; they can cause a fatal renal syndrome.

Macrolides
- The macrolides are used primarily to treat pulmonary infections caused by *Legionella* and gram-positive organisms.
- As a rule of thumb, antibiotics are to be taken on an empty stomach to allow faster absorption into the bloodstream. A few exceptions to this rule exist to avoid GI upset. In most cases, food will not lessen the effect of the antibiotic; it will just slow down the absorption rate. A "Take with food" sticker is placed on some antibiotics because their primary side effect is GI upset, and food intake can minimize this.
- Macrolides should not be administered with theophylline, warfarin, carbamazepine, or cyclosporine.
- Zithromax has had extremely good results. It is to be taken on an empty stomach. The patient takes a loading dose of two 250 mg capsules the first day, then one 250 mg capsule on days 2 through 5. Perhaps this loading regimen and short course, which creates very good compliance, accounts for the success of this drug.

Quinolones
- Quinolones are among the drugs that penetrate bone and thus are good for bone and joint infections. They have many other uses and are especially good for UTIs and upper respiratory infections. They should not be used in persons under 18 years of age or pregnant women. A short course of some of the quinolones can knock out a UTI. Trovan should be reserved for life-threatening infections.
- The primary side effect is GI upset. Antacids should not be taken with these drugs. They are phototoxic and increase the risk of theophylline toxicity.

Streptogrammins
- Streptogrammins are a drug class with side effects similar to the quinolones. They are the alternative for drugs resistant to vancomycin. Since the drugs are such an important advance in antimicrobial therapy, they were approved under the FDA's accelerated approval regulations.

Aminoglycosides
- Aminoglycosides are used to treat very serious infections. They are ototoxic and nephrotoxic and may cause neuromuscular blockade. After initial dosing they should be adjusted according to plasma concentration in the individual patient. Some current evidence supports once-daily dosing; it can be as effective with fewer side effects.

Miscellaneous Antibiotics

- Macrodantin (nitrofurantoin) is often used in sulfa-allergic patients and works much better when taken with food.
- Vancomycin is also ototoxic and nephrotoxic, and neutropenia can be a problem. It is one of the few drugs effective against *Clostridium difficile*, as well as methicillin-resistant *Staphylococcus aureus*.
- Clindamycin has a very broad spectrum, with especially high concentrations in bone. The most serious side effect is pseudomembranous colitis. If diarrhea develops, the drug must be discontinued.
- Metronidazole (Flagyl) is used primarily to treat infections of the vaginal canal, cervix, and male urethra. It may discolor the urine. The warning against alcohol consumption is very important with this drug. It reacts to ethanol in the same way as disulfiram (Antabuse). It makes the drinker very nauseated, causes vomiting, increases blood pressure, and causes a flushing reaction and headache.

- While the literature recommends taking antibiotics on an empty stomach as a general rule, the prudent technician will be aware of exceptions and will place a "Take with Food" label on certain antibiotics. Some of these are doxycycline, some erythromycins, some forms of Augmentin, etc., and certainly Macrodantin. The food in most cases only slows absorption and does not affect the therapeutic index of the antibiotic.
- Pentamidine is used as a second-line drug for pneumonia caused by *Pneumocystis carinii*.

Drug Summary

The following drugs were discussed in this chapter. Each generic drug name is followed in parentheses by one or more brand names. An asterisk (*) indicates drugs frequently written using either brand or generic name. These need to be memorized.

Sulfonamides
sulfamethoxazole (Gantanol)*
sulfamethoxazole-trimethoprim (SMX-TMP) (Bactrim, Septra)*
sulfasalazine (Azulfidine)* *SAS*
sulfisoxazole (Gantrisin)*
sulfisoxazole-phenazopyridine (Azo Gantrisin)

Penicillins
apo Amoxil
amoxicillin (Amoxil, Polymox*)
Clavulin amoxicillin-clavulanate (Augmentin)
ampicillin (Omnipen, Principen)*
ampicillin-sulbactam (Unasyn)
carbenicillin (Geocillin)*
dicloxacillin (Dynapen)*
mezlocillin (Mezlin)
nafcillin (Unipen)*
oxacillin (Bactocill, Prostaphlin)
penicillin G
penicillin V (Veetids)
piperacillin (Pipracil)*
piperacillin-tazobactam (Zosyn)
ticarcillin (Ticar)*
ticarcillin-clavulanate (Timentin)

Cephalosporins and Related Drugs
aztreonam (Azactam)
cefaclor (Ceclor)*
cefadroxil (Duricef)*
cefamandole (Mandol)*
cefazolin (Ancef,* Kefzol)
cefdinir (Omnicef)
cefepime (Maxipime)
cefixime (Suprax)
cefonicid (Monocid)
cefoperazone (Cefobid)
cefotaxime (Claforan)*
cefotetan (Cefotan)
cefoxitin (Mefoxin)*
cefpodoxime (Vantin, Proxetil)
ceftazidime (Fortaz)*
ceftibuten (Cedax)
ceftizoxime (Cefizox)

ceftriaxone (Rocephin)*
cefuroxime (Zinacef, Ceftin)*
cephalexin (Keflex)*
cephalothin (Ceporacin)
cephapirin (Cefadyl)
cephradine (Velosef)*
imipenem-cilastatin (Primaxin)
loracarbef (Lorabid)
meropenem (Merrem)

Tetracyclines
demeclocycline (Declomycin)
doxycycline (Vibramycin)*
minocycline (Minocin)*
tetracycline (Achromycin, Sumycin) *apo-tetra*

Macrolides
azithromycin, Z-Pak (Zithromax)
clarithromycin (Biaxin)
dirithromycin (Dynabac)
erythromycin (A/T/S, EryDerm, T-Stat)*
erythromycin base (Eryc, E-mycin,* Ery-Tab)
erythromycin estolate (Ilosone)*
erythromycin ethylsuccinate (E.E.S., EryPed*)
erythromycin glucaptate (Ilotycin)
erythromycin stearate (Erythrocin)*
erythromycin-sulfisoxazole (Pediazole)

Quinolones
cinoxacin (Cinobac)
ciprofloxacin (Cipro, Ciloxin)*
enoxacin (Penetrex)
gatifloxacin (Tequin)
levofloxacin (Levaquin)
lomefloxacin (Maxaquin)
moxifloxacin (Avelox)
nalidixic acid (NegGram)*
norfloxacin (Noroxin)*
ofloxacin (Floxin,* Ocuflox)
sparfloxacin (Zagam)
trovafloxacin (Trovan)

Streptogrammins
quinupristin-dalfopristin (Synercid)

Aminoglycosides
amikacin (Amikin)*
gentamicin (Garamycin)*
neomycin (Mycifradin)
netilmicin (Netromycin)
streptomycin (none)
tobramycin (Nebcin)   tobrex

Miscellaneous Antibiotics
chloramphenicol (Chloromycetin)
clindamycin (Cleocin) Dalacin
metronidazole (Flagyl)*
nitrofurantoin (Macrodantin)
pentamidine (Pentam, NebuPent)
vancomycin (Vancocin)

Chapter Review

Pharmaceuticals and Body Functions

Select the best answer from the choices given.

1. It is especially important that a person taking sulfa drugs
   a. avoid the sun and drink lots of water.
   b. drink lots of water and get sufficient rest.
   c. get sufficient rest and avoid the sun.
   d. take the medication with food.

2. The primary side effect of Augmentin is *Clavulin (fight Penicillin)*
   a. drowsiness.
   b. rash.
   c. dry mouth.
   d. diarrhea.

3. Penicillin should be taken with
   a. colas.
   b. water.
   c. fruit juices.
   d. all of the above.

4. The drug of choice (DOC) for "strep throat" is
   a. sulfa.
   b. tetracycline.
   c. penicillin.
   d. a cephalosporin.

5. Primaxin is an excellent drug to use against beta-lactamase producing bacteria. The most serious side effect to watch for in this drug is
   a. a rash.
   b. diarrhea.
   c. drowsiness.
   d. seizures.

6. The DOC for Rocky Mountain spotted fever
   a. is penicillin.
   b. are sulfonamides.
   c. are aminoglycosides.
   d. is tetracycline.

7. Which drug is it very important to take with food?
   a. Methenamine
   b. Nitrofurantoin *macrobid , macro dantal*
   c. Sulfasalazine
   d. Sulfamethoxazole

8. You can drink milk with all of the listed drugs except
   a. Macrodantin.
   b. Achromycin.
   c. Vibramycin
   d. Augmentin. *clavulin*

9. Which drug has a large amount of sugar in the oral liquid dosage form?
   a. Suprax
   b. Omnicef
   c. Ceclor
   d. Lorabid

10. Clindamycin has a special affinity for
    a. bone.
    b. the eyes.
    c. the brain.
    d. the heart.

The following statements are true or false. If the answer is false, rewrite the statement so it is true.

_F_ 1. Alcohol has no effect on the patient taking Flagyl.

_F_ 2. Quinolones can be used safely with theophylline and antacids.

_T_ 3. It could be very dangerous to dispense an out-of-date tetracycline.

_F_ 4. Ceclor is the DOC for "strep throat." *Penicillin*   *Kidney & liver.*

_F_ 5. If someone is allergic to penicillin, they will be allergic to cephalosporins. *only 10%*

_F_ 6. A nosocomial infection is community-acquired.

_F_ 7. The onset of fever is always diagnostic of <u>bacterial infection</u>.

_F_ 8. Sulfa drugs may be used for <u>UTIs</u> and <u>GI</u> upset.

_T_ 9. The major side effects of an aminoglycoside are ototoxicity and nephrotoxicity.

_T_ 10. The most common side effect of sulfa is a rash.

Diseases and Drug Therapies

1. List the five ways antibiotics work.

2. Give three combinations of frequently used penicillins, generic and brand names.

3. List five infections the sulfas are used to treat.

4. How do a bactericidal antibiotic and a bacteriostatic antibiotic differ?

5. How do a nosocomial and community-acquired infection differ?

6. Define superinfection.

7. Which auxiliary labels would you put on a sulfa prescription if there is only room for two? (Make a list of all the labels you might need to put on a sulfa drug. Choose the two you think are most important. Defend your choices.)

8. Specifically describe how penicillin kills bacteria.

9. Why is Suprax prescribed frequently for school-age children?

10. Being a prudent technician, which antibiotics would you put a "Take with food" auxiliary label on?

11. Why is Lorabid frequently given to children?

12. If you got Rocky Mountain spotted fever and were given the drug of choice, what would you be sure to have the technician check?

13. If someone picks up a prescription for Flagyl (metronidazole) and is on the way to a New Year's Eve party, what would you be sure to tell them?

14. Why is resistance developing to antibiotics?

15. Describe empirical treatment and when it would be used.

Dispensing Medications

1. You live in a state that allows a CPhT (certified pharmacy technician) to take a prescription over the phone. You take a prescription from the dentist for a patient with mitral valve prolapse. The patient is to have dental work done. The patient is allergic to penicillin, but the dentist does not know this. What do you suggest the dentist substitute for amoxicillin? (Hint: dental prophylaxis)

2. Amoxicillin comes in 500 mg capsules. The next patient the dentist writes for does not have a penicillin allergy. How many capsules will you dispense for the old regimen? the new regimen?

3. You receive a prescription for a Z-pack. You have azithromycin, but not in the pack. How will you dose the drug?

4. It is hard to remember which labels go on certain drugs. Create a chart listing the antibiotics covered in this chapter that should be taken with food and those that cause photosensitivity. Keep it with you in the pharmacy for reference.

Internet Research

Use the Internet to complete the following assignments.

1. Antibiotic resistance is of serious concern to the medical community as well as the society at large. Use Internet resources to write a brief report outlining the current thinking related to antibiotic resistance. Include both popular press as well as more scientific perspectives in your report. Address the following questions: What are the primary concerns about antibiotic resistance? What measures are being taken to address this problem? Is there any difference of opinion between the popular media and the medical community?

2. Research one of the disease states mentioned in this chapter (e.g., Lyme disease, walking pneumonia, or meningitis). Write a short report that describes the disease, its etiology (i.e., causes and origin), signs, symptoms and treatments (including drug therapies). List your Internet source(s).

Antivirals, Antiretrovirals, and Antifungals

Chapter 5

Learning Objectives

◇ Introduce the student to antivirals, antiretrovirals, and antifungals.

◇ Differentiate antivirals, antiretrovirals, and antifungals by their indications, therapeutic effects, side effects, dosages, and administration.

◇ Use antiviral, antiretroviral, and antifungal terminology correctly in written and oral communication.

◇ Define differences in mechanisms of action of antibiotics, antivirals, antiretrovirals, and antifungals.

Viruses and fungi are often confused with each other but are vastly different entities. This is why it takes drugs with very different mechanisms of action to treat them. These infections are often related because patients with debilitating viral infections often contract an equally debilitating fungal infection. When the body's natural defenses or natural bacteria are wiped out by an antibiotic, a fungus often takes over and reproduces in these same areas of the body. Like viral infections, fungal infections can be deadly if left untreated.

VIRUSES AND THEIR CHARACTERISTICS

A virus is a minute infectious agent which is much smaller than a bacterium. Unlike a bacterium, a virus does not have all the components of a cell and thus it is able to replicate only within a living host cell. Viruses, among the most common infectious agents in humans, replicate by using the host cells' metabolic processes. A virus can infect a spectrum of cells including animal, plant, or bacteria cells. Most common viruses are spread by one of the following routes.

◇ direct contact
◇ ingestion of contaminated food and water
◇ inhalation of airborne particles

The individual virus particle, a virion, consists of nucleic acid (nucleoid), either deoxyribonucleic acid (DNA) or ribonucleic acid (RNA) (but not both), and a protein shell (capsid) that surrounds and protects the nucleic acid. Depending on the virus, the capsid may be covered with spikes that attach to the host cell. Binding of the spikes to membrane receptors stimulates a process whereby the cell engulfs the virus. A virus without an envelope covering the capsid is called a naked virus.

Stages of Viral Infection

Within the body, viral infection takes place at the cellular level and in the following stages.

1. The virus attaches to a cell receptor.
2. The cell membrane indents and closes around the virus (endocytosis) and thus the virus penetrates the cell.
3. The virus escapes into cytoplasm.
4. The virus uncoats, sheds its covering, and presents its DNA or RNA to the cell nucleus.
5. This allows the virus to convert the nuclear activity in the cell to viral activity and rapidly reproduce new viral particles. (It uses the energy of the host cell to infect the cell.)

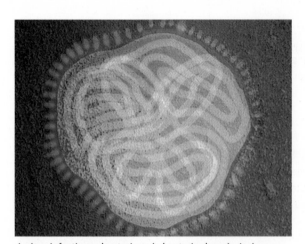

A virus infecting a bacterium (a bacteriophage). A virus does not have all the components of a cell and requires the metabolic and genetic resources of a living cell to replicate itself.

When viruses take over host cell nuclear activity, they synthesize viral enzymes, DNA, and protein, which leads to production of more virus particles. The infected host cell may be so damaged that it disintegrates, releasing bursts of mature virions. If the host cell is not destroyed, the virions are released slowly. During the release process, the virion often receives an envelope, or capsid, from the nuclear or the plasma (cell) membrane. All virus-infected cells have some cellular characteristics different from those of uninfected cells. These differences provide opportunities to target and block viral division with medications without affecting normal cells.

The flu is an example of a common viral infection; it is due to different strains of the influenza virus. Symptoms are usually more severe than those of the common cold and include malaise (vague discomfort and tiredness), myalgia (muscle pain), headache, chills, and fever. Patients with shortness of breath, wheezing, purulent or bloody sputum, fever persisting for more than seven days, or severe muscle pain should be advised to seek medical attention. Those at high risk for complications are elderly persons and patients with cardiovascular disease, renal disease, diabetes, asthma, and immunocompromised patients (such as those with HIV or those who recently received transplants). Annual vaccinations for these patient populations are encouraged.

Viral Classification

Viral infections are classified in two ways. The first classification is the duration or length of time they have been present in the body as well as their severity. The second classification measures the extent of the infections within the body or the parts of the body that are affected.

VIRAL DURATION AND SEVERITY Within the classification of duration and severity there are three categories: acute, chronic, and slow. An acute viral infection quickly resolves with no latent infection. Examples include the common cold, influenza, and various other respiratory tract infections. A chronic viral infection has a protracted course with long periods of remission interspersed with reappearance, such as the herpes virus infection. A slow viral infection maintains a progressive course over months or years, with cumulative damage to body tissues, ultimately ending in the host's death. Examples of this type of destructive viral infection include human immunodeficiency virus (HIV) and diseases affecting the central nervous system (CNS).

VIRAL INFECTION   When evaluating the extent of the viral infection, it must be determined whether the infection is local or generalized. A local viral infection affects tissues of a single system, such as the respiratory tract. A generalized viral infection is one that has spread or is spreading to other tissues by way of the bloodstream or tissues of the CNS.

Latent Viruses

Latency is a problem with some viruses. Some can lie dormant and then, under certain conditions, reproduce and again behave like an infective agent, causing cell damage. Herpes virus and HIV, for example, may remain in the cell in a latent, undetectable form, so the disease may surface years after the initial breakout or transmission of infection. Some viruses can transform normal animal cells into cancer cells.

Virus and Cell Interaction

A virus can have several damaging effects on a host cell. It can kill the host cell, alter the cell, incorporate into the genetic material of the host cell thus becoming part of its nucleic acid pool, or divide when the host cell divides.

Most viruses possess several antigens on their surface that stimulate the host cell to produce immunoglobulins. Immunoglobulins are substances that prevent the virus from attaching to a cell receptor. They can also destroy the virus. Thymus cells (T cells) may also become sensitive to viral antigens, at which time they release chemicals to kill the virus or stimulate other cells, such as macrophages, to destroy the virus or virus-infected cells.

A very significant response of some virus-infected cells is production of a substance called interferon. Although interferon is produced by the viral infection, it is coded by the host cell's DNA. Interferons protect neighboring uninfected cells from viral infection and interfere with viral multiplication. Interferons are host cell-specific, i.e., those made by human cells will work only in human cells. In addition to their antiviral activity, however, interferons act against a number of different viruses by binding to the surface of uninfected cells and stimulating the cell to produce other antiviral proteins.

Vaccination

The prevention of viral infections by providing immunity is the principle of vaccination. The process of vaccination exposes the patient to a component of a virus or a similar viral strain that does not produce infection. The exposure of the body to these harmless materials prepares certain white blood cells to react to the designated virus. Thus, when a vaccinated patient encounters the actual virus, the infection cannot develop because the patient's natural defenses are already primed from the vaccine. Unfortunately, vaccines are available for only a small number of viruses.

An influenza vaccine is developed annually according to the genetic changes that are predicted to occur the following year. The vaccine is only as good as the match it makes with a particular infecting strain of flu. It is made from viral particles that are raised in poultry eggs and then inactivated or killed. The protection from the vaccine lasts for only a year; thus, annual revaccination is needed. The vaccine usually becomes available in September and is given through November. It is recommended for high-risk populations such as healthcare workers, people in contact with patients with influenza, nursing home residents, public safety workers, individuals sixty-five or older, and immunocompromised patients. In certain situations, an antiviral medication may be prescribed to patients who cannot take the vaccine or have been exposed to influenza.

Antivirals

There are fewer medications to treat viral infections than there are for bacterial infections. Part of the difficulty is that antibiotics often disrupt a cellular process that is unique to the bacterium being treated. This allows dosing of the medication without causing toxicity to the patient. However, because viruses use the cellular processes of the host to function and replicate, medications that block the life cycle of the virus are often toxic to the patient. Thus, the antivirals have been formulated to search and destroy the virus cell lodged in its host cell without interfering with the host cell's normal function. Table 5.1 gives an overview of the most-commonly used antiviral agents.

Many of the antivirals are potent drugs used to treat difficult diseases like AIDS. A significant number of antiviral agents have emerged in recent years as a result of the tremendous amount of drug research dedicated to finding treatments for HIV.

Antivirals are among the drugs of choice for the following conditions.

⋄ cytomegalovirus (CMV) retinitis
⋄ genital herpes
⋄ herpes simplex
⋄ herpes simplex keratitis
⋄ herpes zoster (shingles)
⋄ influenza prophylaxis
⋄ organ transplantation
⋄ varicella (chicken pox)

Antiviral side effects can range from mild (headache) to severe (renal disorders). Side effects related to specific agents are outlined in the following section.

Table 5.1	Most-Commonly Used Antivirals		
Generic Name	**Brand Name**	**Dosage Form**	
Systemic Agents			
acyclovir	Zovirax	tablet, capsule, oral suspension, IV, ointment	
amantadine	Symmetrel	capsule, syrup	
cidofovir	Vistide	IV	
famciclovir	Famvir	tablet	
foscarnet	Foscavir	IV	
ganciclovir	Cytovene	capsule, IV	
oseltamivir	Tamiflu	capsule	
ribavirin	Virazole	aerosol inhalant	
rimantadine	Flumadine	tablet, syrup	
valacyclovir	Valtrex	caplet	
zanamivir	Relenza	inhalant	
Ophthalmic Agents			
ganciclovir	Vitrasert	ocular implant	
vidarabine	Vira-A	ointment	

Systemic Agents Zovirax (acyclovir) acts by interfering with viral DNA and inhibiting its replication. It is used to treat genital herpes in certain patients, herpes zoster (shingles), and varicella (chicken pox). The IV form is considered the drug of choice for a form of encephalitis. The dosage regimen changes depending on the type of infection being treated and the patient's status, so manufacturer's charts should be consulted. A range of short- and long-term side effects have been reported. The latest research suggests adding acyclovir to HIV-positive patients' usual antiretroviral for suppression of herpes in patients with multiple outbreaks. HIV seems to grow more quickly when an active herpes infection is present.

Famvir (famciclovir) is used to manage acute herpes zoster (shingles), to treat recurrent herpes simplex in immunocompromised patients, and in genital herpes. The primary side effects are nausea and headache. The advantage of this drug is that it can be dosed less frequently than others in this class. It is a prodrug, and the active compound after biotransformation is penciclover.

Valtrex (valacyclovir) is used to treat herpes zoster in immunocompetent adults and in genital herpes. It should be taken with plenty of water and within 48 hours of the onset of the zoster rash. It shortens the duration of postherpetic neuralgia. Side effects include nausea, vomiting, diarrhea, and constipation. It is better absorbed than acyclovir, and once absorbed, is converted to acyclovir in the liver and gut. The end result is higher blood levels. It is also given less frequently.

Symmetrel (amantadine) prevents absorption of viral particles into the host cell by inhibiting uncoating or removing of the capsid of the virus. It is used in the prophylaxis of influenza A. Sufficient blood levels of the drug are necessary to prevent infection. After infection it still may reduce the severity of symptoms. Amantadine also has some therapeutic effect on parkinsonism. Side effects are rare and relate primarily to the CNS. Concomitant ingestion of antihistamine or caffeine increases neurotoxicity.

Cytovene (ganciclovir) is used in treating cytomegalovirus (CMV) retinitis in immunocompromised patients. It is often used for patients undergoing transplantation and for those with HIV infection. The pharmacist must follow chemotherapy preparation and dispensing guidelines when mixing and labeling this drug. Previously ganciclovir was available only in an IV form, but an oral form has become available. The IV form should not be used for rapid or bolus injection.

Foscavir (foscarnet) is used in treating CMV infections in patients with HIV infection. It is also used in patients undergoing transplantation. Patients must be hydrated, and a prescription for a hydration product should accompany the prescription for both of these drugs. It should be delivered as an IV infusion, rather than as a rapid or bolus injection.

Flumadine (rimantadine) is indicated for prophylaxis and treatment of infections caused by influenza A virus strains. The most frequent side effects involve the GI and nervous systems. It also has CNS-related side effects but fewer than amantadine.

Relenza (zanamivir) is indicated for the treatment of influenza A and B. Therapy with zanamivir must be initiated within forty-eight hours of the onset of symptoms. The drug is inhaled using a breath-activated plastic device called a diskhaler. The recommended dosage is two inhalations daily, administered at twelve-hour intervals for five days. If the patient is also using a bronchodilator, the patient should be instructed to use the bronchodilator immediately prior to the administration of zanamivir. Zanamivir is sometimes prescribed as a prophylactic, especially in nursing homes and other group settings. However, because of the complexities associated with administering the drug, it is prescribed only when necessary.

Tamiflu (oseltamivir) is an oral inhibitor of the enzyme neuraminidase and is indicated for the treatment or prevention of influenza A and B. As with zanamivir, therapy

Warning

Amantadine, rimantadine, and ranitidine can be easily confused. Amantadine is 50 mg and 100 mg. Rimantadine is also 50 mg. They are both antiviral agents. Ranitidine is usually 150 mg and 300 mg. Dosing and indications will help with the latter.

Warning

Cytovene and Cytosar might be confused. Cytosar is chemo and is 10 mg. Cytovene is 250 mg and 500 mg, so dosing should help identify the drug.

Warning

Patients who are given Cytovene or Foscavir IV must be well-hydrated. If hydration orders are not provided, the physician should be contacted. Some institutions have "standing orders" for hydration when these drugs are prescribed.

must be initiated within 48 hours of symptom onset. Food generally improves tolerance and, as such, oseltamivir is generally recommended to be taken at breakfast and dinner. Oseltamivir has been shown to decrease the duration of the flu by three days.

Virazole (ribavirin) is useful in treating viral infections. It is absorbed systemically from the respiratory tract following nasal and oral inhalation. Absorption depends on respiratory factors and the drug delivery system. Maximal absorption occurs with use of the aerosol generator via an endotracheal tube. The highest drug concentrations of ribavirin are found in the respiratory tract and erythrocytes. The most common side effects are fatigue, headache, and insomnia. Nausea and anorexia can also occur. Patients who are pregnant or who are planning to become pregnant should not use this drug.

Vistide (cidofovir) is used for the treatment of CMV. Its advantage is that it can be dosed every two weeks. Cidofovir must be administered with normal saline and probenecid to reduce the incidence of nephrotoxicity.

OPHTHALMIC AGENTS **Vira-A (vidarabine)** is an ophthalmic agent that can prevent viral replication by blocking the viruses' synthesis mechanisms. It is available only as an ophthalmic preparation. Vidarabine can cause burning, lacrimation, and blurred vision. Patients should be told to avoid eye makeup when using this drug. They may also need to wear sunglasses due to photosensitivity. Patients must be instructed to notify their physician if there is no improvement within seven days.

Vitrasert (ganciclovir) is an ocular implant that seems to work better than systemic therapy for CMV retinitis. It does not treat any systemic manifestations of the contralateral eye in this dosage form.

ANTIRETROVIRALS

Antiretrovirals have been developed specifically to limit the progression of the retrovirus HIV. The HIV retrovirus causes acquired immunodeficiency syndrome (AIDS), a dysfunction of the immune system associated with a very high mortality rate. Due to the severity of the disease, FDA approval of AIDS-related drugs has been subject to special accelerated processes.

There are currently three classes of antiretroviral drugs.

- ◇ nucleoside reverse transcriptase inhibitors (NRTIs)
- ◇ non-nucleoside reverse transcriptase inhibitors (NNRTIs)
- ◇ protease inhibitors (PIs)

Nucleoside Reverse Transcriptase Inhibitors (NRTIs)

Neuraminidase is the viral enzyme that facilitates the release of newly formed virus particles. Nucleoside reverse transcriptase inhibitors (NRTIs) bind and inhibit the action of this enzyme to prevent the spread of the virus to healthy cells. They inhibit reverse transcriptase, causing the formation of a defective proviral DNA. This defective proviral DNA is unable to be incorporated into the host cell's nucleus. Table 5.2 gives an overview of the most-common NRTIs in current use.

The NRTIs, with the exception of didanosine, can be taken with or without food and generally do not interfere with other drugs. These agents are usually administered in two to three doses per day. Class side effects of NRTIs include lactic acidosis with hepatic steatosis.

Generic Name	Brand Name	Dosage Form	Side Effects
abacavir	Ziagen	solution, tablet	hypersensitivity reaction; fever, rash, nausea and vomiting, malaise, fatigue, loss of appetite, respiratory symptoms
didanosine, ddI*	Videx, Videx EC	powder, tablet, capsule	pancreatitis, peripheral neuropathy, nausea and vomiting, diarrhea
lamivudine, 3TC*	Epivir	solution, tablet	minimal toxicity
stavudine, d4T*	Zerit	powder, capsule	pancreatitis, peripheral neuropathy
zalcitabine	Hivid	tablet	peripheral neuropathy stomatitis
zidovudine, AZT*	Retrovir	capsule, syrup, IV	anemia, neutropenia, nausea and vomiting, headache
zidovudine-lamivudine	Combivir	tablet	see above
zidovudine-lamivudine-cibacuvir	Trizivir	tablet	see above

* The old research names for these drugs are listed because the technician may receive a prescription with only this name for the drug

Retrovir (zidovudine, AZT) was one of the first drugs developed specifically for the treatment of HIV. With the exception of stavudine, zidovudine can be combined with any of the other NRTIs. The combination of zidovudine with lamivudine, with or without a protease inhibitor, is recommended for the prevention of HIV after a needlestick or sexual exposure. The most common side effects of zidovudine are headache, anorexia, diarrhea, GI pain, nausea, and rash.

Videx (didanosine) is indicated in the treatment of advanced HIV in patients who cannot tolerate zidovudine therapy or who have had significant clinical or immunologic deterioration during therapy with zidovudine. This drug is typically combined with zidovudine or stavudine and should not be combined with zalcitabine due to overlapping toxicities. The patient should allow for an interval of at least two hours between the administration of didanosine and any drug that requires gastric acidity for digestion. The formulation Videx EC has much less GI side effects and does not have to be taken separately from other medications. Both formulations should be taken on an empty stomach. Alcohol consumption will increase the risk of pancreatitis.

Hivid (zalcitabine), the least potent of the NRTIs, is not as frequently prescribed for HIV. These tablets should be dosed every eight hours and must be stored in air-tight containers. Zalcitabine should be taken on an empty stomach.

Zerit (stavudine) is generally prescribed for the treatment of HIV after the failure of zidovudine-containing regimens. This drug is typically well-tolerated. However, it is associated with an increased risk of peripheral neuropathy. Pancreatitis is a side effect when the drug is combined with didanosine.

Epivir (lamivudine) is indicated in the treatment of HIV and chronic Hepatitis B. Epivir must be taken exactly as prescribed. It has the least side effects of any of the NRTIs.

Ziagen (abacavir) is one of the few HIV drugs that penetrates the CNS. This characteristic makes abacavir an invaluable therapeutic weapon, since HIV itself is able to penetrate and proliferate within the CNS. Although abacavir has few reactions with other drugs, the use of alcohol will increase the drug's toxicity and patients must be instructed to avoid alcohol completely. Patients should also be cautioned to be on the alert for any of a number of side effects that could signal an adverse and potentially life-threatening reaction to the drug. Fifty percent of patients experience a hypersensitivity to abacavir that generally occurs in the first six weeks. These side effects include rash, nausea, abdominal pain, malaise, or respiratory symptoms. The patient must be instructed to stop taking abacavir immediately if he or she experiences any of these symptoms.

Non-Nucleoside Reverse Transcriptase Inhibitors (NNRTIs)

Non-nucleoside reverse transcriptase inhibitors (NNRTIs) inhibit the action of the reverse transcriptase neuraminidase by preventing the formation of proviral DNA. Resistance to one NNRTI generally causes resistance to the whole class. NNRTIs can induce or inhibit the cytochrome P-450 system. Drug interactions are common. Table 5.3 gives an overview of the most-commonly used NNRTIs currently on the market.

Sustiva (efavirenz) has a long duration of action relative to other NNRTIs and is only dosed once a day, preferably at bedtime. Patients taking efavirenz should be instructed to avoid high-fat meals. Common side effects include dizziness and headache. The drug may also induce vivid dreams, nightmares, and hallucinations. These typically occur between one and three hours of administration and will generally subside after two to four weeks on the drug. Efavirenz is a cytochrome P-450 mixed inhibitor/inducer.

Viramune (nevirapine) is associated with a high incidence of rash, especially during the early phase of treatment. To mitigate this effect, the drug is typically given at a lower dose during the first two weeks of treatment and then increased to the appropriate therapeutic level. Nevirapine is a cytochrome P-450 inducer. The antibiotic rifampin (a drug used to treat tuberculosis) interferes with the efficacy of nevirapine by reducing its serum concentrations in the body. In turn, nevirapine decreases the serum concentration of the protease inhibitor class of antiretrovirals. As a result, these drugs are not generally prescribed in combination. Nevirapine also decreases the effectiveness of birth control pills. Hepatotoxicity has been reported after one dose. Monitoring liver function tests is imperative.

Rescriptor (delavirdine), a cytochrome P-450 inhibitor, in contrast to nevirapine and many other NNRTIs, can increase the serum levels of some protease inhibitors. This drug is associated with a lower frequency of rash than Viramune. Delavirdine should not be taken in tandem with any antacid. Patients should be instructed to

Table 5.3	Most Commonly Used Non-Nucleoside Reverse Transcriptase Inhibitors (NNRTIs)	
Generic Name	**Brand Name**	**Dosage Form**
delavirdine	Rescriptor	capsule, tablet
efavirenz	Sustiva	capsule
nevirapine	Viramune	capsule, tablet

avoid the ingestion of antacids one hour before and one hour after the administration of delavirdine.

Protease Inhibitors (PIs)

The protease inhibitors prevent the cleavage of certain HIV protein precursors which are necessary for the replication of new infectious virions. This mechanism results in the production of immature, noninfectious virions. These drugs are typically combined with other antiretroviral drugs and their use has led to marked clinical improvement and prolonged survival among AIDS patients. Protease inhibitors are metabolized through cytochrome P-450, thus drug interactions are common and can be severe. Table 5.4 gives an overview of the most-commonly prescribed protease inhibitors.

Class side effects associated with all protease inhibitors include redistribution of body fat, referred to as "protease paunch," characterized by a humped back, facial atrophy, breast enlargement, hyperglycemia, hyperlipidemia, and possible increase in bleeding episodes in patients with hemophilia.

Agenerase (amprenavir) contains a significant quantity—more than the recommended daily allowance (RDA)—of vitamin E to enhance its absorption. Therefore, patients who are taking this drug should be instructed to avoid the use of any other vitamin E supplements. Amprenavir is contraindicated in patients with sulfa allergies. One side effect peculiar to this drug is numbness around the mouth. The most common side effect associated with amprenavir is nausea.

Crixivan (indinavir) has been shown to be less effective when taken in combination with St. John's Wort. Thus, patients who are taking indinavir should be instructed to avoid this herbal remedy. Indinavir is very sensitive to moisture and is always packaged with a desiccant. Patients should be instructed to store the drug in its original container. Indinavir should not be taken with high-fat meals or grapefruit juice. It should be taken on an empty stomach or with a low-fat meal. In order to lower the incidence of kidney stones, the patient should consume 48 oz. of water daily.

Kaletra (lopinavir-ritonavir) can cause nausea and vomiting, diarrhea, and pancreatitis. The solution contains 47% alcohol.

Viracept (nelfinavir) is the most-commonly used protease inhibitor. This drug is well-tolerated with the exception of diarrhea, which generally resolves itself with continued use. Imodium AD and calcium carbonate can help control the diarrhea. Nelfinavir should be taken with food.

Norvir (ritonavir) is prescribed primarily for its ability to increase the serum concentrations and dosage frequency of other protease inhibitors, thereby reducing the side effects of these drugs. As such, ritonavir is generally given at a low dose. Ritonavir should be taken with food. This drug has many side effects including an unusual one, an altered sense of taste. Ritonavir, whether in capsule or solution

Table 5.4	Most-Commonly Prescribed Protease Inhibitors (PIs)	
Generic Name	**Brand Name**	**Dosage Form**
amprenavir	Agenerase	solution, capsules
indinavir	Crixivan	capsule
lopinavir-ritonavir	Kaletra	solution, capsule
nelfinavir	Viracept	powder, tablet
ritonavir	Norvir	solution, capsule
saquinavir	Invirase, Fortovase	capsule

form, should be stored in the refrigerator. It is the most potent inhibitor of cytochrome P-450 and has many drug interactions.

Patients on **saquinavir** should be instructed to avoid sunlight. **Fortovase**, a soft gel preparation, has largely replaced the older formulation **Invirase** because of its improved bioavailability.

Responding to Exposure to HIV

The Centers for Disease Control (CDC) has developed guidelines for the management of healthcare worker exposures to HIV. These guidelines include recommendations for the administration of antiretroviral drugs as post-exposure prophylaxis (PEP). Healthcare worker risks include exposure to the blood and other body fluids of an HIV-positive patient and needle-stick injuries. Following such an exposure, the administration of an appropriate antiretroviral regimen should begin within two hours. Research has shown that prompt treatment can decrease the risk of infection by 80%. Clearly, preventing exposure to HIV through appropriate precautions is the primary means of protection against HIV infection for heathcare workers as well as the public at large. People accidentally exposed to blood with a high virus titer (terminal patients) or to deep needle injury should start immediately (within one to two hours) because they are at high risk. Exposures through unprotected sex or intravenous drug use can be even more risky than accidental exposures.

Combining Antiretrovirals

None of the antiretrovirals currently available can eradicate AIDS, but when used appropriately they can decrease viral replication, improve immunological status, and prolong life. The standard care for the treatment of AIDS is to administer three or more drugs in combination. The regimens are difficult to follow since the drugs must be taken around the clock. As such, patient compliance is frequently poor. Clear, written instructions for taking the medications, as well as adequate warnings about the potential for drug interactions, may encourage better compliance.

Table 5.5 gives an overview of current recommendations for HIV therapy dosing regimens. The following antiretroviral drug combinations should be avoided.

⬥ didanosine with zalcitabine
⬥ zidovudine with stavudine
⬥ lamivudine with zalcitabine
⬥ stavudine with zalcitabine

Table 5.5 **Antiretroviral Dosing Regimens**

Regimen Type	Recommendation	Indications
standard therapy	2 NRTIs + 1 PI 2 NRTIs + 1 NNRTI 2 NRTIs + ritonavir + 1 additional PI	
alternative therapy	1 PI + 1 NRTI + 1 NNRTI abacavir + 2 additional NRTIs	
post-exposure prophylaxis (PEP)	zidovudine + lamivudine + indivavir or nelfinavir	needle sticks and exposure to body fluids or blood of an HIV-positive patient

FUNGI AND THEIR CHARACTERISTICS

A fungus is a single-cell organism similar to a human cell. Both human (animal) and fungal cells are eukaryotic (having a defined nucleus). Fungi include mushrooms, yeasts, and molds. They are marked by the absence of chlorophyll, the presence of a rigid cell wall, and reproduction by spores. Human cell membranes contain cholesterol; fungi contain ergosterol, the basis for antifungal drugs.

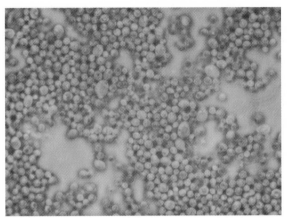

Fungi are multicellular organisms, unlike viruses.

Fungal Diseases

Systemic fungal diseases are most likely to develop in patients whose immune system is depressed by disease, drug therapy (for example, the use of corticosteroids or antineoplastics), or poor nutrition. Often the host is unaware of contracting an active infection. The nails are a common target of fungal infection. Examples of fungal organisms and the diseases they cause are included in Table 5.6.

Antibiotics usually make fungal infections worse by wiping out the body's natural flora, allowing the fungus to take over. A typical scenario is the woman who has been taking an antibiotic and then gets a vaginal infection that has to be treated with an antifungal agent.

Antifungals

Antifungals prevent synthesis of ergosterol, a building block for fungal cell membranes. Humans use cholesterol and therefore human cells are not affected by antifungals. These agents act by inhibiting fungal cytochrome P-450, which is different from human cytochrome P-450. Therefore, antifungals have little effect on human cells. Most of these drugs come in a topical form; these agents will be discussed later in Chapter 16. Many of the topical antifungals are now OTC preparations.

Pulse dosing for fungal nail infections is becoming increasingly common. Each pulse dose is usually one week per month. Because the drug persists in the nail for several months, this regimen works as well as a continuous daily dose. Since patients take much less drug, treatment is safer and costs a lot less. Antifungal agents in this drug class are very expensive, and most health plans do not cover them. Table 5.7 lists the most-commonly used antifungals.

Table 5.6	Examples of Fungal Organisms and the Resulting Disease
Organism	**Disease**
Aspergillus	aspergillosis
Blastomyces	blastomycosis
Candida (yeast)	candidiasis
Coccidioides	coccidioidomycosis
Cryptococcus	cryptococcosis
Histoplasma	histoplasmosis

Table 5.7

Most-Commonly Used Antifungals

Generic Name	Brand Name	Dosage Form
amphotericin B	Fungizone, Amphocin	oral suspension, IV, topical
	Amphotec, Abelcet (ABLC), AmBisome	IV
butenafine	Mentax	topical cream
caspofungin	Cancidus	IV
ciclopirox	Loprox, Penlac	topical (nail polish)
clotrimazole	Mycelex, Lotrimin, FemCare	oral, troche, topical, vaginal
fluconazole	Diflucan	tablet, oral suspension, IV
flucytosine	Ancobon	capsule
griseofulvin	Grisactin, Fulvicin, Gris-PEG	capsule, tablet, oral suspension
itraconazole	Sporanox	capsule, oral suspension
ketoconazole	Nizoral	tablet, topical
miconazole	Monistat, Micatin	topical, vaginal
nystatin	Nilstat	tablet, oral suspension, topical, vaginal
terbinafine	Lamisil	tablet, topical
terconazole	Terazol	vaginal

Antifungals are dispensed in two forms, topical agents and systemic agents. Even though the topical agents seem relatively mild compared to other topical agents, serious side effects have been reported. Close attention to the dosing regimen is needed to avoid overdosing.

Fungizone (amphotericin B) is used for blood-borne, life-threatening fungal infections. Amphotericin B interferes with cell wall permeability, allowing substances and electrolytes to leak out. Certain infections may necessitate four to six weeks of therapy. Cumulative blood levels of the drug should be monitored so as not to exceed 1 g to 4 g over four to six weeks. (These numbers vary depending on the reference source.) The drug must be infused slowly, not mixed or "piggybacked" with other drugs. To avoid precipitation, it should not be mixed with normal saline. Vital signs should be checked every thirty minutes during infusion. The following should be monitored closely: electrolytes (especially potassium and magnesium), BUN (blood urea nitrogen), serum creatinine, liver function, temperature, complete blood count, and fluid input and output. Antiemetics (covered in Chapter 11) can reduce the severity of nausea and vomiting. Frequent change of the IV site is necessary if the patient does not have a central venous catheter, as phlebitis (inflammation of a vein) is common with administration of this drug.

Side effects are fever, chills, shaking, and headache. Prophylaxis with aspirin, acetaminophen, and/or antihistamine are often necessary. A common, serious side effect is renal toxicity; patients may be left with residual kidney damage; potassium, calcium, and magnesium stores are often depleted; and anemia is common.

Abelcet, AmBisome, and **Amphotec (amphotericin B)** are lipid complex injectable forms with less kidney toxicity. They are indicated for treating aspergillosis or any type of progressive fungal infection in patients unresponsive to amphotericin B. Cardiopulmonary resuscitation equipment should be available in case of anaphylactic reaction. A wide range of side effects have been reported. These drugs can be administered IV or IM.

Diflucan (fluconazole) is metabolized through the cytochrome P-450 system. The oral form is used for vaginal or oral candidiasis; the IV form should be reserved for patients unable to tolerate amphotericin B. The most common side effects are headache, rash, and GI upset.

Sporanox (itraconazole) is especially useful for fungal infections under the nails. It can be taken for a much shorter period than the other antifungals with the same results. It should be taken twice a day with a fatty meal but not in conjunction with antacids or H₂ blockers. Because liver toxicity can occur, patients should report any unusual nausea, vomiting, jaundice, or changes in the stool to the physician immediately. Capsules should not be substituted for the oral solution, as the solution is more readily absorbed. Patients should drink a cola when taking this drug, as absorption is improved by increasing stomach acidity.

Lamisil (terbinafine) kills the fungus instead of just inhibiting its growth. It also persists longer in the nail after drug therapy has been stopped. The oral form is taken once daily for six weeks for fingernails and twelve weeks for toenails. Pulse dosing works very well. It may be better than Sporanox. The topical form is for treatment of athlete's foot, jock itch, and ringworm. It is applied to the affected area for at least one week, not to exceed four weeks. It should not be used vaginally.

Mentax (butenafine) is similar to terbinafine. This drug should be applied to the affected area once a day for four weeks. This drug remains effective for up to four weeks after its final application. Thus, symptoms may continue to improve even after the therapy is discontinued.

Ancobon (flucytosine) is synergistic with amphotericin B for *Candida* and *Cryptosporidium* infections. It is usually given in conjunction with another antifungal, such as fluconazole or itraconazole. The most common side effects are rash and GI upset.

Grisactin, Fulvicin, and **Gris-PEG (griseofulvin)** are indicated for fungal infections of the hair, skin, and nails. They can be used safely in children. The drugs bind to human keratin, making it resistant to infection. The dose is taken with a fatty meal. The patient should avoid exposure to sunlight. If headache occurs, it usually goes away. Dizziness and drowsiness may be side effects.

Nizoral (ketoconazole) comes as a shampoo for patients with fungal infection of the scalp. In tablet form, it has the same side effects profile as the other antifungal agents. Side effects are dose dependent and include nausea, anorexia, and vomiting.

Mycelex, Lotrimin, and **FemCare (clotrimazole)**, supplied as a troche, are especially effective against oropharyngeal candidiasis. Oral administration over a long time necessitates periodic monitoring of liver function. This drug is also an OTC vaginal cream. It is the DOC for ringworm in the topical form.

Monistat (miconazole) as IV is used to treat severe systemic fungal infections and fungal meningitis. Topically it is primarily used in the treatment of vulvovaginal candidiasis and is an OTC preparation. If a female patient indicates that she frequently gets vaginitis when on an antibiotic, the technician may alert the pharmacist to suggest an OTC vaginal antifungal.

Nilstat (nystatin) is most often used in liquid form, swish and swallow, for children with candidiasis.

Terazol (terconazole) is a prescription drug. If a patient has a vaginal fungal infection as a result of antibiotic use, it would be prudent to get the doctor to write a prescription for this drug. It works the same as the OTC vaginal antifungals, but since it is prescribed it can be covered by insurance, causing less out-of-pocket expense for the patient.

Loprox and **Penlac (ciclopirox)** are topical antifungals which inhibit the transport of certain elements in the fungal cell, thereby blocking the synthesis of DNA and, subsequently, cellular reproduction. The drug is prescribed either as a cream or as a "nail polish" to treat nail tissue infections and has fewer side effects than oral antifungals. Ciclopirox should not be taken in combination with oral antifungals.

Patients should be instructed to apply this medication at bedtime and to keep the formulation away from light.

Cancidus (caspofungin) is the first of a new class of antifungal drugs, the glucan synthesis inhibitors that inhibit the synthesis of $\beta(1,3)$-D-glucan, an integral component of the fungal cell wall. It is only available in IV form for the treatment of invasive aspergillosis in patients who are refractory to other therapies such as amphotericin B and itraconazole.

Chapter Summary

Viruses and Their Characteristics

◇ Viruses are highly specialized microorganisms that replicate intracellularly by using the cell's metabolic process.

◇ A virus has a spectrum of cells it can infect and only in these can it multiply. These are referred to as host cells; they can be animal, plant, or bacteria.

◇ All virus-infected cells have some characteristics different from uninfected cells. These differences offer ways to block viral division without affecting normal cells.

◇ Latency is a problem with viruses. They can lie dormant and then under certain conditions reproduce and behave once more like an infective agent, causing cell damage. Herpes virus and HIV both have this characteristic.

◇ Some virus-infected cells produce interferon, which protects neighboring uninfected cells from viral infection.

◇ Even though the body has defense mechanisms, such as producing interferons, some viruses can cause normal animal cells to be transformed into cancer cells.

◇ A major problem in the development of antivirals is the intimate relationship between host and virus. The search for selective inhibitors of viral activity that are not too toxic to the human host is still under way. The use of interferons from outside the body is leading the way.

◇ Symmetrel (amantadine) and Flumadine (rimantadine) are often prescribed for influenza prophylaxis. Flumadine has fewer side effects. Symmetrel is also used for Parkinson's disease.

◇ The IV form of acyclovir is the drug of choice for a form of herpes encephalitis and severe herpes in immunocompromised persons.

◇ Famvir, Zovirax, and Valtrex are used to manage acute herpes zoster (shingles).

◇ Symmetrel (amantadine) and Flumadine (rimantadine) are often prescribed for influenza prophylaxis. Flumadine has fewer side effects. Symmetrel is also used for Parkinson's disease.

◇ Cytovene (ganciclovir) is used primarily in treating cytomegalovirus (CMV) retinitis in immunocompromised patients. It is also used for transplantation patients. When mixing this drug, technicians must use chemo precautions, and the drug must be labeled with an appropriate label. It is very important that these patients be hydrated.

◇ Ophthalmic antivirals are Vira-A, and Vitrasert.

◇ An inhalation antiviral is Virazole. Maximum absorption occurs with the use of the aerosol generator via an endotracheal tube. Side effects are fatigue, headache, and insomnia. Virazole is especially for use in patients with respiratory syncytial virus (RSV), which usually occurs in children.

Antiretrovirals

◇ Neuraminidase is the viral enzyme that facilitates the release of newly formed virus particles. Nucleoside reverse transcriptase inhibitors (NRTIs) bind and inhibit the actions of this enzyme.

◇ Retrovir (zidovudine, AZT) was the first drug available specifically to treat the HIV virus.

◇ Non-nucleoside reverse transcriptase inhibitors (NNRTIs) inhibit the action of the reverse transcriptase neuraminidase by preventing the formation of proviral DNA.

- Protease inhibitors (PIs) prevent the cleavage of certain HIV protein precursors, which are necessary for replication of the virus.
- The standard of care for HIV patients involves the combination of three or more antiretroviral drugs. Since these regimens are often complex and difficult to follow, compliance is an issue. None of the current drugs can eradicate the disease but they can improve immunological status and prolong life. Some drug combinations should be avoided.

Fungi and Their Characteristics

- A fungus is a microscopic, eukaryotic protist reproduced by spores such as mushrooms, yeasts, and molds. Human cells contain cholesterol; fungi contain ergosterol, the primary target for antifungal drugs. This selective action is the basis for antifungal drugs.
- Systemic fungus diseases are most likely to develop in patients whose immune system is depressed by disease or drug therapy such as with corticosteroids or antineoplastics.
- Antifungals prevent the synthesis of ergosterol, a building block for fungal cell membranes. Activity is due to inhibiting fungal cytochrome P-450, which is different from human cytochrome P-450; therefore, antifungals have little effect on human cells.
- Amphotericin B can be administered orally, intravenously, intramuscularly, or topically. Intravenous administration necessitates prophylaxis with diphenhydramine, aspirin, or acetaminophen. It causes fever, headaches, shaking, and chills. It must be infused slowly and cannot be piggybacked or mixed with other drugs. The patient should be checked frequently while taking this drug or during infusion. Laboratory tests should also be monitored.
- Diflucan is used primarily for oral or vaginal candidiasis and cryptosporidium.
- Sporanox is for fungus under the nails. It takes a much shorter course of therapy than the older drugs. It should be taken with a fatty meal, and antacids should be avoided. Sporanox is especially toxic to the liver, so signs of jaundice, such as yellowing of the skin, should be monitored.
- Lamisil is an antifungal that works in less time and may be even better than Sporanox for fungus under nails. It kills the fungus instead of just inhibiting its growth. It persists in the nails even after therapy is completed. After therapy it still takes several months for clear nails to grow out. Patients should take the drug six weeks for fingernails and twelve weeks for toenails.
- Pulse dosing for fungal nail infections appears to be very effective and less costly.
- Ancobon is usually given in conjunction with another antifungal.
- Griseofulvin can be used for fungal infections of the hair, skin, and nails. It is often used in children. It is taken with a fatty meal, and sunlight should be avoided.
- Mycelex comes in a troche especially effective for oral candidiasis.
- Liquid Nystatin is often used for candidiasis in children and infants.
- Females taking antibiotics frequently need an OTC antifungal to treat vaginitis, which occurs due to the antibiotic.
- Cancidus is the first in the new class of antifungal drugs. It is approved for use in patients with invasive aspergillosis unresponsive to other therapies.

Drug Summary

The following drugs were discussed in this chapter. Each generic drug name is followed in parentheses by one or more brand names. An asterisk (*) indicates drugs frequently written using *either* brand *or* generic names. These need to be memorized.

Antivirals   ~~virus.~~

Systemic Agents
acyclovir (Zovirax)*
amantadine (Symmetrel)*
cidofovir (Vistide)
famciclovir (Famvir)
foscarnet (Foscavir)
ganciclovir (Cytovene)*
oseltamivir (Tamiflu)
rimantadine (Flumadine)*
valacyclovir (Valtrex)
zanamivir (Relenza)

Ophthalmic Agents
ganciclovir (Vitrasert)
vidarabine (Vira-A)*

Inhalation Agent
ribavirin (Virazole)

Antiretrovirals

NRTIs
abacavir (Ziagen)
didanosine, ddI (Videx, Videx EC)
lamivudine, 3TC (Epivir)
stavudine, d4T (Zerit)
zalcitabine (Hivid)
zidovudine, AZT (Retrovir)
zidovudine-lamivudine (Combivir)
zidovudine-lamivudine-cibacuvir
    (Trizivir)

NNRTIs
delavirdine (Rescriptor)
efavirenz (Sustiva)
nevirapine (Viramune)

PIs
amprenavir (Agenerase)
indinavir (Crixivan)
lopinavir-ritonavir (Kaletra)
nelfinavir (Viracept)
ritonavir (Norvir)
saquinavir (Invirase, Fortovase)

Antifungals
amphotericin B (Fungizone,* Abelcet,
    Amphotec, Amphocin, AmBisome)
butenatine (Mentax)
caspofungin (Cancidus)
ciclopirox (Loprox, Penlac)
clotrimazole (Mycelex,* Lotrimin,
    FemCare)
fluconazole (Diflucan)*
flucytosine (Ancobon)
griseofulvin (Grisactin, Fulvicin, Gris-
    PEG)*
itraconazole (Sporanox)
ketoconazole (Nizoral)*
miconazole (Monistat, Micatin)*
nystatin (Nilstat)*
terbinafine (Lamisil)
terconazole (Terazol)

Chapter Review

Pharmaceuticals and Body Functions

Select the best answer from the choices given.

1. Which one of the listed drugs is used as prophylaxis for influenza and also in treating Parkinson's disease?
   a. AZT
   b. Rimantadine
   c. Symmetrel
   d. Cytovene

2. Which drug listed requires the pharmacy technician to use chemo precautions when mixing?
   a. Zovirax
   b. Cytovene
   c. Famvir
   d. Videx

3. Which drug listed is a lipid complex and less toxic than the older IV form of the drug?
   a. Zovirax
   b. Cytovene
   c. Abelcet
   d. Videx

4. Which drug listed should not be taken in combination with didanosine?
   a. Stavudine
   b. Zalcitabine
   c. Zidovudine
   d. Indivir

5. Which of the following drugs should be stored in its orginal container with a dessicant?
   a. Saquinavir
   b. Indinavir
   c. Zanamivir
   d. Oseltamivir

6. All the organisms listed below are fungi except
   a. *Escherichia coli.*
   b. *Histoplasma.*
   c. *Aspergillus.*
   d. *Candida.*

7. Which drug is synergistic with amphotericin B for Candida?
   a. Ancobon
   b. Nilstat
   c. Mycelex
   d. Sporanox

8. Which two antifungals come in an IV dosage form?
    a. Diflucan and amphotericin B
    b. Diflucan and griseofulvin
    c. Gris-PEG and amphotericin B
    d. Clotrimazole and ketoconazole

9. Which antifungal is especially useful for treating fungal infection under the nails because of the shorter time span needed for treatment?
    a. Gris-PEG
    b. Sporanox
    c. Nilstat
    d. Mycelex

10. Which vaginal antifungal requires a prescription?
    a. Femstat
    b. Gyne-Lotrimin
    c. Mycelex
    d. Terazol   *vaginal suppository or cream that interact with latex condoms.*

The following statements are true or false. If the answer is false, rewrite the question so it is true.

___T___ 1. A virus cannot reproduce outside the cell.

___T___ 2. Host cells can be animal, plant, or bacteria.

___F___ 3. A virus cannot lie dormant and then under certain conditions reproduce and again behave like an infective agent.

___F___ 4. The elderly, patients with cardiovascular or renal disease, and patients with diabetes or asthma are *not* at risk for influenza.

___F___ 5. Zovirax (acyclovir) is available in the following dosage forms: oral, parenteral, topical, and suppositories.

___T___ 6. The most common side effects of fluconazole (Diflucan) are headache, rash, and GI upset.

___T___ 7. Gris-PEG is used for fungal infections of the hair, skin, and nails.

___F___ 8. The patient taking Fulvicin should be told to take the dose on an empty stomach and get plenty of sun.

___T___ 9. Most antiviral and antifungal agents are very expensive.

___F___ 10. Very few antivirals and antifungals are available as topical agents.

Diseases and Drug Therapies

1. Identify two classifications for a virus.
2. Explain why you would not mix amphotericin B with normal saline.
3. Explain how pulse dosing works.
4. What are the most common side effects of Nizoral?
5. Why is latency a problem with some viruses?

Dispensing Medications

1. You receive the following prescription. This is the only one given for this patient.

   Joe Brown
   Amphotericin B 1 mg/kg
   over 6 hr every other day.
   Mix in D_5W.
   a. If Mr. Brown weighs 150 pounds, how much will you mix?
   b. Give at least two reasons for calling the doctor.

2. You receive the following prescription:

   Joe Lee
   Foscarnet 60 mg/kg IV over 1 hr q8h for 2 weeks.
   a. If Mr. Lee weighs 180 pounds, how much will you mix?
   b. This is the only prescription you receive. What has the doctor forgotten?

3. You receive the following prescription:

   Jim Tucker
   Dispense 1 month's supply.
   Septra DS bid # _____
   Rifampin 300 mg qd # _____
   Clotrimazole 10 mg
   (1 troche) 5 times
   daily # _____
   AZT 100 mg q4h
   around the clock # _____
   a. How many will you dispense of each?
   b. What is the patient's diagnosis?

   Sig chart:
   bid = twice a day
   qd = every day
   q4h = every 4 hours

Internet Research

Use the Internet to complete the following assignments.

1. What are the newest drug treatments for AIDS? Create a table listing four to six new drugs, include their generic and brand names, and their side effects. List your Web sources.
2. Find current HIV/AIDS statistics. How many individuals in the United States are HIV-positive? At what rate (individuals per year) is the virus spreading? Make sure to include the date and source of the information in your report. Do you think it is difficult to get an accurate figure? Why or why not? List your Internet sources.

Antihistamines, Decongestants, Antitussives, and Expectorants

Chapter

6

Learning Objectives

◆ Understand the differences in the antihistamines, decongestants, antitussives, and expectorants.

◆ Know how and when each drug class should be used.

◆ Recognize and understand the side effects that may occur with each group.

◆ Know why some drugs are prescribed for their side effects.

The indications for these four classes of drugs include some of the most prevalent diseases, among them the common cold and cough. Only recently did the FDA approve a drug to treat symptoms of the common cold. A large number of drugs in these four groups are available as OTC products. This is an area where technicians can put to use their drug knowledge. While it is still incumbent upon the technician to refer to the pharmacist in areas requiring judgmental decisions, the OTCs have directions printed on the package. The technician will be the person who most frequently directs the patient to the OTC counter. While recommendations should not be made, the technician can definitely make the patient aware of the proper uses and side effects of these drugs.

ANTIHISTAMINES

Histamine is found in all body tissue. It induces capillary dilation and increases capillary permeability, both of which help to decrease blood pressure. It contracts most smooth muscle, increases gastric acid secretion, increases heart rate, and mediates hypersensitivity. Basically, there are two types of drugs that block the histamine receptors. The drugs commonly referred to as antihistamines block the H_1 receptors in the upper respiratory system. The other group of antihistamines are referred to as H_2 blockers and they affect the cells in the gastrointestinal tract. We will discuss the H_1 blockers, commonly referred to as antihistamines, in this chapter.

Antihistamines are well absorbed in tissues and widely distributed across the blood-brain barrier and placenta. Sedation occurs when they penetrate the blood-brain barrier. Pregnant mothers are warned not to take antihistamines because these products can cross the placenta and adversely affect the fetus. Table 6.1 lists the most-commonly used antihistamines.

Therapeutic Uses for Antihistamines

The drugs normally thought of as antihistamines (H_1 blockers) provide symptomatic relief by acting on the H_1 receptors to prevent histamine release. They have many uses including

Table 6.1	Most-Commonly Used Antihistamines		
Generic Name		**Brand Name**	**Dosage Form**
OTCs			
brompheniramine		Dimetane, Dimetapp	tablet, caplet, syrup
chlorpheniramine		Chlor-Trimeton	tablet, capsule, chewable
clemastine		Tavist	tablet, syrup
cyclizine		Marezine	tablet
dimenhydrinate		Dramamine	tablet, capsule
diphenhydramine		Benadryl	tablet, capsule, topical
doxylamine		Unisom	tablet
meclizine		Bonine	tablet, capsule
triprolidine-pseudoephedrine		Actifed	tablet, caplet
Prescription Drugs			
azatadine		Optimine, Trinalin	tablet
azelastine		Astelin	spray
cetirizine		Zyrtec	tablet
cyproheptadine		Periactin	tablet, syrup
diphenhydramine		Benadryl	IM, IV
fexofenadine		Allegra	tablet
hydroxyzine hydrochloride		Atarax	tablet, capsule, syrup, IM, IV
hydroxyzine pamoate		Vistaril	capsule, syrup
loratadine		Claritin	tablet
meclizine		Antivert	tablet, capsule, chewable
promethazine		Phenergan	tablet, syrup, suppository, IM, IV
trimeprazine		Temaril	tablet, syrup

Warning

Cyproheptadine and cyclobenzaprine look alike. Cyproheptadine comes in 4 mg and cyclobenzaprine in 10 mg. One is an antihistamine, and the other is a muscle relaxant.

Warning

Hydroxyzine and hydralazine are easily confused but they are very different drugs for very different indications. Both can be dosed four times a day and have the same dosages.

Warning

Vistaril and Zestril look alike. Zestril is a medication for the heart and Vistaril is an antihistamine. Dosing will help here. Zestril comes in 2.5 mg, 5 mg, 10 mg, 20 mg, and 40 mg. Vistaril comes in 25 mg, 50 mg, and 100 mg.

- ◇ treatment of allergies, insomnia, and rashes
- ◇ symptomatic relief of urticarial lesions (rash), edema, and hay fever
- ◇ control of cough
- ◇ alleviation of vertigo
- ◇ alleviation of nausea and vomiting
- ◇ relief of serum sickness (hypersensitivity reaction that may occur several days to two to three weeks after receiving antisera or following drug therapy)
- ◇ control of venom reactions (venom contains histamine and other substances causing histamine release)
- ◇ mitigation of the extrapyramidal side effects of antipsychotic medication
- ◇ prophylaxis for certain drug reactions
- ◇ prophylaxis for certain drug allergies

Antihistamines can also be used in the treatment of hypersensitivity reactions. Hypersensitivity is a state of altered reactivity in which the body reacts with an exaggerated immune response to a foreign agent. This response can range from quite serious, as in serum sickness, to a slight rash or low-grade fever.

Table 6.2 lists the common indications for the antihistamines listed in Table 6.1. Some antihistamines are promoted for specific indications even though there is a lot of overlap in therapeutic uses of these drugs. The side effect profile is also the same even though there may be varying degrees for each drug. They are more effective at preventing some allergic reactions from occurring than they are in reversing these actions once they have taken place.

Antihistamines' Side Effects and Dispensing Issues

Sedation, the most common side effect of antihistamines, is synergistic with alcohol use. Some antihistamines are actually prescribed to induce sleep. In fact, almost

Table 6.2	Indications for Common Antihistamines

Generic Name	Brand Name	Indication
OTCs		
brompheniramine	Dimetane, Dimetapp	allergies
chlorpheniramine	Chlor-Trimeton	allergies
clemastine	Tavist	allergies (less sedating)
cyclizine	Marezine	nausea
dimenhydrinate	Dramamine	vertigo, motion sickness
diphenhydramine	Benadryl	allergies, insomnia
doxylamine	Unisom	sleep
meclizine	Bonine	vertigo, motion sickness
triprolidine-pseudoephedrine	Actifed	allergies
Prescription Drugs		
azatadine	Optimine, Trinalin	allergies
azelastine	Astelin	allergies
cetirizine	Zyrtec	allergies
cyproheptadine	Periactin	increases appetite
diphenhydramine	Benadryl	allergies, insomnia
fexofenadine	Allegra	allergies (less sedating)
hydroxyzine hydrochloride	Atarax	allergic reactions
hydroxyzine pamoate	Vistaril	induces sleep
loratadine	Claritin	allergies (less sedating)
meclizine	Antivert	vertigo
promethazine	Phenergan	nausea
trimeprazine	Temaril	allergies

every OTC sleeping pill contains the antihistamine **diphenhydramine**. These drugs also have anticholinergic side effects: drying of the mouth and mucosa of the upper respiratory tract, blurred vision, constipation, and urinary retention. Dizziness is also a common side effect. The newer drugs on the market have fewer side effects.

The most common side effects of the currently available antihistamines include

- ◇ hyperactivity in some children
- ◇ anticholinergic (atropine-like dry mouth, blurred vision, constipation, and urinary retention)
- ◇ sedation

Tavist (clemastine) is the only drug approved by the FDA for cold symptoms and is the least sedating OTC antihistamine.

Allegra (fexofenadine) is not as sedating as many of the other antihistamines. Studies have shown no arrhythmias or other serious reactions having occurred with this drug.

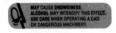

Astelin (azelastine) was the first antihistamine nasal spray. It is indicated in seasonal allergic rhinitis and seems to work as well as the oral antihistamines for itchy, runny nose and sneezing. It tastes bitter. Even though the drug has a low incidence of sedative side effects, the bottle should carry a sticker warning about drowsiness. It is stable for three months after the bottle is opened.

DECONGESTANTS

Vasodilation of blood vessels in the nasal mucosa allow leakage of fluids into these tissues resulting in swelling and stuffiness. Decongestants stimulate the alpha-adrenergic receptors of the vascular smooth muscle, constricting the dilated arteriolar network within the nasal mucosa. This constriction shrinks the engorged mucous membranes, which promotes drainage, improves nasal ventilation, and relieves the feeling of stuffiness. Shrinking the mucous membranes not only makes breathing easier but also permits the sinus cavities to drain. Topical agents are more immediately effective but of shorter duration than systemic agents. Decongestants should not be given to patients who cannot tolerate sympathetic nervous system stimulation. Sympathetic nervous system stimulation causes increased heart rate, increased blood pressure, and increased CNS stimulation. Decongestants are often combined with antihistamines in an effort to offset the side effect of drowsiness of the antihistamine. Most decongestants are OTC drugs.

It is very important that the label directions be followed regarding the frequency and duration of use. Topical nasal application of these drugs is often followed by a rebound phenomenon called *rhinitis medicamentosa*, which results when these agents are used over prolonged periods. It is thought to be caused by severe nasal edema and reduced receptor sensitivity. Patients with this condition use more spray more often with less response. Patients should be counseled on the use of topical decongestants to prevent rhinitis medicamentosa. Duration of therapy of a nasal decongestant should be limited to three to five days.

Table 6.3 describes the most-commonly used decongestants. Decongestants can be administered topically or orally. Topical administration takes the form of drops, sprays, and vapors that are applied nasally. Oral administration takes the form of capsules, syrups, and tablets and are often combined with antihistamines. Administering decongestants orally distributes the drug through the systemic circulation to the vascular bed of the nasal mucosa.

Therapeutic Uses of Decongestants

Decongestants are used for temporary symptomatic relief of nasal congestion due to the common cold, upper respiratory allergies, and sinusitis. They promote nasal sinus drainage and are useful in providing vascular constriction of blood vessels in the nasal mucosa. Vessel constriction allows excess tissue fluids to be carried away in circulation, thus reducing swelling in the mucosa, opening air passageways, and allowing the patient to breathe more freely.

Decongestants' Side Effects and Dispensing Issues

Decongestants should *not* be taken if the patient is using other sympathomimetic drugs. They should also be avoided if the following conditions exist.

- ◇ diabetes
- ◇ heart disease

Table 6.3	**Most-Commonly Used Decongestants**		
Generic Name	**Brand Name**		**Dosage Form**
naphazoline	Privine		nasal drops, ophthalmic
oxymetazoline	Afrin		nasal drops, ophthalmic
phenylephrine	Neo-Synephrine, Neo-Synephrine II		nasal drops, spray, ophthalmic
pseudoephedrine	Sudafed		tablet, capsule, oral solution
tetrahydrozoline	Tyzine		nasal drops, spray, ophthalmic
xylometazoline	Otrivin		nasal drops, spray

- hypertension
- hyperthyroidism
- prostatic hypertrophy
- Tourette's syndrome

Both oral and topical agents have side effects, sometimes just unpleasant, but sometimes serious. These effects differ for oral agents and topical agents. They are listed in Table 6.4.

ANTITUSSIVES

Antitussives are agents that suppress coughing and are indicated when reducing cough frequency is needed, especially when the cough is dry and nonproductive. The mechanism by which the narcotic and nonnarcotic agents affect a cough's intensity and frequency depends on the principal site of action: 1) CNS depression of the cough center in the medulla (cough reflex) or 2) suppression of the nerve receptors within the respiratory tract.

The cough reflex involves two types of receptors found in the lungs and airways. These receptors, when stimulated, can initiate the events leading to a cough.

- stretch receptors: muscle response to elongation
- irritant receptors: coarse particles and chemicals

The cough reflex is a coordinated series of events.

1. An inspiration interrupts regular respiratory rhythm.
2. The thorax and abdominal muscles contract rapidly, compressing the diaphragm against the lungs.
3. The airway closes, compressing airway gas.
4. A peristaltic muscular wave moves over the bronchi and bronchioles.
5. Pressure exceeds 100 mm, the glottis opens, and the laryngeal muscles relax.
6. Air flows outward, carrying mucus and foreign bodies.

Theoretically, the cough reflex can be stopped at several points. The antitussive products are formulated to act on one or more of the events in this series by

- correcting or blocking the irritation of receptors
- blocking transmission to the brain

Table 6.4	Side Effects of Decongestants	
Oral Agents	**Topical Agents**
anxiety	burning sensation
CNS stimulation (can be used to avoid sleep)	contact dermatitis
dizziness	dry mouth
hallucinations	rhinitis medicamentosa
headache	sneezing
increased blood pressure	stinging sensation
increased heart rate	
insomnia	
tremor	

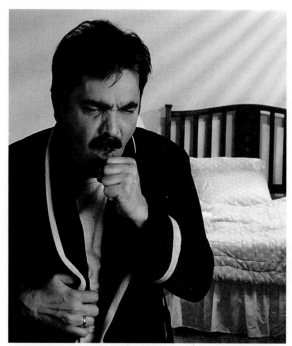
Stimulating receptors in the airways and lungs produces a cough.

◇ increasing the cough center threshold
◇ blocking the action of the expiratory muscles

Table 6.5 lists the most-commonly used antitussives.

Therapeutic Uses of Antitussives

Antitussives are drugs that specifically block or suppress the act of coughing. Coughing is a mechanism for clearing the airways of excess secretions and foreign materials. Excessive intensity and frequency with lack of sputum production can be annoying to the patient.

Antitussives' Side Effects and Dispensing Issues

Codeine is considered the "gold standard" against which the efficiency of other antitussive therapies are measured. Codeine's average adult dose is 15 mg every four to six hours. In addition to being a CNS depressant, codeine is thought to have a drying effect on the respiratory mucosa; this would be detrimental to patients with asthma or emphysema. The most common side effects are nausea, drowsiness, lightheadedness, and constipation, especially if the recommended dose is exceeded. Codeine also has an additive effect if taken with other CNS depressants, such as alcohol. Codeine should be taken with food to decrease stomach upset.

When used at the recommended dosage, codeine has low potential for dependency. Stringent controls have been placed on codeine-containing products as a result of their misuse. They may be purchased in some states without a prescription, but the purchaser must sign for them, be an adult according to state law, and show identification. They may be dispensed only by the pharmacist since it requires the pharmacist to initial by the patient's signature.

Hycodan (hydrocodone-homatropine) is a C-III drug used for symptomatic cough relief. It causes drowsiness and impaired vision. The patient should be

Table 6.5	**Most-Commonly Used Antitussives**		
Generic Name	**Brand Name**	**Classification**	**Dosage Form**
benzonatate	Tessalon Perles	prescription	pearl-shaped capsule
codeine	combined with antihistamines, other antitussives, and expectorants	C-V	syrup
dextromethorphan	Delsym, Robitussin D	OTC	syrup, lozenges, liquid
diphenhydramine	Benadryl, Benylin	OTC	tablet, syrup, lozenges
hydrocodone-homatropine	Hycodan	C-III	syrup

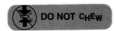 DO NOT CHEW

instructed to notify the physician in the event of difficulty urinating or constipation. This combination drug has a high sugar content, and thus is obviously contraindicated in diabetic patients. Before dispensing it, the pharmacy technician should check the patient profile for a diagnosis or medications indicating diabetes.

Delsym and **Robitussin D (dextromethorphan)** are considered equivalent to codeine, without its analgesic properties, and do not depress respiration or have abuse potential. The average adult dose is 10 mg to 20 mg every four hours. Dextromethorphan interacts with monoamine oxidase inhibitors (MAOIs). It is often combined with other drugs (e.g., diphenhydramine, guaifenesin).

Benadryl and **Benylin (diphenhydramine)** are both antitussives and antihistamines. The usual adult dose is 25 mg every four hours. The main side effect is drowsiness, which is additive if the drug is taken with other CNS depressants.

Tessalon Perles (benzonatate) is a prescription drug used for a nonproductive cough. Its anesthetizing effects are local; it anesthetizes the stretch receptors in the airway, lungs, and pleura but does not affect the respiratory center. The label should indicate "Do not chew," as chewing the drug would cause a very unpleasant effect with pronounced salivation. Fluid intake is especially encouraged to help liquefy sputum. The main side effects are sedation, headache, and dizziness.

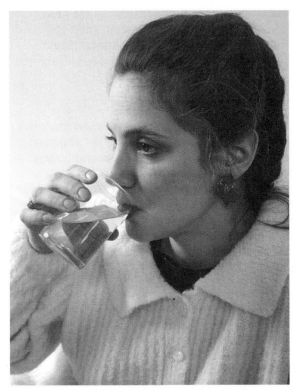

Sometimes maintaining good fluid intake is all that is needed to allow the respiratory tract to clear itself through coughing.

EXPECTORANTS

The purpose of expectorant agents is to enable the patient to rid the lungs and airway of mucus when coughing. Expectorants will produce a cough attended with expiration of material from the bronchi. This type of cough is called a productive cough. Expectorant agents decrease the thickness and stickiness of mucus, decreasing viscosity and increasing expectoration of mucus. If a patient is well hydrated, it is no problem to cough up mucus. Fluid intake and adequate humidity in the inspired air are important to liquefy mucus in the respiratory tract and, therefore, are essential in cold therapy. This can be accomplished by drinking six to eight glasses of water a day, which can be as, or more, effective than an expectorant.

For the patient who prefers using an expectorant, the most-commonly used OTC expectorant is **guaifenesin**. It can be taken in caplet, capsule, liquid, syrup, tablet, or sustained release form. A common brand name is **Robitussin**.

Guaifenesin is especially indicated in patients with a persistent or chronic cough (from smoking, asthma, or emphysema) with excessive secretions. It comes in many combinations. For example, **Humibid** is a tablet form of guaifenesin. It comes in chewables and alternate brand names as well. Expectorants liquefy secretions and decrease thickness and stickiness of mucus; therefore, they are used for both dry, unproductive coughs and productive coughs. The side effects include vomiting, nausea, GI upset, and drowsiness.

Chapter Summary

Antihistamines

◇ Antihistamines, decongestants, antitussives, and expectorants each have a different mechanism of action and purpose. They are often confused. Most are OTC products.

◇ Antihistamines are used primarily to combat allergic reactions, nausea, vertigo, and insomnia. They prevent binding of histamine to the receptor sites.

◇ The most common side effects of antihistamines are sedation and anticholinergic responses (dry mouth, constipation, urinary retention).

◇ Many antihistamines are sold OTC.

◇ Diphenhydramine is the major ingredient in OTC sleep medications.

◇ Phenergan (promethazine) and Antivert and Bonine (meclizine) are the antihistamines used primarily for nausea and motion sickness. Phenergan and Antivert require a prescription; Bonine does not.

◇ Dramamine (dimenhydrinate) and Bonine (meclizine) are used for vertigo and motion sickness.

◇ Claritin and Allegra are prescription antihistamines that are less sedating than others currently available. Tavist is the least-sedating OTC antihistamine.

◇ Tavist is the OTC antihistamine with the least drowsiness effect. It has been approved by the FDA for treatment of symptoms of the common cold.

◇ Histamine release is implicated in anaphylactic reactions, hay fever, allergic rhinitis, allergic dermatitis or eczema, contact dermatitis, and urticaria (hives).

Decongestants

◇ Decongestants stimulate the alpha-adrenergic receptors of the vascular smooth muscle, constricting the dilated arteriolar network and shrinking the engorged mucous membranes. This promotes drainage of the sinus cavities and makes breathing easier. This sympathetic stimulation also increases heart rate and blood pressure and stimulates the CNS. Patients sometimes take decongestants to overcome drowsiness; these drugs should not be taken by those who cannot tolerate sympathetic stimulation.

◇ Topical application of decongestants (nasal sprays and drops) can cause a rebound phenomenon, *rhinitis medicamentosa.*

Antitussives

◇ The cough reflex can be stopped at several points in the reflex pathway.

◇ Antitussives are indicated to reduce the frequency of a cough, especially when dry and nonproductive. Codeine is the antitussive with which all others are compared, commonly referred to as the "gold standard of antitussives."

◇ Dextromethorphan may be as effective as codeine, without the addictive side effect profile.

Expectorants

◇ Expectorants decrease thickness and stickiness of mucus by decreasing viscosity.

◇ Guaifenesin is the most-used expectorant, but water may work as well.

Drug Summary

The following drugs were discussed in this chapter. Each generic drug name is followed in parentheses by one or more brand names. An asterisk (*) indicates drugs frequently written using *either* brand *or* generic name. These need to be memorized.

Antihistamines

OTCs
brompheniramine (Dimetane, Dimetapp)
chlorpheniramine (Chlor-Trimeton)
clemastine (Tavist)*
cyclizine (Marezine)
dimenhydrinate (Dramamine)
diphenhydramine (Benadryl)*
doxylamine (Unisom)
meclizine (Bonine)*
triprolidine-pseudoephedrine (Actifed)

Prescription
azatadine (Optimine, Trinalin)
azelastine (Astelin)
cetirizine (Zyrtec)
cyproheptadine (Periactin)*
diphenhydramine (Benadryl)
fexofenadine (Allegra)
hydroxyzine hydrochloride (Atarax)*
hydroxyzine pamoate (Vistaril)*
loratadine (Claritin)*
meclizine (Antivert)*
promethazine (Phenergan)*
trimeprazine (Temaril)

Decongestants
naphazoline (Privine)
oxymetazoline (Afrin)
phenylephrine (Neo-Synephrine, Neo-Synephrine II)
pseudoephedrine (Sudafed)*
tetrahydrozoline (Tyzine)
xylometazoline (Otrivin)

Antitussives
benzonatate (Tessalon Perles)
codeine
dextromethorphan (Delsym, Robitussin D)*
diphenhydramine (Benylin, Benadryl)
hydrocodone-homatropine (Hycodan)

Expectorants
guaifenesin (Robitussin, Humibid)*

Chapter Review

Pharmaceuticals and Body Functions

Select the best answer from the choices given.

1. The following drugs can be bought over the counter, without a prescription *except*
   a. meclizine.
   b. promethazine.
   c. diphenhydramine.
   d. clemastine.

2. The OTC antihistamine that causes the least sedation is
   a. chlorpheniramine.
   b. diphenhydramine.
   c. clemastine.
   d. brompheniramine.

3. The drug most used in OTC sleep medications is
   a. pseudoephedrine.
   b. diphenhydramine.
   c. guaifenesin.
   d. dextromethorphan.

4. A controlled substance used to relieve cough is
   a. codeine.
   b. Hycodan.
   c. a and b.
   d. Robitussin.

5. The most used antitussive is
   a. dextromethorphan.
   b. diphenhydramine.
   c. benzonatate.
   d. codeine.

6. All the following are antihistamines, *except*
   a. cyclizine.
   b. oxymetazoline.
   c. brompheniramine.
   d. Dramamine.

7. All the following are decongestants, *except*
   a. azatadine.
   b. Sudafed.
   c. Neo-Synephrine
   d. Afrin.

8. All the following are antitussives, *except*
   a. Tessalon.
   b. Benylin.
   c. Delsym.
   d. hydroxyzine.

9. All the following are expectorants, *except*
   a. guaifenesin.
   b. water.
   c. a and b.
   d. Temaril.

10. Diphenhydramine is often prescribed for its
   a. diuretic effects.
   b. decongestant effects.
   c. sedating qualities. sleep
   d. ability to help students remain alert and test better.

The following statements are true or false. If the answer is false, rewrite the statement so it is true.

T 1. Nasal decongestants can cause a rebound phenomenon. The nasal mucous membranes become even more congested and edematous as the drug's vasoconstrictor effect subsides. This leads to a cycle of more frequent use of the agent causing the problem.

T 2. Cough involves two types of receptors—stretch and irritant.

T 3. Drinking eight glasses of water a day may be more effective than an expectorant.

T 4. Astelin is stable for three months after the bottle is opened.

F 5. Antihistamines work better at treating allergies than preventing them.

T 6. It is important for patients with high blood pressure to understand that decongestants only make the blood pressure increase.

F 7. Allegra (fexofenadine) has been shown to cause arrhythmias.

F 8. If a patient is taking an expectorant or antitussive, he or she does not need to bother with fluids.

F 9. An expectorant is used only for a dry, nonproductive cough.

F 10. Antihistamines are prescribed for many reasons, including vertigo, insomnia, allergic reactions, and birth control.

dizziness

Diseases and Drug Therapies

1. Explain the difference in antihistamines, decongestants, antitussives, and expectorants.
2. Which drug is approved by the FDA for treating symptoms of the common cold?
3. Explain cough reflex, step by step. Where does Tessalon Perles interfere with this cascade?
4. Explain how an antitussive works.

Dispensing Medications

1. A truck driver wants an OTC antihistamine that will not make him sleepy. Which one would be recommended? Would it be safe to take this drug and drive?
2. The physician orders Vistaril 100 mg IM q4h prn How much will you draw up per dose?

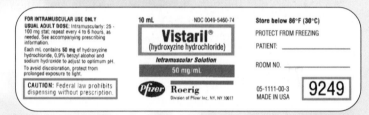

3. Identify a drug prescribed for its side effects. Explain.
4. When is the best time to take an antihistamine for an allergy? Why?
5. Astelin is opened on August 1. When would the drug expire?

Internet Research

Use the Internet to complete the following assignments.

1. Select three OTC antihistamines discussed in this chapter. Locate the manufacturer's Web site for each. Describe your process for finding the manufacturer: Did you need to go to another Web site first or did a search on the drug name lead you directly to the site? What type of information was available on the manufacturer's site? Did it list side effects? Did it list indications and contraindications? Create a table with the drugs you selected, the manufacturer's Web site address, and a brief description of the site's information related to that particular drug.
2. Create a similar table for three prescription medications discussed in the chapter. What strikes you most in terms of the difference of the Internet coverage between OTC and prescription drugs? What factors, in your opinion, might account for this difference?

Narcotic Pain Relievers and Other Nervous System Drugs

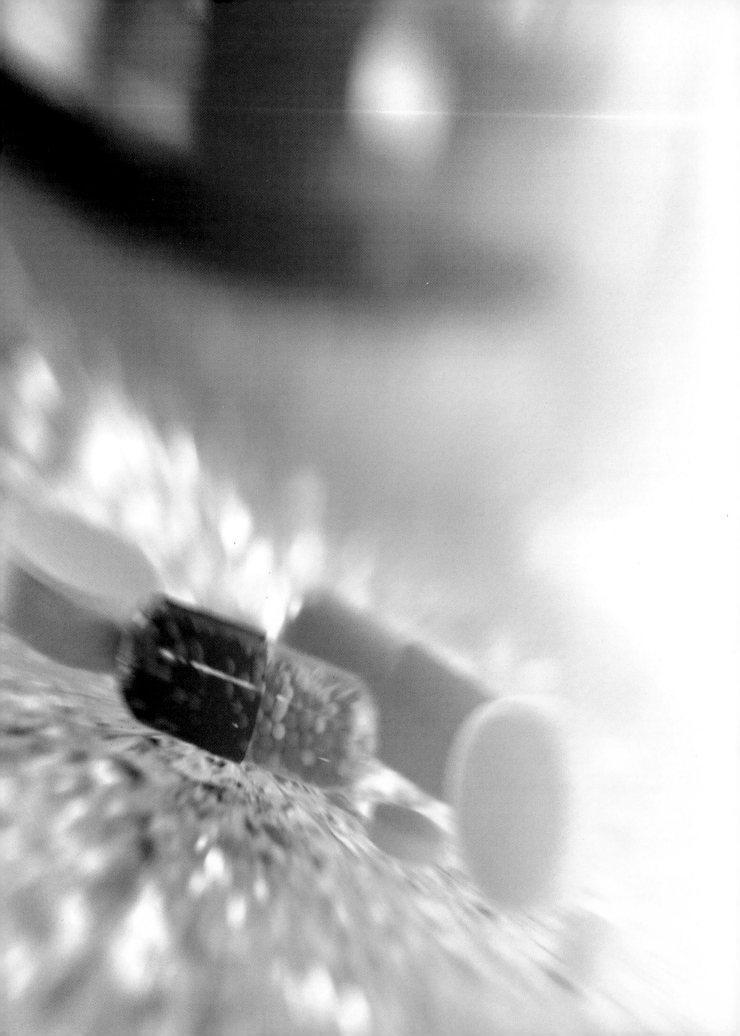

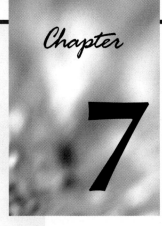

Anesthetics, Analgesics, and Narcotics

Chapter

7

The nervous system coordinates the other body systems and is the body's link with the outside world. It works continuously to preserve homeostasis, that is, to keep the other physiologic systems of the body in a normal state. The neurotransmitters (chemical messengers), an integral part of this system, control the behavior of most drugs in the body. Their activity determines the reactions of anesthetics, analgesics, and narcotics as well as their interaction with each other and the other body chemicals and systems.

Learning Objectives

- ◇ Understand the central and peripheral nervous systems, their functions, and their relationship to drugs.
- ◇ Become aware of the role of neurotransmitters.
- ◇ Learn how drugs affect body systems and where they work in the body.
- ◇ Understand the concept of general and local anesthesia, and know the functions of these agents.
- ◇ Define the action of neuromuscular blocking agents in reducing muscle activity.
- ◇ Distinguish between narcotic and nonnarcotic analgesia.
- ◇ Become familiar with the various types of agents for migraine headaches.

THE NERVOUS SYSTEM

The nervous system has two components: the central nervous system (CNS) and the peripheral nervous system (PNS). Neurotransmitters, chemical substances that are selectively released from neurons, are important to the study of drugs and drug actions. Neurotransmitters stimulate or inhibit activity in their target cells, especially other neurons.

The Central Nervous System

The CNS consists of the brain and the spinal cord, the two organs that evaluate incoming information and determine responses. The CNS coordinates and controls the activity of other body systems as well. Sense organs throughout the body detect heat, cold, pain, and the presence of chemicals, and convert that information into a chemical/electrical message. The message is transmitted to the spinal cord, to the brainstem, and to the cerebral cortex. As the impulses pass through the memory and emotional areas of the lower brain, they are compared with previous experiences on the basis of "like, dislike, or do not care." The thought process is a series of chemical reactions from the sense organs. The process involves the neurotransmitters; some are stimulatory and others are inhibitory. When the balance between the two is disturbed, the person may experience many of a number of physical, mental, or emotional disorders. The primary CNS transmitters are acetylcholine, norepinephrine, dopamine, GABA, and serotonin.

The Peripheral Nervous System

The PNS consists of the afferent system, nerves and sense organs that bring information to the CNS, as well as the efferent system, nerves that dispatch information out from the CNS. The efferent system has two parts, the autonomic nervous system (ANS) and the somatic nervous system. The primary PNS transmitters are acetylcholine, norepinephrine, and dopamine.

THE AUTONOMIC NERVOUS SYSTEM The ANS (Figure 7.1) regulates activities of structures not under voluntary control, i.e., below the level of consciousness. The ANS controls respiration, circulation, digestion, body temperature, metabolism, blood glucose, pupil dilation, GI motility, sweating, and certain glandular functions. By means of these unconscious adjustments, the ANS maintains internal balance. In the ANS, there are two neurons between the CNS and the muscle tissue it innervates. The ANS has two major components, the sympathetic nervous system and the parasympathetic nervous system. The major transmitters of the sympathetic system are norepinephrine, dopamine, and epinephrine. The major transmitter of the parasympathetic system is acetylcholine.

THE SOMATIC NERVOUS SYSTEM The second part of the PNS, the somatic nervous system, is concerned with skeletal muscles. There is only one neuron between the CNS and the skeletal muscles.

Major Neurotransmitters

The major neurotransmitters have the following actions.

- ◇ Acetylcholine (ACh) acts on receptors in smooth muscle, cardiac muscle, and exocrine glands; anticholinergics block these receptors.

Figure 7.1

The Autonomic Nervous System

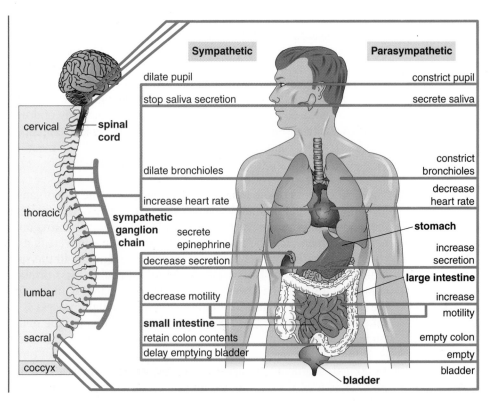

- Dopamine acts on receptors in the CNS and kidneys. Dopamine receptors are blocked by specific dopamine-blocking drugs.
- Epinephrine acts on cardiac receptors and bronchodilator adrenergic receptors. It is also referred to as adrenaline, the fight-or-flight chemical.
- Norepinephrine acts on alpha and beta receptors and is blocked by drugs classified as alpha and beta blockers.
- Serotonin acts on receptors in smooth muscle and gastric mucosa. It produces vasoconstriction.

Drug Effects on the Nervous System

Numerous drugs mimic or influence the action of chemical mediators. For example, some drugs have anticholinergic effects. This means the drug is blocking the acetylcholine receptors, and the physiologic result is just the opposite of that produced by ACh. ACh produces major effects on several organs. In the cardiovascular system, ACh reduces heart function and lowers arterial pressure through vasodilation. In the smooth muscles, ACh increases motility in the gastrointestinal and urogenital systems, bronchial constriction in the respiratory system, and pupil constriction (miosis) of the eyes. In the glands, it increases secretions.

The anticholinergic drugs can have important side effects in certain groups of patients. Some reactions to watch for include

- decreased GI motility
- decreased sweating
- decreased urination
- dilated pupil
- dry eyes
- dry mouth

Receptors are in most instances proteins within the cell membrane. Transmitters bind to the receptors. When a transmitter binds to a receptor, a molecular change occurs in the receptor compound, causing the membrane to be more permeable to various ions. Ions will then directly affect the receptor cell (cell receiving stimulation). Receptors may also activate enzyme systems which promote chemical reactions within the cell.

The following are some especially important receptors in the study of drugs.

- **Alpha receptors** control contraction of blood vessels, dilation of pupils (mydriasis), and relaxation of the GI tract smooth muscle. The most important action of the alpha adrenergic receptors is to cause vasoconstriction, raising blood pressure, but they also cause decongestion. (This is why the decongestants should not be taken by someone with high blood pressure.)
- **Beta-one receptors** (β_1) increase heart rate and contractive force of the heart.
- **Beta-two receptors** (β_2) dilate blood vessels (vasodilation) to skeletal muscles, increase skeletal muscle contractility (muscle tremors), and relax smooth muscle of bronchioles, the GI tract, and the uterus. The most important actions of the beta adrenergic receptors are bronchodilation and heart stimulation.

ANESTHESIA

Before 1846, surgical procedures were uncommon. The understanding of the pathophysiology of disease and of its surgical treatment was simplistic. Aseptic technique and prevention of wound infection were almost unknown. The lack of satisfactory anesthesia was also a major deterrent to surgery. Typically, an operation was done only in emergency situations (e.g., amputating a limb).

Some pain relief methods were available. Drugs like alcohol, hashish, and opium derivatives were taken by mouth. Physical methods were sometimes used, such as packing the limb in ice or inducing ischemia with a tourniquet before amputation. Unconsciousness was achieved by a blow to the head or strangulation. The most common method was simple restraint of the patient by force. No wonder surgery was a last resort!

General Anesthetics

Drugs that allow painless and controlled surgical, obstetric, and diagnostic procedures constitute the cornerstone of modern pharmacological therapy. The hallmark of anesthetic drugs is controllability. For this reason, most potent anesthetics are gases or vapors.

General anesthesia is the unique condition of reversible unconsciousness and absence of response to otherwise painful stimuli. It is characterized by four reversible actions:

- ◇ unconsciousness (unawareness)
- ◇ analgesia
- ◇ skeletal and muscle relaxation
- ◇ amnesia on recovery

These drugs are classified as general or local, according to the type of anesthesia they induce. They are provided in a variety of dosage forms and strengths. One anesthetic may be superior to another, depending on the clinical circumstances. Final selection is based on the drugs and anesthetic techniques judged safest for the patient.

The physiologic effects of anesthesia involve many systems.

- ◇ **Nervous System** All nerve tissue is depressed in the peripheral system.
- ◇ **Respiratory System** Function is depressed, and the anesthesiologist controls oxygen concentration and ventilation. Inhalation anesthetics generally irritate the respiratory tract and salivary glands, causing increased mucous secretion, coughing, and spasm.
- ◇ **Endocrine System** Some anesthetics cause pituitary secretion of antidiuretic hormone (ADH), which may cause postoperative urinary retention. The adrenal medulla may release epinephrine and norepinephrine, which can counter depression caused by inhibited nerves.
- ◇ **Cardiovascular System** The activity of cardiac muscle in the myocardium is reduced, and the resultant loss of tone reduces blood pressure. Vagus inhibition increases the heart rate. Some drugs make the heart sensitive, which may cause arrhythmias.
- ◇ **Skeletal Muscular System** Anesthesia depresses systems within the brain and spinal reflexes, causing some muscle relaxation.
- ◇ **GI System** Common GI effects are nausea and vomiting.
- ◇ **Hepatic System** Some medications are suspected of causing liver changes.

The goals of balanced anesthesia are

- ◇ amnesia—to eliminate the patient's memory of the procedure
- ◇ adequate muscle relaxation—to provide a quiet, relaxed operative field

- adequate ventilation—to maintain adequate oxygen concentration
- pain control—to eliminate or greatly reduce the patient's pain

The indicators used to assess the degree of general anesthesia are

- blood pressure
- hypervolemia, hypovolemia
- oxygen level
- pulse
- respiratory rate
- tissue perfusion
- urinary output (reduction in urine volume sends more blood to the brain)

PREANESTHETIC MEDICATIONS Medication is sometimes used preoperatively to help control the effects of anesthesia. The purpose is to control sedation, postoperative pain, provide amnesia, and decrease anxiety. Review of the medication history is important in determining which anesthetic to use for an individual patient.

Several classes of drugs offer agents to be used before anesthesia.

- Narcotics alleviate pain and depress the respiratory center. (As will be explained later in this chapter, morphine is the most important narcotic analgesic. It is the standard against which all others are measured.)
- Barbiturates depress respiration about as much as does normal sleep and also lessens cardiovascular depression.
- Drugs such as benzodiazepines are the most used preoperative sedatives. They can cause retrograde amnesia, which is a desirable quality in a drug when anesthetizing a patient. They relieve anxiety as well as act as an anticonvulsant. Phenothiazines are often prescribed for their anti-emetic properties as well as sedative effects.

INHALANT ANESTHETICS All inhalant anesthetics reduce blood pressure. Fluids are often given before surgery to help counter this drop in blood pressure. These agents also make the patient hypervolemic. The respiratory system excretes 80% to 90% of inhalation anesthetics. A reduction in renal function is common after anesthesia. This is caused by a decreased renal blood flow with reduced glomerular filtration. Nausea and vomiting may also occur. Table 7.1 lists the most-commonly used inhalant anesthetics. They are marketed as compressed gases in the liquid or gaseous state under high pressure in steel cylinders.

Nitrous oxide is not a potent anesthetic and usually is used with other agents. It will reduce blood pressure. Activity includes analgesia only, with no amnesia or skeletal muscle relaxation. It may be used alone as in dental procedures. It has a tremendous advantage of being rapidly eliminated; its disadvantage is that it may cause hypoxia. In balanced anesthesia it is supplemented with hypnotics (barbiturate or benzodiazepine), analgesics (intravenous narcotic), and muscle relaxants. It is administered with more powerful anesthetics, such as halothane, to hasten the uptake of the more powerful agent.

Ethrane (enflurane) has the advantages of rapid induction and recovery. A short-acting barbiturate is usually infused first to render the patient unconscious. It is a mild stimulant of bronchial and salivary secretions. The disadvantages are excessive depression of the respiratory and circulatory systems. High concentrations may stimulate seizures in susceptible patients, and malignant hyperthermia is a possibility. Uterine relaxation prohibits its use during labor.

Table 7.1	Most-Commonly Used Inhalant Anesthetics	
Generic Name	**Brand Name**	
desflurane	Suprane	
enflurane	Ethrane	
halothane	Fluothane	
isoflurane	Forane	
nitrous oxide (N₂0)		

Forane (isoflurane) produces rapid induction and recovery, with no excessive tracheal or salivary secretions. The disadvantages are progressive respiratory and blood pressure depression, with possible malignant hyperthermia. It may cause less renal and hepatic toxicity than any other commonly employed anesthetic.

Suprane (desflurane) is a controlled anesthetic with rapid onset and rapid recovery. It is often used in ambulatory surgery. It reduces the required dose of neuromuscular blocking agents. It produces a high incidence of irritation for children and is therefore not recommended for use in the pediatric population.

MALIGNANT HYPERTHERMIA Malignant hyperthermia is a rare, but serious, side effect of anesthesia associated with a marked increase in intracellular calcium levels. This syndrome, which involves a sudden and rapid rise in body temperature with accompanying irregularities in heart rhythms and breathing, must be treated immediately. Other symptoms include a greatly increased body metabolism, muscle rigidity, and fever of 110°F or more. Malignant hyperthermia is potentially life-threatening. Death may result from cardiac arrest, brain damage, internal hemorrhaging, or failure of other body systems. This syndrome must be identified and treated early for a good outcome.

Treatment involves the IV infusion of the drug **Dantrium (dantrolene)**. Dantrium is not an anesthetic. It is a skeletal muscle relaxant used to treat multiple sclerosis (MS), stroke, cerebral palsy, and spinal cord injury. Dantrium is thought to reduce muscle tone and metabolism by either preventing the ongoing release of calcium from the storage sites in the muscle or by enhancing the reuptake of calcium. All hospitals require that a drug kit for the treatment of malignant hyperthermia be immediately accessible whenever anesthesia is administered.

It is often the responsibility of the pharmacy technician to ensure that the correct drugs are available and have not expired. Dantrium, in particular, has a very short shelf life and, as such, must be replenished frequently. A malignant hyperthermia kit generally contains the following components.

◇ dantrolene
◇ sterile water
◇ procainamide
◇ furosemide
◇ glucose
◇ sodium bicarbonate, 7.5%

INJECTABLE ANESTHETICS The injectable anesthetics include the ultrashort-acting barbiturates and benzodiazepines. The intravenous (IV) products are very lipid-soluble. Initially they are distributed to the brain, liver (where they are metabolized), kidneys, and other organs with high-volume blood flow, and later to fat and muscle.

Body distribution lowers concentrations that maintain anesthesia. Most of the injectable anesthetics are administered by an IV drip but some do have other dosage forms. Table 7.2 lists the most-commonly used injectable general anesthetics.

The barbiturates **Pentothal (thiopental)** and **Brevital (methohexital)** are primarily for induction of short procedures. Respiratory depression, yawning, coughing, or laryngospasm may occur. In the awake patient, these agents may cause excitement or delirium in the presence of pain. Brevital is the shortest acting of the two. These agents can be used to induce anesthesia prior to administration of another agent or alone for short procedures. The big advantages of the barbiturates are rapid induction, fast recovery, and little postanesthetic excitement or vomiting.

The benzodiazepines **Valium (diazepam)**, **Ativan (lorazepam)**, and **Versed (midazolam)** are used for induction, short procedures, and dental procedures. They are metabolized to active products, so they work longer than the barbiturates. The onset of action is shorter, potency is greater, and elimination more rapid with Versed, so it is the preferred agent. Benzodiazepines are useful to control and prevent seizures induced by local anesthetics.

Ketalar (ketamine) produces a sort of anesthesia known as dissociative amnesia: the patient appears to be awake but neither responds to pain nor remembers the procedure. This agent enhances muscle tone and increases blood pressure, heart rate, and respiratory secretions. Onset is quick (within thirty seconds) and effects last five to ten minutes.

Amidate (etomidate) is used to supplement a weak anesthetic (e.g., nitrous oxide) or for short procedures such as gynecologic ones (e.g., dilation and curettage). It may cause transient involuntary muscle contractions. Nausea and vomiting are common during the recovery period.

Diprivan (propofol) is used for maintenance of anesthesia, for sedation, or for treatment of agitation of patients in the intensive care unit. It has demonstrated

Table 7.2   **Most-Commonly Used Injectable Anesthetics**

Generic Name	Brand Name	Dosage Form
Barbiturates		
methohexital	Brevital	IV
thiopental	Pentothal	IV, rectal
Benzodiazepines		
diazepam	Valium	IM, IV, capsule, solution, tablet
lorazepam	Ativan	IM, IV
midazolam	Versed	IM, IV
Others		
etomidate	Amidate	IV
fentanyl	Sublimaze	IV
	Oralet	lozenge (raspberry lollipop)
	Duragesic	transdermal patch
fentanyl-droperidol	Innovar	IM
ketamine	Ketalar	IM, IV
morphine	various	IM, IV
propofol	Diprivan	IV
sufentanil	Sufenta	IV

Warning

Diprivan and Diflucan might be confused. This could be life threatening if an ICU patient needed Diflucan for an infection and received Diprivan instead.

antiemetic properties. The side effects are drowsiness, respiratory depression, motor restlessness, and increased blood pressure. It changes urine color to green. Any unused drug must be discarded after twelve hours. It should be administered by slow infusion and mixed only with 5% dextrose. It is a white emulsion, stable in glass containers, and should be stored at room temperature.

Innovar (fentanyl-droperidol) can be given IM as a preoperative medication. **Sublimaze** IV, **Oralet** lollipop, and **Duragesic** patch are all forms of **fentanyl**. Fentanyl can be used as a preoperative medication and a narcotic-analgesic. It is used extensively for open-heart surgery procedures because it lacks some of the cardiac depressant actions of other anesthetics. It is used as a supplement in balanced anesthesia. The Oralet raspberry lollipop is used extensively with children.

ANTAGONISTS Antagonists are used to reverse narcotic overdoses whether seen in surgery or not. All operating rooms and emergency rooms will maintain an adequate, quickly accessible supply of these drugs.

Romazicon (flumazenil) antagonizes benzodiazepines by competing at receptor sites. It blocks sedation, recall, and psychomotor impairment. It is used for complete or partial reversal of sedative effects of the benzodiazepines used as general anesthesia or to reverse the effects of a benzodiazepine overdose. Adverse reactions are headache, nausea, vomiting, dizziness, and agitation.

Narcan (naloxone) is an antagonist that competes for the opiate receptor sites. Although it has a greater affinity for the receptor, the action of this drug is much shorter than that of the competing narcotic. Thus, when the naloxone wears off, the opioid will reattach to the receptor. Consequently, naloxone must be given repeatedly until the opioid is cleared from the patient's system. Naloxone must be stored away from light.

Revex (nalmefene) partially or completely reverses the effects of opiate, including respiratory depression. The half-life is about ten hours compared with one hour for Narcan. (The half-life of heroin and morphine is two hours; that of meperidine is four hours.)

Neuromuscular Blocking Agents

Neuromuscular blocking, an important adjunct to general anesthesia is often used to facilitate endotracheal intubation. Endotracheal intubation, the insertion of a tube into the trachea, enables the administration of general anesthesia and also helps to maintain an open airway. The administration of neuromuscular blocking agents results in immediate skeletal muscle paralysis.

There are two mechanisms to achieve neuromuscular blocking. **Anectine (succinylcholine)** is the only agent that works via a depolarizing mechanism. All other neuromuscular blocking agents are considered to be non-depolarizing agents. Succinylcholine works as an agonist of the nicotinic cholinergic receptors. This action causes a persistent depolarization at the motor endplate and results in a sustained flaccid skeletal muscle paralysis. Bradyarrhythmias are reversed with atropine. The nonpolarizing agents work as competitive antagonists to acetylcholine at the nicotinic cholinergic receptors.

Table 7.3 gives an overview of the most-commonly used neuromuscular blocking agents. As noted in the table, many of these agents must be stored in a refrigerator.

Agents to Reverse Neuromuscular Blocking Agents

To reverse the effects of a nondepolarizing blocking drug requires the administration of one of several anticholinesterase agents, including **neostigmine**, **edrophonium**,

Table 7.3   **Most-Commonly Used Neuromuscular Blocking Agents**

Generic Name	Brand Name	Storage	Dosage Form
Short Duration			
succinylcholine	Anectine	refrigerate	IM, IV
Intermediate Duration			
atracurium	Tracrium	refrigerate	IV
cisatracurium	Nimbex	refrigerate	injection
rocuronium	Zemuron	refrigerate	IV, injection
vecuronium	Norcuron	room temperature	injection
Extended Duration			
doxacurium	Neuromax	room temperature	injection
mivacurium	Mivacron	room temperature	IV, injection
pancuronium	Pavulon	refrigerate	injection
pipecuronium	Arduan	room temperature	injection
tubocurarine	(none)	refrigerate	injection

and **pyridostigmine**. These drugs inhibit the destruction of acetylcholine by acetylcholinesterase and thereby restore the transmission of impulses across the myoneural junctions.

There are additional uses of atropine. It is administered preoperatively to decrease secretions and salivation during surgery. It is used to treat sinus tachycardia and bronchospasms. As an ophthalmic preparation, it is used for eye exams. Many of the anticholinesterase agents are also used in the treatment of myasthenia gravis.

Table 7.4 gives an overview of the most-commonly used pharmacologic agents prescribed to reverse neuromuscular blockers.

Local Anesthetics

Local anesthetics produce a transient and reversible loss of sensation in a defined area of the body. They relieve pain without altering alertness or mental function. The introduction of cocaine as a topical ophthalmologic anesthetic in 1884 opened the first era in history of local anesthesia. Cocaine was used for procedures on the eye and nasal mucosa. The second era began in 1904 with the introduction of procaine, the first local anesthetic suitable for injection. Lidocaine, introduced in the 1940s, is the most widely used drug.

Local anesthetics are available in a variety of dosage forms for use in a range of conditions. These dosage forms and applications are

Table 7.4   **Most-Commonly Used Agents to Reverse Neuromuscular Blocking**

Generic Name	Brand Name	Dosage Form
edrophonium	Enlon	injection
neostigmine	Prostigmin	injection
pyridostigmine	Mestinon, Regonol	injection, syrup, tablet

- topical (drops, sprays, lotions, ointments): to treat sunburn, insect bites, hemorrhoids
- infiltration (superficial injection): to suture cuts, to perform dental procedures, and to block small nerves
- nerve block (injection): to prevent transmission of the pain impulse
- IV: for reasons other than anesthesia
- epidural (injection into the space between the dura of the vertebral canal): to block afferent pain nerve impulses to provide regional anesthesia
- spinal (subarachnoid or intrathecal injection): to block afferent pain nerve impulses from the lower part of the body

Local anesthetics decrease the neuronal membrane's permeability to sodium ions. This results in inhibition of depolarization with resultant blockade of conduction.

Local anesthesia is advantageous because all types of nervous tissue are affected—somatic and autonomic. The action is reversible, with recovery and no residual nerve damage. In response to the activity of the anesthetic, function is lost in the following order.

1. pain perception
2. temperature
3. touch sensation
4. proprioception (recognition of body position/posture and joint positions)
5. skeletal muscle tone

Nerve fibers (cells) determine the degree and speed with which a local anesthetic acts.

Local anesthetics depress the small, unmyelinated fibers first and the larger, myelinated fibers (fibers surrounded by a myelin sheath of Schwann cells) last. The time of onset of action is shorter for smaller fibers, and the concentration of drug required is smaller. Systemic action depends on the time the drug is in contact with nerve tissue. Inflammation reduces pH, thereby reducing drug activity. Vasodilation caused by the agent itself ties in with action duration. Many local anesthetics cause vasodilation, resulting in the drug being absorbed more rapidly into the bloodstream and diluted. Addition of a vasoconstrictor (epinephrine) slows absorption of a drug into the bloodstream (1:200,000 concentration). Epinephrine, as a vasoconstrictor, should *not* be used in areas of fingers, toes, ears, nose, or external genitals because cutting blood flow may result in ischemia and subsequent gangrene. Alkalization enhances drug penetration and onset of activity.

Local anesthetics are classified by their chemistry into two classes, esters and amides. Esters are short-acting and are metabolized mainly by pseudocholinesterase of the plasma and tissue fluids; metabolites are excreted in urine. Amides are longer-acting, metabolized by liver enzymes, and metabolites are excreted in urine. Table 7.5 lists the most-commonly used local anesthetics and presents them according to these two classes.

Local anesthetics are given to produce a pharmacologic response in a well-defined area of the body. Occasionally the anesthetic is absorbed into the blood from the administration site, and it can affect organs along the way, with most serious effects on blood vessels, heart, and brain. Other side effects are CNS stimulation, with anxiety, apprehension, nervousness, confusion, and seizure followed by depression, sedation, unconsciousness, and respiratory arrest. The excitement phase is treated with Valium. The depressed phase is treated by providing life support. After high doses, cardiovascular effects can be direct: myocardial depression, arterial vasodilation, bradycardia (autonomic blockade), arrhythmias, hypotension, and cardiac arrest.

Table 7.5	Most-Commonly Used Local Anesthetics	
Generic Name	**Brand Name**	**Dosage Form**
Esters		
benzocaine	Americaine	lubricant, ear drops
chloroprocaine	Nesacaine	epidural
dyclonine	Dyclone	topical
procaine	Novocain	SC, IM, IV
tetracaine	Pontocaine	SC, IM, IV
	Cetacaine	spray, liquid, ointment
Amides		
bupivacaine	Marcaine	injection
etidocaine	Duranest	SC, IV, dental cartridge
levobupivacaine	Chirocaine	injection, IV
lidocaine	Xylocaine	SC, IM, IV, topical, oral solution
lidocaine-epinephrine	Otocaine	dental cartridge
lidocaine-prilocaine	EMLA	cream
mepivacaine	Carbocaine	SC, IM, IV, single- and multi-dose vial

All local anesthetics except cocaine cause relaxation of vascular smooth muscle and can lead to vascular collapse. Hypersensitivity or an allergy to a particular local agent can cause histamine release at the injection site. The most common reactions are skin rashes, edema, and asthma (most associated with the ester type). This hypersensitivity usually develops when the agent is used frequently or for prolonged periods. An amide can generally be substituted for an ester to avoid these hypersensitivity reactions.

Local anesthetics that are derivatives of para-aminobenzoic acid (PABA), such as benzocaine, procaine, and tetracaine, may antagonize the activity of sulfonamides (Gantrisin, Gantanol, Bactrim, Septra), which compete with the antibiotic for sites of action on the receptor of a bacterial cell.

The smallest dosage and lowest concentration required to produce the desired effect should be used.

PAIN MANAGEMENT

Pain is the activation of electrical activity in afferent neurons with sensory endings in peripheral tissue with a higher firing threshold than those of temperature or touch. These neurons are activated by stimulation sufficient to cause tissue damage. Pain is primarily a protective signal to warn of damage or presence of disease. It is also part of the normal healing process. This process involves inflammation, where protective cells move into the injured area releasing chemical mediators that cause fluids and plasma proteins to leak into the surrounding tissue. The result is repair, healing, and stimulation of pain nerve endings. Pain perception arises from the transmission of nerve impulses. Sharp, acute pain is transmitted by large fast-myelinated fibers. Pain itself can be a disease.

The challenges in pain management are to assess the patient properly and to select the most successful and cost-effective therapy for the patient and the patient's family. Goals of management include enhancing functionality and productivity in order to improve the patient's quality of life.

In January of 2001, the Joint Commission on the Accreditation of Healthcare Organizations (JCAHO) issued its pain management standards. JCAHO uses the standards to evaluate the performance of healthcare providers. The new pain management standards emphasize the right of patients to receive appropriate pain management and education. The standards define pain as the "fifth" vital sign along with temperature, pulse, respiration, and blood pressure. As such, healthcare providers are encouraged to make regular pain intensity assessments.

Pain is classified as acute, chronic nonmalignant, and chronic malignant.

◇ **Acute** This type of pain is associated with trauma or surgery; patients show anxiety. It is usually easy to manage by identifying and treating the cause, and it disappears when the body heals.

◇ **Chronic Nonmalignant** This type of pain may have a diagnosed or an undiagnosed cause, such as a nonmalignant disease. The pain lasts for more than three months and may respond poorly to treatment. Patients may not appear to be in pain, but have signs and symptoms of depression. The neurotransmitters involved in pain transmission are the same as those involved with depression (norepinephrine, dopamine, serotonin). A form of this type of pain is chronic pain syndrome, in which pain lasts longer than three months, may or may not have an anatomic basis, creates an overwhelming lifestyle for the patient, and does not respond to medication.

◇ **Chronic Malignant** This type of pain accompanies malignant disease and often increases in severity as the disease progresses.

Physiologic responses to pain are as varied as the patients themselves. These responses include

◇ catabolism (tissues, such as muscle, and substances break down)
◇ delayed stomach and bowel function
◇ impaired immune response
◇ increased autonomic activity (heart rate and blood pressure)
◇ increased metabolism
◇ muscle rigidity
◇ negative emotional response (depression)
◇ shallow breathing
◇ water retention

Inadequate treatment of pain can have adverse physiological, psychological, and immunological effects. Good clinical care must be based on the optimization of risk/benefit considerations. The major sources of pain, the pain characteristics, and their treatment are listed in Table 7.6.

Sympathetically mediated pain occurs from oversensitivity to a pain stimulus; that is, pain occurs when no pain should be felt. Nerve damage usually occurs as a result of trauma to the area. Hair, nail, and skin changes result (e.g., color, overgrowth of hair); swelling and changes in skin temperature are common.

The pain receptors in the CNS are the limbic system, thalamus, hypothalamus, midbrain, and spinal cord. Natural pain-relieving chemicals are also present in the body, primarily in the brain. The brain produces these chemical substances (enkephalins and endorphins) in response to the pain stimulus. As pain increases, the levels of these chemicals also increase. In order to achieve adequate pain control, pain medication should be administered around the clock.

Table 7.6	Major Sources of Pain			
Source	**Areas Involved**	**Characteristics**	**Treatment**
somatic	body framework (bones, muscles, ligaments)	throbbing, stabbing, well-localized	narcotics, NSAIDs, nerve blockers
visceral	kidneys, intestines, liver	aching, throbbing, sharp, gnawing, crampy, deep-squeezing; associated with sweating, nausea, vomiting	narcotics, NSAIDs, nerve blockers, antiemetics
neuropathic	nerves (destruction)	burning, aching, numbing, tingling, viselike, knifelike, constant	antidepressants, anticonvulsants
sympathetically mediated	overactivity in sympathetic system	occurrence when no pain should be felt	nerve blockers

Narcotics and Opiates

Warning
Codeine and Lodine can look alike depending on the handwriting.

A narcotic is a pain-modulating chemical derived from opium (e.g., morphine, codeine) or synthetically produced that produces insensibility or stupor. Opioid agonists are a group of natural, semisynthetic, and synthetic drugs that interact with specific receptor sites having their main effects on the CNS, GI tract, and to a lesser extent in peripheral tissues.

All narcotics have the potential to induce tolerance and dependence. The prototype is morphine; all other narcotics are evaluated against it. Narcotics have the following reactions.

- **Analgesia** Narcotics reduce pain from most sources (organs, trauma, myocardial infarction, terminal illness, and following surgical procedures). Some pain is unresponsive to opiates.
- **Sedation** Narcotics allay anxiety and cause drowsiness.
- **Euphoria and Dysphoria** Narcotics produce feelings of well-being and feelings of disquiet, restlessness, or malaise, respectively.

Narcotics also reduce the cough reflex and respiratory drive; they increase mental clouding; and can cause nausea, vomiting, and constipation.

Patients can develop tolerance to pain therapy within days or weeks. As a result, patients may need to be titrated every day or two. A good rule of thumb is to increase the current dose by 50% when needed, based on evaluation of pain control. After long-term treatment and disease regression, dosage reduction is often possible, without signs of withdrawal or recurrence of pain. Patients in pain have activated endorphin systems and are pharmacologically, physiologically, and biochemically different from drug abusers. Patients with medical reasons for their pain who are treated with appropriate opiates rarely become addicted.

Although opioids will frequently impair judgment and psychomotor function for a period following the onset or acceleration of therapy, after a few days these adverse effects usually diminish markedly. Opioids are associated with a high incidence of constipation. Thus, an opioid regimen often requires a clinically prescribed bowel program.

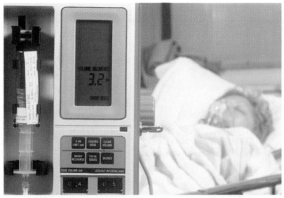
A patient-controlled analgesia pump can allow the patient to regulate the amount of pain medication she receives. This results in better pain control with less drug used.

An effective means of controlling pain in hospitalized patients is the patient-controlled analgesia (PCA) pump. The patient regulates, within certain limits, the amount of drug received. This provides better pain control with less drug when patients administer the drug on pain onset. Once pain has been ongoing for a long time, it is much more difficult to control. Another remarkable development in pain control is the transdermal fentanyl patch (Duragesic). By providing stable blood levels of drug, this seems to control pain and allow the patient to remain more alert than other forms of delivery.

A simple scheme for analgesic selection is known as the analgesic ladder.

1. Mild to moderate pain is treated with a nonsteroidal anti-inflammatory drug (NSAID) (prototype: aspirin) and an adjuvant analgesic.
2. If adequate relief is not achieved, a nonnarcotic analgesic (e.g., NSAID) is given with a "weak" opioid (prototype: codeine).
3. If this fails, the patient is given a strong opioid (prototype: morphine), with an adjuvant analgesic if indicated.

Symptoms of narcotic overdose are respiratory depression, decreased body temperature, decreased blood pressure, tachycardia, and coma. The treatment is assisted ventilation and a narcotic antagonist. Methadone, an opioid analgesic, used in addiction treatment provides patients with a longer-lasting and legal alternative to narcotic addiction.

Addiction and Dependence

Underprescription of opioids for nonmalignant pain is not uncommon because of physician fear of regulatory authorities and the possibility of the patient becoming addicted. Now awareness is increasing that chronic pain is not being adequately treated and that opioids are appropriate when other treatments fail or are not tolerated. Chronic opioid therapy has a low risk of addiction when used appropriately for pain.

Although patients undergoing chronic opioid therapy do become physically dependent, addiction must not be confused with dependence. Dependence is a physical phenomenon. Patients who are dependent will experience an abstinence syndrome (withdrawal) when drug therapy is discontinued or when the dose is reduced substantially.

Addiction, on the other hand, is a compulsive disorder leading to continued use of the drug despite harm to the user. Symptoms of addiction include preoccupation with the drugs, refusal of medication tapers, a strong preference for a specific opioid (usually for short-acting over long-acting drugs), and a general decrease in the ability to function. An addicted patient does not generally take the medication as prescribed. Opioid addicts have a tendency to rely on multiple prescribers and pharmacies to cover their behavior. The pharmacy technician must be alert to these signs of addiction when dispensing opioids, as it is their legal and moral responsibility to notify the pharmacist and/or prescribing physician if drug-seeking behavior is suspected.

Combination Drugs for Managing Pain

The combination of a narcotic and a nonnarcotic oral analgesic often results in analgesia superior to that produced by either agent alone. Attacking pain on two fronts (peripherally and centrally) enhances relief and facilitates use of lower doses of each agent. This produces a more favorable side effect profile.

A real risk often overlooked with the combination drugs, however, is aspirin or acetaminophen toxicity. When a prescription is filled, the pharmacy technician should check to make sure the patient is not getting over 4 g of aspirin or 4 g to 5 g acetaminophen per day. Often prescribers are concerned only with the addiction potential of the narcotic and overlook this important toxicity. The technician who checks this possibility performs a valuable service for the patient. The technician must constantly be on the alert regarding C-III, C-IV, and CV drugs. They may be refilled for no more than six months. After this time, the patient must get a new prescription. C-IIs have absolutely no refills.

Narcotic Analgesics

Table 7.7 describes the most-commonly used narcotic analgesics. Many of the narcotic agents are narcotics in combination with nonnarcotics. Table 7.8 gives an overview of pharmacotherapeutic options for moderate to severe pain.

Narcotics may produce a range of side effects in individual patients. Some common effects are mental confusion, reduced alertness, nausea, vomiting, dry mouth, constipation, urinary retention, histamine release (flush, wheal, and flare), vessel dilation, inflammatory process, and bronchial constriction (especially in asthmatics).

Narcotics inhibit normal peristalsis, causing local spasms (reduced linear movement). Stool softeners and increased fluid intake may be of benefit. The patient can experience postural hypotension. Urinary retention can result because of spasmodic activity of the ureter and major sphincter of the bladder. This can last from twenty-four to forty-eight hours and is most pronounced in patients over fifty-five years of age.

Warning

Lortab and Lorabid can be confused. The dosing should help identify the drug prescribed.

| Table 7.7 | **Most-Commonly Used Narcotic Analgesics** |

Generic Name	Brand Name	Dosage Form
acetaminophen-codeine	Tylenol with Codeine	capsule (C-III)
		tablet, IM, IV, SC (C-III), elixir (C-V)
hydrocodone-acetaminophen	Lortab (C-III), Vicodin (C-III), Vicodin Tuss	tablet, expectorant, elixir
hydromorphone	Dilaudid (C-II)	tablet, syrup, liquid, IM, IV, SC, suppository
	Dilaudid-HP (C-II)	IV
meperidine	Demerol (C-II)	tablet, syrup, IM, IV, SC
morphine	Roxanol (C-II)	oral solution, IM, IV, SC, suppository
	MS Contin (C-II)	tablet
oxycodone	Oxycontin (C-II), OxyIR	capsule, liquid, tablet
oxycodone-acetaminophen	Percocet (C-II)	tablet
	Tylox (C-II)	capsule
oxycodone-aspirin	Percodan (C-II)	capsule
pentazocine	Talwin (C-IV)	IM, IV, SC
pentazocine-naloxone	Talwin NX (C-IV)	tablet
propoxyphene	Darvon (C-IV)	capsule
propoxyphene-acetaminophen	Darvocet-N 100 (C-IV)	tablet

Table 7.8   Pharmacotherapeutic Options for Moderate to Severe Pain

Indication	Pharmacotherapeutic Options for Treatment
bone pain	calcitonin dexamethasone prednisone NSAIDS
cancer pain	opioids
fibromyalgia	antidepressants opioids
lower back pain	muscle relaxants opioids
neuropathic pain	antidepressants anticonvulsants
osteoarthritis	NSAIDS glucocorticoid injections

Respiratory depression is dose-related. Care should be used in patients with chronic obstructive pulmonary disease (COPD), asthma, bronchitis, or emphysema. Any narcotic should be used with caution in patients with COPD or asthma; reduction of the dosage is necessary.

Narcotics act on an area identified as the chemotrigger zone (CTZ), which in turn acts on the vomiting center to produce emesis. This can be very dangerous in a patient heavily sedated with narcotics as it can result in aspiration of vomitus into the airway. Antiemetics may be given to prevent or offset this reaction.

Narcotics can also stimulate seizures in patients with convulsive disorders. They can mask signs of head injury. Most narcotics are metabolized by the liver; thus serious liver disease may cause the patient to become comatose. Reduced doses must be used in these patients.

Dose requirements vary with the severity of pain; individual response to pain, age, weight, and the presence of concomitant disease. Table 7.9 provides the comparative doses of common narcotic analgesics and provides dosage equivalents to 10 mg of morphine. Narcotics have no set or optimal dose. Morphine is the most important narcotic analgesic. It is the standard against which all others are measured. The right dose is the dose that controls pain without excessive or intolerable adverse side effects.

Pain medication is often administered around the clock. Acute pain has a beginning and an end and warns of a problem. Chronic pain has no end. The suffering includes a sense of helplessness and hopelessness. Total pain has physical, psychological, social, and spiritual components. Adequate sleep, mood elevation, diversion, sympathy, and understanding all can raise an individual's pain threshold. Alternatively, fatigue, anxiety, fear, anger, sadness, depression, and isolation can lower the pain threshold. Uncontrolled pain is a potent factor in lowering the pain threshold.

Patient comfort is the goal, and the response of the patient should be the basis for dosage adjustments. The key to effective pain management is constant reassessment. Doses should be titrated, and the dose should be repeated at a time *before* the pain recurs (adjusted to each individual).

Table 7.9

Comparative Doses of Narcotic Analgesics

Generic Name	Brand Name	Dose Equivalent to 10 mg IM Morphine
morphine	(many)	10 mg
codeine	(many)	130 mg, IM
meperidine	Demerol	300 mg, po
fentanyl	Sublimaze	0.1 mg, IV
methadone	Dolophine	10–20 mg, po
oxycodone	Percodan, Percocet	30 mg, po
oxymorphone	Numorphan	1.5 mg, IV
pentazocine	Talwin	120–180 mg, po
propoxyphene	Darvon	130–250 mg, po
buprenorphine	Buprenex	0.3 mg, IM
hydromorphone	Dilaudid	1.5 mg, IM

Note: These equivalents will vary slightly depending on reference.

Warning

Morphine sulfate and magnesium sulfate are often confused, especially when the prescriber uses the abbreviations of MSO_4 or $MgSO_4$.

No drug is more effective than morphine. Some are more potent, but none are more effective when given in equianalgesic doses. Oral doses of most drugs are essentially equivalent to rectal suppository doses, and intramuscular doses are essentially equivalent to subcutaneous (SC) doses. Intravenous doses are usually more potent than intramuscular or subcutaneous doses. The subcutaneous dose of morphine is two to three times as potent as the oral dose. When patients cannot tolerate oral medications (e.g. due to nausea or vomiting), the rectal suppository route should be considered.

Another alternative is SC or IV infusion. Narcotic side effects should be anticipated and minimized so pain relief is not offset by creating other distressing symptoms. All patients taking regular doses of narcotic become constipated and should be maintained on some form of bowel preparation from the outset of narcotic therapy. Another side effect, especially of morphine, is nausea due to the drug's stimulatory effect on the CTZ and the inhibitory effect on GI motility. Appropriately prescribed narcotics rarely cause clinically significant respiratory depression.

MIGRAINE HEADACHES

Migraine headaches are severe, throbbing, vascular headaches. They are characterized by recurrent unilateral head pain combined with neurologic and GI disturbances that can severely affect the quality of life and daily function. The headache comes from dilation of cerebral surface vessels. Nausea is reported by approximately 90% of all migraine sufferers. Photobia (sensitivity to light) and phonophobia (sensitivity to sound) are also common. Lying down in a dark room often helps. Sedative, antiemetic, and narcotic agents are helpful. Oral contraceptives can exacerbate migraine, partly because of their estrogen component. Patients should be educated to initiate treatment promptly, before a headache develops into a full migraine.

Classic migraine has five components: prodrome, aura, headache, headache relief, and postdrome. Other symptoms may occur. Nausea, vomiting, and anorexia are common. Photophobia, phonophobia, and hyperesthesia may occur. The aura results from neurologic symptoms related to visual and sensory disturbances, or both: flashing lights; shimmering heat waves; bright lights; dark holes in the visual field; blurred, cloudy vision; or even a transient loss of vision. The headache generally dissipates in six hours, but may last one to two days.

The pathogenesis of the migraine is not completely understood. One well known theory—referred to as the vascular theory—proposes that migraines are caused by vasodilation and the concomitant mechanical stimulation of sensory nerve endings. Researchers now suspect the mechanism is more complicated than this. About 30% of migraine attacks are immediately preceded by an aura of sensory or visual change. These migraines are classified as migraine with aura. All other migraines are classified as migraine without aura.

Serotonin (5-HT) appears to be involved in the pathogenesis of migraine. Serotonin is a potent vasoconstrictor; the level in platelets increases before migraine attacks and decreases afterward. Changes in serotonin level parallel the migraine symptoms. There are subclasses of serotonin receptors; it has been theorized that stimulating the 5-HT$_1$ and 5-HT$_2$ receptors in the cerebral and temporal arteries will cause vasoconstriction, which inhibits neural transmission, thereby alleviating migraine due to excessive dilatation of cranial arteries. Diet, stress, sleep habits, certain medications, hormonal fluctuations, depression, atmospheric changes, and environmental irritants have all been implicated as causative factors that lower the threshold for neural transmission in the trigeminal system.

The initial treatment for migraine should focus primarily on nondrug interventions. Identifying and eliminating trigger factors may be effective in many patients. For example, a quiet environment and sleep may help as many as 25% of patients during an acute attack. When symptoms are severe or debilitating and attacks are frequent, drug therapy may be indicated.

The medications used in migraine therapy can be divided into two classes: prophylactic therapy and abortive therapy. Prophylactic therapy attempts to prevent or reduce recurrence. Abortive therapy treats acute migraine headaches after they occur. The abortive drugs should be taken at the first sign of a headache. Patients must be educated to understand the importance of treating the attack as soon as possible—long before it develops into a full migraine, at which point the treatment is much less effective. Prophylaxis of migraines is indicated in any of the following situations: when headaches occur more than twice a month, when headaches become refractory to acute therapy, and when the pattern is predictable.

Abortive therapy treatment is most effective when it begins at the first sign of aura or headache. The traditional therapies for acute migraine are simple analgesics, NSAIDs, ergotamine-containing medications, and other drugs.

To be effective, ergotamine therapy should be initiated early in the attack. Ergotamine has significant adverse effects that limit its usefulness. The most common, regardless of the administration route, are nausea and vomiting. These effects may be exacerbated if a rectal suppository is used, since absorption is enhanced. Ergotism (a syndrome of progressive vasoconstriction and ischemia of vital organs) and ergot headache (a medication-headache cycle occurring with daily use of ergotamine) have been reported. To avoid these adverse effects, patients should be instructed regarding the maximum daily and weekly dosages, and the importance of avoiding ergotamine use on consecutive days or more than twice a week.

Prophylaxis is indicated if migraines occur more than twice a month, they occur in predictable patterns, or they become refractory to acute therapy. Inderal (propranolol) is the drug of choice for prophylaxis for migraines. Prophylactic therapies for migraines include the following classes of drugs:

◇ anticonvulsants
◇ beta blockers
◇ calcium channel blockers
◇ NSAIDS
◇ tricyclic antidepressants

Table 7.10 gives an overview of the most-commonly used agents for migraine headaches.

Selective 5-HT Receptor Agonists

Imitrex (sumatriptan) binds to serotonin receptors causing vasoconstriction of blood vessels in the dura. It first entered the market as a subcutaneous injection and now is in tablet form also. When injected, it is effective in about fifteen minutes. It may cause tingling, warm sensation, chest discomfort, dizziness, vertigo, and discomfort at the injection site. It has little or no activity on dopamine, beta, and alpha-adrenergic receptors; therefore, there is the relative absence of side effects such as nausea and vomiting and peripheral vasoconstriction. No drug interactions with sumatriptan have been identified. The use of alcohol, of course, should be avoided since alcohol is a major contributor to migraines. The maximum recommended adult dose (subcutaneous route) is two 6 mg doses in twenty-four hours. A second dose may be administered at least one hour after the first dose if some improvement occurs but the migraine is still not relieved. The subcutaneous administration route is especially beneficial to patients with diminished gastric absorption or nausea and vomiting. The autoinjector is very easy to use. The patient should receive an injection at the first sign of a headache.

Zomig (zolmitriptan) is a drug similar to sumatriptan. It constricts cerebral blood vessels and reduces inflammation of sensory nerves. The dose can be repeated in two hours but never more than 10 mg should be taken in twenty-four hours.

Maxalt-MLT (rizatriptan) oral tablets are quickly absorbed and have the most rapid onset of action among all the migraine therapies. Many patients experience

Table 7.10   Most-Commonly Used Agents for Migraine Headaches

Generic Name	Brand Name	Dosage Form
Selective 5-HT Receptor Agonists		
naratriptan	Amerge	tablet
rizatriptan	Maxalt-MLT	sublingual tablet
	Maxalt	tablet
sumatriptan	Imitrex	SC, tablet, nasal spray
zolmitriptan	Zomig	tablet
Ergot Preparations		
dihydroergotamine	Migranal	nasal spray, injection
ergotamine	Ergomar	sublingual tablet
ergotamine-belladonna-phenobarbital	Bellergal-S	tablet
ergotamine-caffeine	Wygraine, Cafergot	tablets, rectal suppositories
Antiemetic Agents		
chlorpromazine	Thorazine	capsule, rectal suppositories, injection, syrup, tablet
metoclopramide	Reglan	injection, solution, tablet
prochlorperazine	Compazine	capsule, tablet, solution, rectal suppository, injection
Opioid Analgesics		
butorphanol	Stadol	IM, IV
	Stadol NS	nasal spray
tramadol	Ultram	tablet
Beta Blocker		
propranolol	Inderal	tablet, capsule, solution, injection
Other		
isometheptene-dichloralphenazone-acetaminophen	Midrin	capsule

relief as soon as thirty minutes after taking this drug. The tablet is dissolved under the tongue. **Maxalt** is not absorbed as rapidly as Maxalt-MLT.

Stadol NS and **Stadol (butorphanol)** are mixed narcotic agonist-antagonists. The NS drug form is an inhalant with central analgesic actions. Both are used to manage moderate to severe pain. They can be addictive and are scheduled in several states. Each bottle of the nasal spray delivers only fourteen doses and fewer if it is primed before each use. The nasal spray is most-commonly used; however, it comes as an injection which can be given either IV or IM.

Ergot Preparations

Migranal (dihydroergotamine) is a nasal spray that constricts peripheral and cranial blood vessels. This drug does not work as quickly as sumatriptan (Imitrex) but lasts longer. Patients should administer one spray in each nostril, repeating in fifteen minutes for a total of four sprays. The head should not be tilted while spraying so it remains in the nostril for absorption. Any drug not used within twenty-four hours should be discarded from the nasal sprayer. Once the ampule is broken, the drug becomes less potent.

Wygraine and **Cafergot (ergotamine)** are a direct vasoconstrictors of smooth muscle in cranial blood vessels and are used to treat migraines. The dose should be titrated to each patient. The patient should be told to initiate treatment at the first sign of an attack and not to exceed the recommended dose.

Antiemetic Agents

Reglan (metoclopramide) can be used to reduce nausea and vomiting and enhance the absorption of other antimigraine products by reducing gastritis. Currently, many physicians are prescribing aspirin and Reglan in place of oral Imitrex. The combination seems to have fewer side effects. Reglan tends to cause drowsiness, but Imitrex is more likely to cause nausea, fatigue, and weakness. Physicians are prescribing 1,000 mg of aspirin with 10 mg of Reglan.

Thorazine (chlorpromazine) has been found effective in some migraines unresponsive to ergotamines. It has antiemetic properties. The side effects include drowsiness, extrapyramidal effects, and orthostatic hypotension.

Opioid Analgesics

Warning
Ultram and Voltaren could be confused.

Ultram (tramadol) when given in combination with an NSAID such as ibuprofen has a high success rate in treating migraines. Because the drug has a slow onset, it was being promoted as a non-addictive substance. However, recent evidence suggests that there is, in fact, some potential for addiction with this drug.

Other Anti-Migraine Agents

Midrin (isometheptene-dichloralphenazone-acetaminophen) has fewer side effects than ergotamine, but is less effective for some people. The patient should take two capsules at the beginning of an attack and then one every one to two hours until cessation of headache, up to five capsules in twelve hours. It is a combination analgesic (acetaminophen), sedative (dichloralphenazone), and vasoconstrictor (isometheptene). It has been effective for mild to moderate migraine attacks. Sedation and gastrointestinal distress occur frequently, but rebound headache is not common. The most frequent side effects are dizziness, insomnia, nausea, vomiting, and transient numbness.

Chapter Summary

The Nervous System

- The primary CNS transmitters are acetylcholine, norepinephrine, dopamine, and serotonin.
- The primary PNS transmitters are acetylcholine, norepinephrine, and dopamine.
- The major transmitter of the parasympathetic system is acetylcholine.
- The major transmitters of the sympathetic system are norepinephrine, dopamine, and epinephrine.
- If a drug is classified as an anticholinergic, some effects will be decreased GI motility, decreased urination, pupil dilation, decreased sweating, dry eyes, and dry mouth.

Anesthesia

- Drugs that allow painless, controlled surgical, obstetric, and diagnostic procedures constitute the cornerstones of modern pharmacologic therapy. The hallmark of anesthetic drugs is controllability. For this reason, most potent anesthetics are gases or vapors.
- General anesthesia is a state of deep sleep in which there is no response to stimulation.
- Anesthesia is characterized by four reversible actions: unconsciousness, analgesia, skeletal muscle relaxation, and amnesia on recovery.
- One anesthetic may be superior to another, depending on the clinical circumstances. Final selection is based on those drugs and anesthetic techniques judged safest for the patient, drugs and techniques that facilitate performance of the surgical procedure, and techniques most acceptable to the patient.
- The purposes of premedication are sedation, helping with pain relief postoperatively, and anxiety reduction.
- The tremendous advantage of nitrous oxide is that it is rapidly eliminated.
- Dantrium acts on skeletal muscle beyond the neuromuscular junction; it is the drug of choice to treat malignant hyperthermia.
- Thiopental is often the preferred induction agent because it rapidly and pleasantly produces hypnosis.
- Sublimaze (fetanyl) is a combination drug used extensively as a narcotic-analgesic for open-heart procedures because it lacks some of the cardiac depressant actions of other anesthetics.
- Fentanyl is also manufactured as a lollipop (Oralet) and a patch (Duragesic).
- Narcan, Revex, and Romazicon are given to reverse overdoses of specific drugs.
- Neuromuscular blocking is important as an adjunct to general anesthesia to ensure motionless muscles during surgery.
- Neuromuscular blocking agents help to intubate patients in both surgical and non-surgical settings. Cholinergic agents reverse neuromuscular blockers.
- Blocking agents act as a depolarizing substance or as an antagonist for receptor sites on the muscle cell.
- Local anesthetics are advantageous because they affect all types of nervous tissue. They relieve pain without altering alertness or mental function.

Pain Management

◇ Pain itself can be a disease; it is classified as acute, chronic nonmalignant, or chronic malignant.

◇ All narcotics have the potential to induce tolerance and dependence.

◇ The effects of narcotics differ on different individuals.

◇ The patient-controlled analgesia (PCA) pump is an effective means of controlling pain, by which the patient can regulate, within certain limits, the amount of drug received. This has provided better pain control with less drug.

◇ The transdermal fentanyl patch Duragesic provides patients with pain control and allows the patient to remain more alert than do most other methods.

◇ Narcan and Revex are the two drugs given for an overdose of narcotics.

◇ It is as important to watch the aspirin or acetaminophen dose in narcotic and nonnarcotic combination analgesics as it is to watch the narcotic dose.

◇ Narcotics act on an area of the brain identified as the chemotrigger zone, which in turn stimulates the vomiting center.

◇ Morphine is the standard against which all other narcotic analgesics are measured.

Migraine Headaches

◇ Patients with migraine headaches should be taught to initiate therapy immediately at the first hint of an episode.

◇ Treatments for migraine headaches are divided into two groups: abortive and prophylactic therapies.

◇ Imitrex (sumatriptan) is an injection for the relief of migraine headaches. It should be used at the first sign of headache. If it brings partial, but not total, relief, the patient should receive a second injection at least one hour after the first dose.

◇ Midrin is a combination drug with fewer side effects than ergotamine. The patient should take two capsules at the onset of headache and then one every one to two hours until the pain stops, up to five capsules in twelve hours.

Drug Summary

The following drugs were discussed in this chapter. Each generic drug name is followed in parentheses by one or more brand names. An asterisk (*) indicates drugs frequently written using *either* brand *or* generic name. These need to be memorized.

Inhalant Anesthetics
desflurane (Suprane)
enflurane (Ethrane)
halothane (Fluothane)
isoflurane (Forane)
nitrous oxide

Benzodiazepines
diazepam (Valium)*
lorazopam (Ativan)*
midazolam (Versed)

Injectable Anesthetics
etomidate (Amidate)
fentanyl (Sublimaze, Oralet, Duragesic)*
fentanyl-droperidol (Innovar)*
ketamine (Ketalar)
methohexital (Brevital)*
morphine
propofol (Diprivan)*
sufentanil (Sufenta)
thiopental (Pentothal)

Antagonists
flumazenil (Romazicon)
nalmefene (Revex)
naloxone (Narcan)*

Neuromuscular Blocking Agents
atracurium (Tracrium)
cisatracurium (Nimbex)
doxacurium (Neuromax)
mivacurium (Mivacron)
pancuronium (Pavulon)
pipecuronium (Arduan)
rocuronium (Zemuron)
succinylcholine (Anectine)
tubocurarine (none)
vecuronium (Norcuron)

Agents to Reverse Neuromuscular Blocking
edrophonium (Enlon)
neostigmine (Prostigmin)
pyridostigmine (Mestinon, Regonol)

Local Anesthetics
benzocaine (Americaine)*
bupivacaine (Marcaine)*
chloroprocaine (Nesacaine)
dyclonine (Dyclone)
etidocaine (Duranest)
levobupivacaine (Chirocaine)
lidocaine (Xylocaine)*
lidocaine-epinephrine (Octocaine)
lidocaine-prilocaine (EMLA)
mepivacaine (Carbocaine)*
procaine (Novocain)
tetracaine (Pontocaine, Cetacaine)

Narcotic Analgesics
acetaminophen-codeine, (Tylenol with Codeine)*
hydrocodone-acetaminophen (Lortab, Vicodin, Vicodin Tuss)*
hydromorphone (Dilaudid, Dilaudid-HP)*
meperidine (Demerol)*
morphine (Roxanol, MS Contin)*
oxycodone (Oxycontin, OxyIR)*
oxycodone-acetaminophen (Percocet, Tylox)*
oxycodone-aspirin (Percodan)*
pentazocine (Talwin)
pentazocine-naloxone (Talwin NX)*
propoxyphene (Darvon)
propoxyphene-acetaminophen (Darvocet-N 100)*

Skeletal Muscle Relaxant
dantrolene (Dantrium)

Agents for Migraine Headaches

butorphanol (Stadol, Stadol NS)
chlorpromazine (Thorazine)*
dihydroergotamine (Migranal)
ergotamine (Ergomar)*
ergotamine-belladonna-phenobarbital (Bellargal-S)
ergotamine-caffeine (Wygraine, Cafergot)
indomethacin (Indocin)*
isometheptene-dichloralphenazone-acetaminophen (Midrin)
metoclopramide (Reglan)*
naratriptan (Amerge)
prochlorperazine (Compazine)
propranolol (Inderal)*
rizatriptan (Maxalt, Maxalt-MLT)
sumatriptan (Imitrex)
tramadol (Ultram)
zolmitriptan (Zomig)

Chapter Review

Pharmaceuticals and Body Functions

Select the best answer from the choices given.

1. If a drug is classified as an anticholinergic, it would have all the following effects *except*
   a. decreased urination.
   b. watery eyes.
   c. pupil dilation.
   d. decreased sweating.

2. The purpose of preanesthetic medications is
   a. sedation.
   b. to help with pain relief.
   c. anxiety reduction.
   d. all of the above.
   e. none of the above.

3. Someone has been given too much Versed in the OR. The surgical resident cannot recall the name of the drug that should be given but sends a stat order to the pharmacy for an antagonist. You should notify the pharmacist and prepare
   a. diazepam.
   b. dantrolene.
   c. flumazenil.
   d. thiopental.
   e. nitrous oxide.

4. This drug is usually reserved for children because of its dosage form.
   a. Innovar
   b. Diprivan
   c. Amidate
   d. Oralet
   e. Dantrium

5. A patient who had outpatient surgery the previous day awakens in the morning and urinates. The urine is green. The patient's caretaker calls, wanting to know if any drugs dispensed to the patient would cause this. Which drug did the patient receive?
   a. Ketalar
   b. Amidate
   c. Diprivan
   d. Innovar
   e. Dantrium

6. The patient is being prepared for open-heart surgery. Which anesthetic will the doctor probably want to use?
   a. Ketalar
   b. Amidate
   c. Diprivan
   d. Innovar
   e. Dantrium

7. Which is the most widely used local anesthetic?
   a. Cocaine
   b. Lidocaine
   c. Chloroprocaine
   d. Tetracaine
   e. Dyclonine

8. Which inhalation anesthetic causes no amnesia or skeletal muscle relaxation and is frequently used in dental procedures?
   a. Methoxyflurane
   b. Nitrous oxide
   c. Halothane
   d. Ethrane
   e. Isoflurane

9. Which drug prevents and/or is used to treat malignant hyperthermia?
   a. Dantrium
   b. Romazicon
   c. Flumazenil
   d. All of the above
   e. None of the above

10. Which drug is a combination drug?
    a. Prozac
    b. Midrin
    c. Xanax
    d. Elavil
    e. None of the above

The following statements are true or false. If the answer is false, rewrite the statement so it is true.

____ 1. The central nervous system consists of the sense organs and nerves that communicate to the CNS.

____ 2. The peripheral nervous system consists of the brain and spinal cord.

____ 3. The primary CNS transmitters are acetylcholine, norepinephrine, dopamine, and serotonin.

____ 4. The primary PNS transmitters are norepinephrine, acetylcholine, and dopamine.

____ 5. Alpha-adrenergic receptors cause vasoconstriction.

____ 6. The hallmark of anesthetic drugs is controllability.

____ 7. Inhalation anesthetics have specific receptors.

____ 8. Local anesthetics depress the small, unmyelinated fibers first and the larger, myelinated fibers last.

_____ 9. Pain itself can be a disease.

_____ 10. All narcotics have the potential to produce tolerance and dependence.

Match the following brand names with their generic names.

1.	Inderal _____	a.	succinylcholine
2.	Anectine _____	b.	pentazocine
3.	Reglan _____	c.	metoclopramide
4.	Talwin _____	d.	propranolol

Classify the following drugs.

a. schedule II   b. schedule III   c. schedule IV   d. not controlled

5. Demerol _____		19.	Duragesic _____
6. Anectine _____		20.	Xylocaine _____
7. fentanyl _____		21.	Americaine _____
8. naloxone _____		22.	Phenaphen _____
9. ergotamine _____		23.	Reglan _____
10. propoxyphene _____		24.	Percocet _____
11. MS Contin _____		25.	Percodan _____
12. Indocin _____		26.	Dilaudid _____
13. Revex _____		27.	Midrin _____
14. Lortab _____		28.	Imitrex _____
15. Tylenol III _____		29.	Darvocet-N 100 _____
16. Vicodin _____		30.	dantrolene _____
17. nitrous oxide _____		31.	hydrocodone-acetaminophen _____
18. diazepam _____		32.	propoxyphene-acetaminophen _____
		33.	Innovar _____

Diseases and Drug Therapies

1. List (a) the goals of balanced anesthesia and (b) indices to assess the degree of general anesthesia.
2. Discuss local anesthetics. Include (a) advantages and (b) order of function loss.
3. Discuss pain. Include (a) classification and (b) major sources and areas involved.
4. Discuss narcotics. Include (a) reactions and (b) analgesic ladder.

Dispensing Medications

1. Outline a stepwise approach to treating migraines. Include the drug of choice for prophylaxis of migraines and the drug of choice for treatment.
2. The patient needs to have an ingrown toenail treated. She is taking Bactrim for a kidney infection. Which three local anesthetics cannot be used?

3. You are the patient and are going to have the following operations. Choose the appropriate anesthetic.
   a. tooth extraction
   b. open-heart surgery

Internet Research

Use the Internet to complete the following assignments.

1. Research current news stories related to the Controlled Substances Act. Find two articles related to pharmaceuticals and summarize each in two or three sentences. List your Internet sources.
2. Research the use of narcotics in the management of chronic pain. Look up the JCAHO pain management standards and compare JCAHO's treatment of the subject to two or three other sites. Define the main controversies surrounding this issue. Why do you think it is important to have standards and guidelines in place? List your Internet sources and comment on the usefulness of each site.

Antidepressants, Antipsychotics, and Antianxiety Agents

Learning Objectives

◇ Differentiate the antidepressant, antipsychotic, and antianxiety agents.

◇ Be prepared to discuss the antidepressant classes, their uses, and their side effects.

◇ Know why and how lithium and other drugs are used in treating bipolar disorders.

◇ Be familiar with antipsychotics and the drugs that prevent their side effects.

◇ Define anxiety, learn its symptoms, and know the drugs used in its treatment.

◇ Recognize the course and treatment of panic disorders, insomnia, and alcoholism.

Diseases based in physical and mental disorders are among the most disabling conditions that healthcare professionals see. Many have their cause in the interaction of central nervous system chemicals. For the patient and the patient's family, these diseases can be overwhelming and frightening. Often, control of symptoms is the only treatment that can be offered. These states include depression, bipolar disorder, psychotic disorders, anxiety, panic attacks, sleep disorders, and alcoholism.

ANTIDEPRESSANTS

Clinical depression is the most common severe psychiatric disorder, affecting 10% of the United States' population. Women are more likely than men to have depression, with peak years usually from ages thirty-five to forty-five. Depression occurs in men later in life.

Depression is characterized by feelings of pessimism, worry, intense sadness, loss of concentration, slowing of mental processes, and problems with eating and sleeping. The patient feels life has no meaning. Changes in neurotransmitters in the brain have an effect on depression.

The three types of mood disorders are mania, bipolar depression, and unipolar depression. Mania is a mood of extreme excitement, excessive elation, hyperactivity, agitation, and increased psychomotor activity. Bipolar patients have mood swings that alternate between periods of major depression and periods of mild to severe chronic agitation (mania). Unipolar depression is major depression with no previous occurrence or mania.

The symptoms of depression are a dysphoric mood or loss of interest in almost all usual activities, low self-esteem, pessimism, self-pity, significant weight loss or gain, insomnia or hypersomnia, extreme restlessness, loss of energy, feelings of worthlessness, diminished ability to think, feelings of guilt, recurrent thoughts of death, and suicide attempts. Most episodes are self-limiting and resolve without treatment within one year.

Antidepressants are classified as selective serotonin reuptake inhibitors (SSRIs), tricyclic antidepressants (TCAs), and monoamine oxidase inhibitors (MAOIs). SSRIs block the reuptake of serotonin, with little effect on norepinephrine. They have the benefit of fewer side effects than the older antidepressants. TCAs act by preventing neuron reuptake of norepinephrine and/or serotonin. The choice of TCAs depends on adverse effects, cost, and patient response to a particular agent. MAOIs inhibit enzymes that break down catecholamines, therefore allowing norepinephrine to build up in the synapse.

Another form of treatment is electroconvulsive therapy (ECT), which has had good success. The patient is anesthetized for comfort and to alleviate anxiety and receives a neuromuscular blocker to reduce the chance of muscle injury or bone fracture during the procedure. The electrical stimulation, administered to the brain, is sufficient to induce seizures. ECT is a most effective therapy for major depressive disorders. It is especially useful in and indicated for treating delusional depression and depression resistant to drug therapy. ECT can be life-saving for patients who otherwise would not recover from their depressive illness.

Unlike most other drugs, antidepressants generally have a delay of onset of relief of ten to twenty-one days. They should never be used on an "as needed" basis to treat depression.

Selective Serotonin Reuptake Inhibitors (SSRIs)

The most-commonly used SSRIs in the treatment of depression are listed in Table 8.1.

Prozac (fluoxetine) is the most established agent in this drug class. It is indicated for major depression and obsessive-compulsive disorder. Adverse effects include nervousness, insomnia, drowsiness, anorexia, nausea, and diarrhea. Most patients lose weight, but a few may gain weight. Patients should avoid alcohol. Pharmacists should be alert for possible interaction with Dilantin (phenytoin). This interaction can raise the serum phenytoin to toxic levels. Patients should take the drug in the morning to avoid insomnia.

Warning

Prozac and Proscar can look almost exactly alike.

Sarafem is a brand of fluoxetine specifically targetted for women suffering from premenstrual dysphoric disorder (PMDD), which is a severe form of premenstrual syndrome (PMS). Serotonin levels are thought to influence the hormonal fluctuation that occurs just prior to the onset of menstruation. Although some women will benefit by taking the drug only during the week prior to menses, most will need to take it daily to achieve the desired effect. It comes in a seven-day pack containing 10-mg or 20-mg capsules.

Luvox (fluvoxamine) is effective for major depression and may be useful in managing anxiety; it is also approved for treatment of obsessive-compulsive disorders. The primary side effect is nausea. Alcohol should be avoided, as should administration with Dilantin (phenytoin). Hard candy can relieve the side effect of dry mouth.

Table 8.1	Most-Commonly Used SSRIs in Depression	
Generic Name	**Brand Name**	**Dosage Form**
citalopram	Celexa	tablet, liquid
fluoxetine	Prozac, Sarafem	capsule, liquid
fluvoxamine	Luvox	tablet
paroxetine	Paxil	tablet
sertraline	Zoloft	tablet
venlafaxine	Effexor	tablet

The indications for **Paxil (paroxetine)** are depression, obsessive-compulsive disorder, and panic disorder. Side effects are nausea, headache, ejaculatory disturbances, and sweating.

Effexor (venlafaxine) blocks both serotonin and norepinephrine and is indicated as therapy for depression. Some refer to it as "Prozac with a punch." A sustained increase in blood pressure may result from its use, and it may actuate manic episodes. Side effects are sweating, headache, somnolence, nausea, vomiting, dry mouth, blurred vision, and abnormal ejaculation or orgasm.

Zoloft (sertraline) is indicated for depression and obsessive-compulsive disorder. The primary side effect reported by patients is nausea when they first begin to take the drug; it may also cause drowsiness. It should be taken once daily without regard for food. Patients should respond in the first eight weeks of therapy.

Celexa (citalopram) is considered to be an SSRI, although it is structurally different from the other drugs in this class. This drug has relatively few drug interactions because it is metabolized through an alternative pathway. It is ideal for patients who are required to take a number of different prescriptions concurrently. Celexa is approved for obsessive-compulsive disorder and is not prescribed for other forms of depression.

Tricyclic Antidepressants (TCAs)

TCAs produce a response in 65% to 70% of patients. Usually, a therapeutic course of ten to twenty days is needed before improvements are apparent. Once the acute phase has subsided, the patient should continue to take the drug for six to twelve months to reduce risk of relapse. TCAs are also used in children with bed-wetting problems. The anticholinergic side effects can decrease urinary urgency. Table 8.2 lists the most-commonly used TCAs. Table 8.3 lists the anticholinergic and sedative properties of the TCAs.

The TCAs can be cardiotoxic in high doses, and this primary side effect needs to be monitored. Patients, particularly the elderly age group, may have postural hypotension and electroencephalographic (EEG) changes or arrhythmias. Deaths have occurred due to these cardiac arrhythmias. Treatment should begin with a low dose, increased as needed to attain a response. Sedation, another side effect, occurs especially in the first few days and may last several weeks; however, most patients become tolerant to this effect. It is usually prudent to advise the patient to take these drugs at bedtime. Dry mouth, blurred vision, constipation, and urinary retention may all resolve within a few weeks. Patients also need to avoid prolonged sun exposure.

Ludiomil (maprotiline) is indicated for treating depression accompanied by neurosis or anxiety. Side effects are similar to those of the other TCAs. It has a high

Warning

Zoloft and Zocor have been mistakenly dispensed one for the other.

Warning

Celexa is often confused with Cerebyx and Celebrex; be careful in dispensing.

| Table 8.2 | **Most-Commonly Used TCAs in Depression** |

Generic Name	Brand Name	Dosage Form
amitriptyline	Elavil	tablet, injection
amoxapine	Asendin	tablet
desipramine	Norpramin	tablet
doxepin	Sinequan	capsule, oral liquid, cream
imipramine	Tofranil	capsule, injection, tablet
maprotiline	Ludiomil	tablet
nortriptyline	Pamelor, Aventyl	capsule, oral solution
protriptyline	Vivactil	tablet
trimipramine	Surmontil	capsule

Table 8.3   **TCA Anticholinergic and Sedative Properties**

Drug	Properties Anticholinergic	Sedative
amitriptyline	+ + + + +	+ + + +
desipramine	+ +	+ +
doxepin	+ + +	+ + + +
imipramine	+ + +	+ + +
nortriptyline	+ + +	+ + +
protriptyline	+ + +	+
trimipramine	+ + + +	+ + + +

Note: The greater the number of + signs, the stronger the property.

seizure profile and may cause seizures in patients without a history of these disorders. The effects may not be felt for three to six weeks after initiation of therapy. The drug should not be discontinued abruptly.

Asendin (amoxapine) is used to treat endogenous depression and mixed symptoms of anxiety and depression. Extrapyramidal effects, including tardive dyskinesia (rare), have significantly reduced consideration of this drug.

Monoamine Oxidase Inhibitors (MAOIs)

MAOIs inhibit the activity of the enzymes that break down catecholamines, thus allowing these transmitters to build up in the synapse. MAOIs are a second-line treatment because of their many interactions with foods and other drugs, but these drugs may be effective for certain patients. They are most beneficial in atypical depression. They are similar in efficacy and adverse effects, but they are not as cardiotoxic as TCAs and may offer some advantages to patients with angina and conduction defects. Table 8.4 lists the most-commonly used MAOIs.

Eldepryl (selegiline) is primarily used in Parkinson's disease as an adjunct in the management of patients in which levodopa/carbidopa therapy is deteriorating. There is some use in Alzheimer's disease as well.

When dispensing any of these drugs, the pharmacist should check the patient profile for interactions with other drugs. If a patient is taking an MAOI and the physician changes to another class of antidepressant, the patient must wait at least two weeks for the MAOI to clear the system (washout period) before starting the second drug. MAOIs generally cause weight gain and edema.

Severe hypertensive reactions have occurred when an MAOI has been taken with food containing a high level of tyramine. The clinical result is sudden onset of a painful, throbbing, occipital headache, which if severe may progress to severe hypertension, profuse sweating, pallor, palpitation, and occasionally death.

Table 8.4   **Most-Commonly Used MAOIs in Depression**

Generic Name	Brand Name	Dosage Form
phenylzine	Nardil	tablet
selegiline	Eldepryl	tablet
tranylcypromine	Parnate	tablet

In addition to providing full disclosure on the drug prescribed, the pharmacist should give the patient detailed instructions on foods and other drugs to be avoided. Patients taking these drugs must absolutely *not* ingest aged cheeses, concentrated yeast extracts, pickled fish, sauerkraut, or broad bean pods due to high levels of tyramine. Severe interactions may occur when someone taking an MAOI takes ephedrine, amphetamine, methylphenidate, levodopa, or meperidine.

Other Antidepressants

Table 8.5 presents the most-commonly used miscellaneous antidepressants.

Desyrel (trazodone) and **Serzone (nefazodone)** exert their effect by preventing the reuptake of serotonin and norepinephrine. They have a much better side effect profile than the TCAs. They have no anticholinergic effects and no effects on cardiac conduction. They may cause orthostatic hypertension, which can be offset by taking them with food. They should be given at bedtime because they can cause drowsiness. Patients should avoid alcohol and sun exposure.

Cases of abnormal penile erection (priapism) have been reported with Desyrel (trazodone), some even requiring surgical intervention. This makes it a drug to avoid in young males, but it is very effective in older men to relieve depression. Serious interactions result when given with Halcion (triazolam) or Xanax (alprazolam).

Wellbutrin and **Zyban (bupropion)** are dopamine-uptake inhibitors with no direct effect on norepinephrine, serotonin, or monoamine oxidase; they are devoid of anticholinergic, antihistaminic, and adrenergic effects. Bupropion has been approved as an aid to smoking cessation. A single dose of the drug should not exceed 150 mg. It may take three to four weeks for the full effects to be realized. The drug should not be discontinued abruptly.

Bupropion has negligible anticholinergic effects. It does not cause sedation, blood pressure effects, or electrocardiographic (ECG) changes. Effects that may occur are headache, impairment of cognitive skills, nausea and vomiting, dry mouth, constipation, seizures, and impotence. There is a significant interaction between bupropion and haloperidol, MAOIs, or trazodone.

Remeron (mirtazapine) is not a reuptake blocker like the SSRIs or TCAs. It actually blocks specific serotonin receptors. This decreases some side effects often seen with SSRIs (i.e., anxiety, insomnia, and nausea). It seems to have some antianxiety effects like the TCAs. It causes drowsiness, increased appetite, and weight gain. A "May cause drowsiness" auxiliary label should be applied.

Drugs Used in Bipolar Disorders

Lithium compounds are the drugs of choice for bipolar mood disorders. If a patient is experiencing three or more of the following symptoms or signs of increased neurological activity, the diagnosis could be mania.

Table 8.5	Most-Commonly Used Miscellaneous Antidepressants		
Generic Name		**Brand Name**	**Dosage Form**
bupropion		Wellbutrin, Zyban	tablet
mirtazapine		Remeron	tablet
nefazodone		Serzone	tablet
trazodone		Desyrel	tablet

- decreased need for sleep
- distractibility
- elevated or irritable mood
- excessive involvement in pleasurable activities with a big potential for painful consequences (e.g., buying sprees, sexual indiscretions, foolish business investments, or reckless driving)
- grandiose ideas
- increase in activity (socially, at work, or sexually)
- pressure to keep talking (emotional labity)
- racing thoughts

The first episode of bipolar disorder typically occurs about age thirty, may last several months, and usually remits spontaneously. Without treatment, however, many patients experience one or more subsequent episodes.

The objective of therapy is to treat acute episodes and prevent subsequent attacks. The specific mechanism of lithium is unknown, but it is believed to alter levels of specific brain chemicals (neurotransmitters) or cause changes in the brain receptors' sensitivity.

Lithium is the drug of choice for treating acute mania and for prophylaxis of unipolar and bipolar disorders. An antipsychotic agent may be added initially to the regimen to control the hostility and agitation that sometimes accompany mania. When the blood level of lithium reaches therapeutic levels, the antipsychotic can be discontinued. Prophylactic therapy is indicated for patients with a family history of this illness and for those who have had two or more episodes within the preceding two years.

LITHIUM AND ITS COMPOUNDS (LITHONATE, ESKALITH, LITHOBID, LITHOTABS) Lithium may indirectly interfere with sodium transport in nerve and muscle cells. It also affects the synthesis and storage of CNS neurotransmitters. Lithium promotes norepinephrine reuptake and increases the sensitivity of serotonin receptors. The usual dosage of lithium is 300 mg, two to three times daily. Therapeutic blood levels are usually attained within five to ten days after the start of therapy. Levels of 0.6 to 0.8 mg/L are effective for most patients. To avoid toxicity, the patient must have blood tests regularly and take the medication at a specific time the day before the test. Even if the patient is taking a therapeutic dosage, slight tremor, especially of the hands, may occur. Salt intake should remain constant during treatment because it can affect lithium blood levels. Alcohol intake increases the potential for toxicity.

Lithium causes a range of effects in many body systems.

- **Gastrointestinal** Bloating and slight abdominal pain are usually transient, but nausea, vomiting, and anorexia are more severe. Most serious are loose and occasionally bloody stools, which could lead to water and electrolyte disturbances. Nausea may be reduced by dividing the doses, taking the dose with meals, or using a slow-release dosage form.
- **Dermatologic** Skin eruptions may occur within the first to third weeks but may clear spontaneously. Acne lesions may appear or worsen and may require decrease or discontinuation of the drug. Psoriasis may be initiated or aggravated.
- **Hematologic** Leucocytosis is apparent the first week and peaks during the second week. It persists throughout treatment.
- **Neuromuscular** When therapeutic levels of the drug in the blood are reached, a fine hand tremor appears. Tremors spread to other body parts, indicating impending toxicity. These tremors may occur at rest or while moving, be aggravated by delicate hand movements, and worsen with emotional stress or caffeine intake.

- ◇ **Weight** Increased tissue mass and sodium and water retention contribute to weight gain.
- ◇ **Renal** Polyuria (increased urination) and polydipsia (increased thirst) are common and usually well tolerated by patients. Polyuria may become a nuisance, with nocturia (bed-wetting), or lead to a serious fluid and electrolyte disturbance.
- ◇ **Teratogenic** If taken in the first trimester of pregnancy, lithium causes abnormal development of the head. It is not recommended during breast-feeding, since it could enter the mother's milk.

OTHER BIPOLAR DRUGS **Tegretol (carbamazepine)** affects the sodium channels which regulate nerve cells. This drug is indicated in bipolar disorders and is also used as an anticonvulsant. It is considered a second-line treatment to lithium and is used for patients who do not respond to lithium or cannot tolerate its side effects. It produces a response in a majority of manic patients within ten days. Side effects, which may be alleviated by briefly decreasing the dose to slow the rate of accumulation in the blood, include dizziness, ataxia, clumsiness, slurred speech, double vision, and drowsiness.

Depakote (divalproex) and **Depakene (valproic acid and its derivatives)**, referred to as *valproates*, are particularly effective among patients with rapid changes of mood (rapid cyclers) and the elderly. They also work well as an adjunct to lithium. They should be taken with food or milk but not with carbonated drinks. Sore throat, fever, fatigue, bleeding, or bruising should be reported to the physician. These are symptoms of thrombocytopenia, which can be a side effect of this drug. They may also cause drowsiness and impair judgment or coordination.

ANTIPSYCHOTICS

Antipsychotics, or neuroleptics, as they are sometimes referred to, reduce symptoms of hallucinations, delusions, and thought disorders but rarely eliminate them. Their primary indication is schizophrenia. Schizophrenia is a chronic psychotic disorder manifested by retreat from reality, delusions, hallucinations, ambivalence, withdrawal, and bizarre or regressive behavior.

Antipsychotic drugs are chosen on the basis of cost, limited adverse effects, and a patient's response history. Drugs do not alter the natural course of schizophrenia. They do, however, reduce, but rarely eliminate, symptoms, such as thought disorders, hallucinations, and delusions. Symptoms such as emotional and social withdrawal, ambivalence, and poor self-care usually do not respond to drug treatment. Most therapeutic gains occur in the first six weeks, but may take up to twelve to eighteen weeks. Discontinuation of these drugs leads to relapse of symptoms. Evidence shows that drug therapy does not reverse memory impairment, confusion, or intellectual deterioration.

Table 8.6 lists the antipsychotics that are most frequently prescribed. In low doses, Compazine and Sparine are commonly used as antiemetics. However, in high doses, they can be used as antipsychotics. They are rarely prescribed this way, but in unusual circumstances it can occur, and the technician needs to be aware of this usage of these drugs. The only antipsychotics that have a ceiling dose are thioridazine, which should not exceed 800 mg per day because abnormal pigment deposits in the retina may result in blindness, and promazine, which should not exceed 1,000 mg per day.

Table 8.6 — Antipsychotics

Generic Name	Brand Name	Dosage Form
clozapine	Clozaril	tablet
fluphenazine	Prolixin	tablet, liquid, IM, SC
haloperidol	Haldol	tablet, liquid, IM
loxapine	Loxitane	capsule, liquid, IM
mesoridazine	Serentil	tablet, liquid, IM
molindone	Moban	tablet, liquid
olanzapine	Zyprexa	tablet
perphenazine	Trilafon	tablet, liquid, IM
prochlorperazine	Compazine	tablet, capsule, liquid, suppository, IM, IV
promazine	Sparine	tablet, IM
risperidone	Risperdal	tablet, liquid
thioridazine	Mellaril	tablet, liquid
thiothixene	Navane	capsule, IM
trifluoperazine	Stelazine	tablet, liquid, IM

Warning

Prochlorperazine and chlorpromazine are easily confused.

Antipsychotics' Side Effects

Side effects of antipsychotics run the gamut from minor annoyances to serious problems that may not be reversible. Common side effects include sedation lasting up to two weeks. Tolerance develops, which is minimized by administering the total daily dose at bedtime. The patient may experience the following side effects.

- **Anticholinergic** Dryness of the mouth, eyes, and throat; blurred vision; and constipation. Problems occur at the beginning of treatment, but tolerance develops.
- **Cardiovascular** Postural hypotension (blood pressure decrease of 20 mm Hg); increase in pulse rate of about 20 bpm (beats per minute) with a change in position. These events may cause fainting or falling, most often in the elderly.
- **Dermatologic** Excessive tanning or burning and a steely gray appearance to the skin after years of therapy, due to drug accumulation in melanocytes. This a rare occurrence with increased usage of the newer drugs.
- **Endocrine** May cause hyperglycemia, lack of menses, lactation in nonpregnant females, breast enlargement in males, change in sex function and drive (females, increases; males, decreases).
- **Hematologic** Some reversible or non-reversible bone marrow depression.
- **Ophthalmologic** Deposit of melanin-drug complex in lens and retina, resulting in blindness.
- **Withdrawal** Relapse.
- **Neurologic** Extrapyramidal side effects (EPSEs) are due to imbalance of cholinergic and dopaminergic transmitters. Dopaminergic blockade results in excessive cholinergic effects. Side effects develop in forty to sixty percent of patients. Early onset symptoms develop within the first four weeks; anticholinergics can balance out some of this. The following muscle coordination conditions develop from the cholinergic and dopaminergic imbalance as early onset symptoms.
  - **Dystonia** Involuntary tonic contraction of skeletal muscles, mostly of head, face, and shoulders.
  - **Akathisia** Motor restlessness. Patients complain of inability to sit or stand still and of a compulsion to pace. While standing, the patient may rock to and fro or shift weight from one leg to the other. This occurs most frequently in the middle-aged, especially women.

- **Pseudoparkinsonism** Tremor, rigidity, and slow movement; apathy with little facial expression; difficulty in walking. The treatment is dose reduction, changing to an agent with less likelihood to produce EPSEs, or giving anticholinergics.

Late onset neurologic side effects are those occurring after six months of treatment. Tardive dyskinesia involves involuntary movements of the mouth, lips, and tongue that is sometimes accompanied by involuntary movements of the limbs or trunk. These actions are made worse by emotional upsets but disappear during sleep. Onset can be insidious and often occurs while the patient is taking the drug. The condition is potentially irreversible, even if the drug is discontinued. Drug withdrawal reveals the presence and severity of tardive dyskinesia. Once it appears, it is rarely progressive and usually either becomes static or slows, improving gradually over weeks or months. Currently there is no satisfactory treatment. Anticholinergics make the condition worse.

Drugs that Minimize the Side Effects of Antipsychotics

Anticholinergics may produce an immediate, but not necessarily a complete response to excess muscle activity resulting from antipsychotic administration. The anticholinergics used to help prevent or minimize some of the side effects are

- ◇ Dramamine (dimenhydrinate)
- ◇ Cogentin (benztropine)
- ◇ Benadryl (diphenhydramine)
- ◇ Artane (trihexyphenidyl)
- ◇ benzodiazepines

Antipsychotics' Dispensing Issues

Risperdal (risperidone) is indicated for the management of psychotic disorders (e.g., schizophrenia) and dementia in the elderly. It is a mixed serotonin-dopamine antagonist and binds to serotonin receptors in the CNS and the periphery with a very high affinity and binds to dopamine receptors with less affinity. The binding of serotonin receptors and dopamine receptors is thought to improve negative symptoms of psychosis and reduce the incidence of EPSEs. The primary side effects are hypotension, sedation, and anxiety.

Clozaril (clozapine), a weak blocker of dopamine$_1$ and dopamine$_2$ receptors, is indicated for managing schizophrenic patients. It also blocks serotonin$_1$, alpha-adrenergic, and histamine CNS receptors. Medication should not be stopped abruptly. Leukocyte counts should be done weekly for the duration of therapy, and frequent blood samples *must* be taken and these results documented by the pharmacy. The patient should report any lethargy, fever, sore throat, flulike symptoms, or indications of infection.

Zyprexa (olanzapine) is used for schizophrenia and is hoped to prove as effective as Clozaril without the need for frequent blood monitoring. Like Clozaril (clozapine) and Risperdal (resperidone), it is atypical. It blocks dopamine and serotonin receptors. It causes fewer movement disorders and is more effective than either drug. Side effects are dizziness, drowsiness, constipation, dry mouth, and weight gain. Patients *must* avoid alcohol.

Warning

Clozaril and Clinoril have been confused.

Warning

Zyprexa looks and sounds like Zyrtec; be careful in dispensing.

ANTIANXIETY AGENTS

Anxiety is a state of uneasiness characterized by apprehension and worry about possible events. Anxiety is a common complaint made to physicians. It is a collection of unpleasant feelings identical to the fearful feelings experienced under conditions of actual danger. The patient feels generalized tension and apprehension and startles easily. Other symptoms include uneasiness and nervousness at work or with people or vague, nagging uncertainty about the future, which may lead to chronic fatigue, headaches, and insomnia.

Exogenous anxiety develops in response to external stresses. The response may be appropriate if conditions warrant apprehension and fear. Endogenous anxiety is not related to any identifiable external factors but occurs spontaneously as a result of a defined abnormality in cellular function in the CNS. The most common self-prescribed treatment for all anxious states is alcohol. Excessive use of alcohol is common in panic patients.

The antianxiety agents include both noncontrolled and controlled substances (see Table 8.7). By far the most-used drugs are the benzodiazepines, also effective in insomnia, panic disorders, alcohol withdrawal syndrome, convulsive disorders, and muscle spasms. When used short-term, they can be effective in controlling anxiety. They are used in the lowest possible doses that control the symptoms while minimizing side effects.

Warning

Xanax and Zantac often look alike. Xanax is for anxiety, and Zantac is for the stomach.

These drugs may cause physical or psychologic dependence, or both. **Xanax (alprazolam)**, **Ativan (lorazepam)**, and **Serax (oxazepam)** produce no active metabolites and thus clear the body more quickly. Patients should understand that continued dosing may cause physical dependence and that stopping the drug abruptly may result in withdrawal side effects. The onset of withdrawal usually occurs one to two days after discontinuing the drug.

Patients taking antianxiety drugs should be monitored closely for onset of depression, which occurs in about one third of cases. Patients who discontinue medication have a high rate of relapse. The drug must be tapered to avoid withdrawal reactions.

Among the side effects of the benzodiazepines are

⬥ dependence if duration of therapy exceeds three months (in general, a patient should not remain on the drug more than six months)
⬥ drug accumulation during multiple dosing (fat soluble)
⬥ link to birth defects if taken early in pregnancy

Table 8.7	**Most-Commonly Used Antianxiety Agents**		
Generic Name		**Brand Name**	**Dosage Form**
Noncontrolled Substances			
amoxapine (TCA)		Asendin	tablet
buspirone (antianxiety)		BuSpar	tablet
hydroxyzine (antihistamine)		Vistaril	capsule, syrup, injection
propranolol (beta blocker)		Inderal	tablet, capsule, injection
trifluoperazine (antipsychotic)		Stelazine	tablet, solution, injection
Controlled Substances			
alprazolam (benzodiazepine)		Xanax	tablet
chlordiazepoxide (benzodiazepine)		Librium	capsule, injection
clorazepate (benzodiazepine)		Tranxene	capsule, tablet
diazepam (benzodiazepine)		Valium	tablet, injection
lorazepam (benzodiazepine)		Ativan	tablet, IM, IV
meprobamate (antianxiety)		Equanil, Miltown	tablet
oxazepam (benzodiazepine)		Serax	tablet, capsule

- muscle relaxation, reduced muscle coordination, impaired reflexes
- paradoxical excitement (hostility, rage, destructive behavior)
- sedation

Inderal (propranolol) is a nonspecific beta blocker widely used in anxiety but currently not approved for that indication. It reduces heart rate and thereby decreases symptoms such as stage fright and test anxiety. It is useful for tremors in these situations.

Vistaril (hydroxyzine), used for some anxious patients, has sedating qualities and is widely used as a preoperative sedative and sleeping pill. This drug is thought to depress subcortical areas of the CNS.

BuSpar (buspirone) acts by selectively antagonizing serotonin receptors without affecting the receptors for benzodiazepine and gamma-aminobutyric acid (GABA). It should be taken with food, and the patient should report any changes in the senses (hearing, smell, or taste). It takes about two weeks to see the full effect of the drug. This drug has few side effects, nausea and headache being the most common. It has shown little potential for abuse.

Asendin (amoxapine) is a TCA frequently prescribed to treat mixed symptoms of anxiety and depression. It is best to take this drug at bedtime to avoid daytime sedation.

Stelazine (trifluoperazine) has been effective in treating nonpsychotic anxiety. It has a high potential for pseudoparkinsonism, dystonias, and tardive dyskinesia, so it is usually given with an antihistamine or benztropine. It blocks dopaminergic receptors. Therapy requires several weeks before the full effects can be seen. The patient should avoid sunlight.

Equanil (meprobamate), when used as an anxiety agent, acts primarily on the hypothalamus, thalamus, limbic system, and spinal cord. Meprobamate also has value in treating muscle rigidity and contractions. Sedation is the primary side effect.

Panic Disorders

Panic is a form of intense, overwhelming, and uncontrollable anxiety. It is neither a voluntary or controllable emotion nor a condition that can be avoided by ignoring it or wishing it away.

Panic attacks have a definite onset and end spontaneously. They occur in public or at home, sometimes interrupting sleep. They are characterized by a sense of fear, apprehension, a premonition of serious illness, and fear of a life-threatening attack. The criteria for diagnosis are three attacks in a three-week period, not stimulated by physical exertion, life-threatening situations, or exposure to phobic stimulus and at least four of the following symptoms: dyspnea, palpitations, chest pain or discomfort, choking sensation, dizziness, feelings of unreality, tingling in hands or feet, hot or cold flashes, sweating, numbness, and trembling.

PATHOPHYSIOLOGY Panic disorders appear to result from a neurochemical defect in part of the brain. In some persons, the brain stem functions abnormally. This abnormality, often characterized by progressive oversensitivity, can develop at any point in life and occurs in the locus ceruleus, which comprises a group of synapses in the brain stem at the level of the pons and medulla. The locus ceruleus determines the organism's level of arousal. Sensory information arriving from all parts of the body passes through this major neurologic junction before distributing to other parts of the brain.

If this abnormality is located in the locus ceruleus, incoming signals are affected, depending on both the current state of the organism and the nature of the arriving messages. If incoming messages are inappropriately amplified to signal a life-threatening stress, the organism is aroused to defense or flight. Excessive amplification of incoming messages gives rise to a state of excessive arousal, excessive autonomic discharges, and increased respiratory drive.

If the incoming message is calm and non-threatening, the stimuli are toned down and the locus does not overreact. Panic patients are unusually sensitive to the stimulant effects of low doses of caffeine and sodium lactate that, when infused, alter intracellular pH and increase impulse transmission through the brain, causing panic symptoms. These patients also experience symptoms from administration of beta-adrenergic agonists, such as norepinephrine.

TREATMENT The panic attack is of neurochemical origin and has both emotional and physical components. Antianxiety and psychotherapeutic measures have proven inadequate, since neither type of drug restores normal neurochemical function to the locus ceruleus. The most successful treatment combines anti-panic medication and behavioral therapy.

Psychotherapy is the preferred treatment in panic disorders for patients whose symptoms cause significant discomfort or impairment; however, short-term administration of an antianxiety agent (i.e., tranquilizer) may be indicated. The benzodiazepines, buspirone, and to a lesser extent, the beta-adrenergic blocking agents are the most appropriate pharmacologic alternatives. Diphenhydramine, hydroxyzine, and other antihistamines are sometimes prescribed, especially for elderly patients. The TCA **Tofranil (imipramine)** and the MAOI **Nardil (phenelzine)** have proven effective.

Patients should try to remember where they were and what they were doing when an attack occurred in order to try to avoid similar situations in the future. However, the attack was not caused by the place or action. Panic disorder has a true biochemical basis and can be effectively treated. These disorders should be viewed with the same objectivity as other chronic, incurable, but drug-controllable diseases.

Sleep Disorders

One third of Americans eighteen years old and over have trouble sleeping in a given year. About 6% seek a physician's help. Indications for using hypnotics (drugs that induce sleep) are the symptoms of insomnia; that is, difficulty in falling or staying asleep or not feeling refreshed on awakening, or both.

The causes of some types of sleep disorders include several types of events or conditions. The causes can be

- ◇ situational: job stress, hospitalization, or travel
- ◇ medical: pain, respiratory problems, or GI problems
- ◇ psychiatric: schizophrenia, depression, or mania
- ◇ drug intake: alcohol, caffeine, or sympathomimetic agents

Diagnosis and effective treatment of the cause can usually eliminate the need for using hypnotic drugs. Treating only the symptoms of insomnia can lead to difficulty in recognizing and treating the underlying illness and may subject the patient to potentially habitual or physical dependence on the drugs.

STAGES OF SLEEP Sleep occurs in four stages.

- ◇ **Stage I (NREM)** Nonrapid eye movements; subject is somewhat aware of surroundings but relaxed (4% to 5% of sleep time).
- ◇ **Stage II (NREM)** Nonrapid eye movements; subject is unaware of surroundings but can be easily awakened (50% of sleep time).

◊ **Stages III and IV (REM)** Subject's sleep is characterized by increased autonomic activity and by episodes of rapid eye movements (REM sleep) with dreaming if possible (> 90 minutes), occurring four to five times a night. This deep sleep (20% to 25% of sleep time) is important to physical rest.

TYPES OF INSOMNIA Transient insomnia is not really a sleep disorder. It is usually a response to an acute stressful event and can normally be expected to improve with time as the person adapts to the stress. Chronic insomnia is most often of multifaceted origin. The first evaluation of patients should include sleep, drug, medical, and psychiatric histories.

TREATING INSOMNIA Effective treatment necessitates both pharmacologic and nonpharmacologic measures. Pharmacologic treatment consists primarily of the adjunctive use of hypnotics in patients with clearly defined insomnia. Nonpharmacologic treatment includes supportive counseling and behavioral treatment. The components of this therapy are

◊ normalizing the sleep schedule as to bedtime and waking time
◊ increasing physical exercise during the daytime
◊ discontinuing use of alcohol as a sedative
◊ sleeping a total of only seven to eight hours in a twenty-four-hour period
◊ reducing caffeine intake
◊ eliminating any drug (e.g., decongestant) that could lead to insomnia

A person facing a clearly identified external stress (grief reaction) may become anxious and have difficulty sleeping. A one- to three-week course of treatment with a hypnotic agent may be justified in such instances. Hypnotic drugs should be used only as an adjunct to medical therapeutic measures.

There are three specific criteria guides for prescribing a hypnotic drug.

◊ The agent must have low addiction and suicide potential.
◊ The agent must minimally alter EEG pattern and not depress REM sleep.
◊ The agent must have minimum interaction with other drugs.

These criteria suggest the benzodiazepine class of drugs. Several are specifically approved for this use. Benzodiazepines are currently the preferred hypnotics, primarily because of their somewhat long duration of effectiveness and lower risk of fatal overdose. Therapy with hypnotic agents decreases the time it takes to fall asleep, reduces early morning awakenings, increases total sleep, and improves quality of sleep.

Most barbiturates and nonbenzodiazepine hypnotics lose their efficacy as hypnotics after one to two weeks of continuous use. REM sleep is reduced by all hypnotics except the benzodiazepines and chloral hydrate; as a result, patients may not feel well rested and significant REM rebound may occur after discontinuation of these agents.

Table 8.8 lists the most-commonly used hypnotic agents for sleep disorders.

Patients should be informed of hypnotic agents' limitations. The drugs should be taken as needed, rather than every night, to reduce the risk of habituation and increase the duration of effectiveness. It is easy to slip into the habit of taking these drugs every day and the patient may not be able to sleep without them. Therapy should be started with a small dose, to be increased only if the initial dose is ineffective. Hypnotics are best administered one hour before bedtime.

The primary side effects of hypnotic medications (seen more often with high doses) are CNS depression (dizziness, confusion, next-day drowsiness, and

Table 8.8 **Most-Commonly Used Agents for Sleep Disorders**

Generic Name	Brand Name	Dosage Form
Benzodiazepines		
alprazolam	Xanax	tablet
chlordiazepoxide	Librium	capsule, injection
clorazepate	Tranxene	tablet
diazepam	Valium	tablet, IM, IV
estazolam	ProSom	tablet
flurazepam	Dalmane	capsule
lorazepam	Ativan	tablet, IM, IV
oxazepam	Serax	tablet, capsule
quazepam	Doral	tablet
temazepam	Restoril	capsule
triazolam	Halcion	tablet
Barbiturates		
amobarbital (C-II)	Amytal	capsule, tablet, IM
butabarbital (C-III)	Butisol	tablet, capsule, elixir
secobarbital (C-II)	Seconal	capsule, IM
Antihistamines		
diphenhydramine	Benadryl	tablet, capsule, syrup, cream, IM, IV
hydroxyzine pamoate	Vistaril	tablet, capsule, syrup, IM
Hypnotics		
chloral hydrate	Noctec	syrup, capsule, suppository
zaleplon	Sonata	capsule
zolpidem	Ambien	tablet

Warning

Diazepam, lorazepam, and alprazolam can all be misread.

impaired reflexes). A side-effect phenomenon, particularly in the elderly, is paradoxical reactions (excitation, irritability, and occasionally, aggressive behavior). Anterograde amnesia (impaired memory for the event) after taking a hypnotic dose may also occur. Patients using a hypnotic should use it only a limited number of times each week, and that use should be restricted to a four- to six-week period.

Sonata (zaleplon) is the shortest acting hypnotic. It has a relatively short duration of action, four hours. It can be taken in the middle of the night. Depending on when the drug is taken, there should be little left-over morning grogginess.

Ambien (zolpidem) is like the benzodiazepines, but it is structurally dissimilar. It has a high affinity to the benzodiazepine receptors, especially the omega$_1$ receptor. It retains hypnotic and many of the anxiolytic properties of the benzodiazepines, but has reduced effects on skeletal muscle and seizure threshold. Rarely is mechanical ventilation required in overdose. It is used for short-term treatment of insomnia. The side effects are dizziness, headache, nausea, diarrhea, and next-day drowsiness.

Some barbiturates are hypnotics, among them **Amytal (amobarbital, C-II)**, **Butisol (butabarbital, C-III)**, and **Seconal (secobarbital, C-II)**. Barbiturates work by depressing the sensory cortex, decreasing motor activity, altering cellular function, and producing drowsiness, sedation, and hypnosis. The C-IIs and C-IIIs are used only for short-term therapy. Use is rare because of the side effect profile which includes significant abuse potential, tremors, and confusion; REM rebound; high suicide potential; and hangover.

Noctec (chloral hydrate), a hypnotic, has quick onset, with no rebound. Dependence is a problem. It also interacts with warfarin. The antihistamines are the safest drugs for treating insomnia. They can be given to children and the elderly. There is no addiction. Even if patients become accustomed to taking a dose at night to fall asleep, they can still sleep without one if tired enough. **Vistaril (hydroxyzine pamoate)** and **Benadryl (diphenhydramine)** are both used for sleep.

ALCOHOLISM

The American Medical Association recognizes alcoholism as a disease that can be arrested but not cured. Alcoholism is a lifetime disease. Alcoholics are in emotional pain and use alcohol to kill that pain. It is the nature of the disease that the alcoholics do not believe they are ill (denial). Hope for recovery lies in their ability to recognize a need for help, their desire to stop drinking, and their willingness to admit that they cannot cope with the problems by themselves.

Alcohol (ethanol) is an anesthetic. Intake of a large quantity of ethanol causes loss of consciousness, with anesthesia. However, the margin between loss of consciousness and medullary paralysis is smaller than with general anesthesia. The emetic action usually prevents death by preventing absorption of lethal concentrations. Most deaths are due to aspiration of vomitus during unconsciousness.

Alcohol's Effects on Metabolism and Excretion

The habitual drinker has an increased ability to metabolize ethanol more rapidly, which increases tolerance. Neurons in the CNS adapt to the presence of ethanol. The drinker learns to compensate to some extent for the depressant action. Heavy beer drinking may lead to the serious complication of obesity coupled with vitamin deficiency. In the later stages of alcoholism, gastritis, and loss of appetite, organic brain damage, alcoholic psychosis, and dementia occur. Cirrhosis of the liver (irreversible damage) results from fatty synthesis and excessive buildup of lipid compounds.

Alcohol withdrawal can be severe and even life-threatening. Benzodiazepines are considered the standard of care for detoxification. The dosage of these drugs must be adjusted according to the needs of individual patients. Benzodiazepines will also prevent detoxification-related seizures.

About forty percent of hospitalized trauma patients have alcohol in their blood when first examined. The first signs of alcohol withdrawal appear within a few hours. In mild withdrawal, symptoms may disappear in one to two days; in severe withdrawal, symptoms may last one to two weeks. Therapy may necessitate administering a sedative, anticonvulsant, beta blocker, or antipsychotic drugs, or a combination of these.

Chemical dependence is the inability to control the use of some physical substance; that is, not being able to quit use or limit the amount taken. A person can be chemically dependent without showing obvious signs. Genetic makeup may affect the chance of becoming dependent, which is often a physical condition that cannot be cured by willpower.

Alcoholism is an incurable and potentially fatal disease. It can be controlled but never cured. Persons usually take a chemical substance for pleasure or to avoid pain. Alcoholism is linked to genetics. The abuser has a different level of brain chemicals, different levels of enzymes, or altogether different enzymes that metabolize the alcohol at different rates and quantities than nonalcoholics. When an alcoholic enters a treatment program, comes to an emergency room, or is admitted into the hospital, the alcoholic is usually given Folvite (folic acid), thiamine (B$_1$), and a multi-purpose vitamin. This particular drug regimen can usually be associated with alcoholism.

Symptoms of dependence are listed in Table 8.9. To resolve their problem, alcoholics must take four steps toward recovery.

1. Acknowledge the problem.
2. Limit the time spent with substance users.
3. Seek professional help.
4. Seek support from recovering alcoholics.

Abrupt withdrawal of alcohol can precipitate some serious, life-threatening symptoms. Table 8.10 lists these symptoms.

Alcohol Antagonists

Only two drugs have been approved for treating alcohol addiction (see Table 8.11).

Antabuse (disulfiram) stops the metabolism of alcohol at the acetaldehyde stage, allowing the latter to accumulate in body tissues. When a patient on disulfiram consumes alcohol, violent side effects are almost instantaneous. These are known as Antabuse-like reactions. The patient usually becomes exhausted and sleeps for several hours after symptoms have worn off. Antabuse (disulfiram) produces a cluster of side effects within minutes of alcohol ingestion. These include

⬧ blurred vision
⬧ confusion
⬧ difficulty breathing
⬧ face becoming hot and scarlet
⬧ intense throbbing in head and neck
⬧ may have chest pain

Table 8.9	Symptoms of Dependence on Alcohol

⬧ blackouts or lapses of memory
⬧ concerns of family, friends, and employers about the substance use
⬧ doing things that cause regret afterwards
⬧ financial or legal problems from substance use
⬧ loss of pleasure without the substance
⬧ neglecting responsibilities
⬧ trying to cut down or quit using a substance but failing
⬧ using alone; hiding evidence
⬧ using to forget about problems
⬧ willingness to do almost anything to get the substance

Table 8.10	Alcohol Withdrawal Symptoms

⬧ agitation	⬧ mental disturbances
⬧ circulatory disturbances	⬧ nausea and vomiting
⬧ convulsions	⬧ restlessness
⬧ delirium tremens (DTs)	⬧ sweating
⬧ digestive disorders	⬧ temporary suppression of REM sleep
⬧ disorientation	⬧ tremor
⬧ extreme fear	⬧ weakness
⬧ hallucinations	

Table 8.11	**Most-Commonly Used Alcohol Antagonists**		
Generic Name		**Brand Name**	**Dosage Form**
disulfiram		Antabuse	tablet
naltrexone		ReVia	tablet

◇ nausea
◇ severe headache
◇ severe vomiting
◇ thirst
◇ uneasiness

Patients who are taking Antabuse must examine food labels to be sure they do not inadvertently ingest alcohol in an everyday product (e.g., cough medicines, mouth washes, flavorings, salad dressings, and wine vinegars).

ReVia (naltrexone) is a pure opiate antagonist that blocks the effects of endogenous opioids released as a result of alcohol consumption, making alcohol consumption less pleasurable. It is used to treat alcohol dependence. ReVia (naltrexone) can cause an acute withdrawal syndrome in opiate-dependent patients, including nausea, dizziness, headache, and weight loss. The patient should be stable after alcohol withdrawal before starting this drug. Those with a history of opiate intake must be opiate-free before starting the drug to prevent withdrawal symptoms.

Chapter Summary

Antidepressants

- Antidepressants are not controlled substances.
- Antidepressants are classified as SSRIs (serotonin-specific reuptake inhibitors), TCAs (tricyclic antidepressants), MAOIs (monamine oxidase inhibitors), lithium (mechanism unknown in bipolar disorders), and miscellaneous (do not fit any of the above categories).
- SSRIs block the reuptake of serotonin with little effect on norepinephrine. They have fewer side effects than the other antidepressant medications.
- TCAs can be cardiotoxic in high doses; watch carefully before dosing.
- MAOIs are a second-line treatment because of their many interactions with drugs and foods.
- A single dose of Wellbutrin (bupropion) should not exceed 150 mg.
- It may take at least two weeks for some of the antidepressants to be effective.
- Lithium is the drug of choice for bipolar manic-depressive disease.
- A patient taking lithium *must* have frequent blood tests to assess lithium levels and maintain a therapeutic range.
- Tegretol (carbamazepine) or Depakote (divalproex) may be substituted if patients cannot tolerate lithium.

Antipsychotics

- Atypical antipsychotics that have a ceiling dose are thioridazine, which should not exceed 800 mg/day, and promazine, which should not exceed 1,000 mg/day.
- The antipsychotic drugs' side effects can be minimized by anticholinergics.

Antianxiety Agents

- Anxiety is a state of uneasiness characterized by apprehension and worry about possible events.
- The most common self-prescribed treatment for anxiety is alcohol.
- The benzodiazepines, buspirone, and, to a lesser extent, the beta blockers are the most appropriate pharmacologic treatments for panic attacks.
- A sedative is an antianxiety drug; a hypnotic induces sleep. Some drugs fit both descriptions.
- REM sleep is reduced by all hypnotic agents except the benzodiazepines and chloral hydrate.
- Benzodiazepines FDA-approved for hypnotic use are Dalmane, Restoril, Halcion, ProSom, and Doral.
- Hypnotics should be administered one hour before bedtime.
- Ambien is a C-IV drug structurally dissimilar to benzodiazepines.
- Patients should take hypnotics only a limited number of times each week, and the duration of use should be restricted to a four- to six-week period.
- Sonata (zalepon) is the shortest-acting benzodiazepine with a duration of action of four hours. Therefore it may be taken in the middle of the night.
- Antihistamines are the safest drugs to use in treating insomnia.

Alcoholism

◆ Alcoholism is an incurable and potentially fatal disease. It can be controlled through behavioral changes.

◆ Alcohol causes effects on body temperature, GI tract, kidneys, and CNS.

◆ Alcoholics have additional enzymes for metabolism and neuronadaption.

◆ Alcoholism is a family disease.

◆ Only two drugs have been approved for treatment of this disease and they are Antabuse (disulfiram) and ReVia (naltrexone).

Drug Summary

The following drugs were discussed in this chapter. Each generic drug name is followed in parentheses by one or more brand names. An asterisk (*) indicates drugs frequently written using *either* brand *or* generic name. These need to be memorized.

Antidepressants
SSRIs
citalopram (Celexa)
fluoxetine (Prozac, Sarafem)*
fluvoxamine (Luvox)
paroxetine (Paxil)
sertraline (Zoloft)*
venlafaxine (Effexor)

TCAs
amitriptyline (Elavil)*
amoxapine (Asendin)*
desipramine (Norpramin)
doxepin (Sinequan)
imipramine (Tofranil)*
maprotiline (Ludiomil)
nortriptyline (Pamelor, Aventyl)*
protriptyline (Vivactil)
trimipramine (Surmontil)

MAOIs
phenelzine (Nardil)
selegiline (Eldepryl)
tranylcypromine (Parnate)

Antihistamines
benztropine (Cogentin)*
dimenhydrinate (Dramamine)*
diphenhydramine (Benadryl)*
hydroxyzine pamoate (Vistaril)*
trihexyphenidyl (Artane)

Antipsychotics
clozapine (Clozaril)
fluphenazine (Prolixin)
haloperidol (Haldol)
loxapine (Loxitane)
mesoridazine (Serentil)
molindone (Moban)
olanzapine (Zyprexa)
perphenazine (Trilafon)
prochlorperazine (Compazine)
promazine (Sparine)*

risperidone (Risperdal)
thioridazine (Mellaril)
thiothixene (Navane)

Antianxiety
buspirone (BuSpar)
meprobamate (Equanil)*
trifluoperazine (Stelazine)

Benzodiazepines
alprazolam (Xanax)*
chlordiazepoxide (Librium)
clorazepate (Tranxene)
diazepam (Valium)*
estazolam (ProSom)
flurazepam (Dalmane)*
lorazepam (Ativan)*
oxazepam (Serax)
quazepam (Doral)
temazepam (Restoril)*
triazolam (Halcion)

Beta Blocker
propranolol (Inderal)*

Barbiturates
amobarbital (Amytal)
butabarbital (Butisol)
secobarbital (Seconal)

Alcohol Antagonists
disulfiram (Antabuse)
naltrexone (ReVia)

Hypnotics
chloral hydrate (Noctec)
zaleplon (Sonata)
zolpidem (Ambien)

Miscellaneous Antidepressants
bupropion (Wellbutrin, Zyban)
mirtazapine (Remeron)
nefazodone (Serzone)
trazodone (Desyrel)*

Drugs for Bipolar Disorders
carbamazepine (Tegretol)*
divalproex (Depakote)*
lithium (Lithonate, Eskalith, Lithobid, Lithotabs)
valproic acid (Depakene)

Chapter Review

Pharmaceuticals and Body Functions

Select the best answer from the choices given.

1. The drug of choice for bipolar disorders is
   a. Prozac.
   b. Serzone.
   c. lithium.
   d. amoxapine.

2. If the patient is taking a therapeutic dose of lithium, there will be a slight tremor of the
   a. hand.
   b. foot.
   c. eyes.
   d. head.

3. Which drug can be safely taken with alcohol?
   a. Lithium
   b. Valium
   c. Ativan
   d. None of the above

4. Which of the listed drugs is/are used in the treatment of bipolar disorders?
   a. Lithium
   b. Carbamazepine
   c. Depakote
   d. All of the above

5. Which drug is said to be replacing lithium for treating bipolar depression, especially in patients with rapid changes of mood and the elderly?
   a. Tegretol
   b. Depakote
   c. Carbamazepine
   d. None of the above

6. Antipsychotic drugs are chosen on the basis of
   a. cost.
   b. side effects.
   c. the patient's history of response.
   d. all of the above.

7. The antipsychotic with a ceiling dose is
   a. chlorprothixene.
   b. loxapine.
   c. thioridazine.
   d. trifluoperazine.

8. An adverse effect of the antipsychotics is
   a. dry mouth.
   b. constipation.
   c. blurred vision.
   d. All of the above

9. Which drug is recommended to treat pseudoparkinsonism?
   a. Diphenhydramine
   b. Dramamine
   c. Cogentin
   d. Eldepryl

10. Which drug is recommended to treat tardive dyskinesia?
    a. Benadryl
    b. Hydroxyzine
    c. Bonine
    d. None of the above

The following statements are true or false. If the answer is false, rewrite the statement so it is true.

_____ 1. The most-used drugs to treat anxiety are the SSRIs.

_____ 2. The only drug approved by the FDA for panic disorder is Valium.

_____ 3. The most successful treatment of panic attacks is behavioral therapy and anti-panic medication.

_____ 4. Withdrawal symptoms in alcoholics may be treated by anticonvulsants, sedatives, and beta blockers.

_____ 5. Alcohol withdrawal symptoms are nausea, uneasiness, and confusion.

_____ 6. Two drugs specifically used to treat alcoholism are Valium and Stelazine.

_____ 7. Sometimes alcohol addiction has no physical signs.

_____ 8. Benzodiazepines are the best hypnotics, and there is no reason that they should not be used as the first-line treatment for sleeplessness.

_____ 9. An MAOI might be a good choice for an antidepressant in a patient with Parkinson's disease.

_____ 10. Desyrel is a good antidepressant in a young male, but a poor choice in an elderly man.

Diseases and Drug Therapies

1. List at least five symptoms of depression.
2. List five symptoms of bipolar disorders.
3. List four noncontrolled medications for anxiety.
4. Which three benzodiazepines used to treat anxiety clear the body most quickly?
5. Which five benzodiazepines are approved for hypnotic use?
6. List the four steps toward recovery for an alcoholic.
7. List the effects of alcohol when combined with Antabuse.
8. List some practical methods of inducing sleep other than drug use.
9. List the side effects of antipsychotics.
10. List three types of depression.

Dispensing Medications

You receive the following incorrect prescriptions. Identify the error in each.

1. Ativan 2 mg
   tid #90
   refills 12

2. Mellaril 400 mg
   tid #90
   refills 12

3. Ambien 5 mg #30
   qd at bedtime
   refills 12

Internet Research

Use the Internet to complete the following assignments.

1. Find Internet sources listing potential drug and food interactions for three of the antidepressants discussed in this chapter. Do you think the information provided on these sites is reliable? Why or why not? Create a table listing the drugs you researched along with their corresponding drug and food interactions.
2. Research bipolar manic-depressive disorder. What are the modes of treatment for this disease (including drug treatment)? What are the most common signs and symptoms of this disorder? List your Internet sources.

Anticonvulsants and Drugs to Treat Other CNS Disorders

Chapter 9

Learning Objectives

- ◇ Develop an understanding of the physiologic processes that occur in epilepsy.
- ◇ Classify seizures and the goals of their therapy.
- ◇ Understand that specific drugs are used in different classes of seizures.
- ◇ Be familiar with Parkinson's disease and the drugs used in its treatment.
- ◇ Know the symptoms of myasthenia gravis, the attention-deficit disorders, ALS, MS, and Alzheimer's and their treatments.

The central nervous system (CNS) disorders cause a range of complex distressing and life-threatening symptoms, some of which are nonresponsive to treatment. They often leave the patient unable to function normally. The chemicals involved in the thought process and motor activity form the basis of some of these diseases and the rationale for their treatment. These diseases include epilepsy in its various forms, Parkinson's disease, myasthenia gravis, attention-deficit disorders, amyotrophic lateral sclerosis, and multiple sclerosis. For some of these diseases, we are still searching for definitive treatment.

EPILEPSY

Epilepsy is a common neurologic disorder defined as paroxysmal, recurring seizures. It involves disturbances of neuronal electrical activity that interfere with normal brain function. These abnormal discharges may occur only in a specific area of the brain or may spread extensively throughout the brain. They may not provoke obvious clinical symptoms, yet seizures may nevertheless be taking place.

Epilepsy is a symptom of brain dysfunction. In the United States 2.5 million persons are affected, and 125,000 new cases are diagnosed each year. All epilepsy patients have seizures, but not all patients with seizures have epilepsy. About 8% of Americans have a single unprovoked seizure in their lifetime; 1% to 2% have chronic epilepsy.

Seizures

Seizures are caused by disordered abnormal electrical discharges in the cerebral cortex, causing a change in behavior of which the patient is not aware. Conscious periods may or may not be accompanied by loss of control over movements or distortion of the senses. When body movement is lost, it may be in only one area of the body or in the entire body.

Seizures result from the sudden, excessive firing of a small number of neurons, often without an exogenous trigger, and the spread of the electrical activity to adjacent neurons. The balance between excitatory and inhibitory impulses determines whether a neuron fires. Healthy persons have a balance between excitement and inhibition. In persons with epilepsy, there is an imbalance between excitement and inhibition and the neurotransmitters. Glutamate, an excitatory amino acid neurotransmitter, and gamma-aminobutyric acid (GABA), an inhibitory neurotransmitter, play the greatest role in seizures. Other contributors are the CNS chemicals involved in the thought process and motor activity. These CNS chemicals are

- acetylcholine (ACh)
- aspartate
- dopamine
- glycine
- norepinephrine
- serotonin

The levels of neurotransmitters are determined by levels of the enzymes that produce them. Upsetting the enzymes disrupts the balance and leads to seizures, especially in a high glutamate-GABA ratio. The causes of seizures are

- alcohol or drug withdrawal
- cardiovascular disease (stroke, transient ischemic attacks)
- congenital disorders (brain lesion at birth)
- electric shock
- epilepsy
- genetic factors
- high fever
- hypocalcemia (reduced calcium in serum)
- hypoglycemia, hyperglycemia (low and high sugar in serum, as from diabetes)
- hyponatremia (reduced sodium in serum)
- hypoxia (reduced oxygen to brain)
- infection (meningitis)
- metabolic abnormalities
- neoplasm (brain tumor)
- toxic substances
- trauma (head, hematoma)
- uremia (renal failure)

The two major types of seizures are partial and generalized. Each is subdivided into additional types, according to their manifestations.

PARTIAL SEIZURES Partial seizures are localized in a specific area of the brain, almost always result from injury to the cerebral cortex, and are the most common. Approximately 65% of epileptics suffer from this type of seizure. Partial seizures occur in two distinct types, which can progress to generalized seizures. In a simple-partial seizure, the patient does not lose consciousness, may have some muscular activity manifested in twitching, and may have sensory hallucinations (visual or auditory phenomena). In the other type of partial seizure, the complex-partial seizure, the patient experiences impaired consciousness, often with confusion, blank stare, and post-seizure amnesia.

GENERALIZED SEIZURES Generalized seizures have no local origin but instead involve both hemispheres simultaneously. They are not due to injury or known structural abnormality. They occur in four types: tonic-clonic, absence, myoclonic, and atonic.

- **Tonic-Clonic (Grand Mal)** The tonic portion of the seizure begins with the body becoming rigid, and the patient may fall. This lasts for a minute or less. The clonic portion is initiated with muscle jerks, accompanied by shallow breathing, loss of bladder control, and excess salivation (foaming at the mouth). Jerking continues for a few minutes. After the attack, the patient is drowsy and confused for moments or hours.
- **Absence (Petit Mal)** This seizure type begins with interruption of the patient's activities by some or all of the following signs: blank stare, rotating eyes, uncontrolled facial movements, chewing, rapid eye blinking, twitching or jerking of an arm or leg, but no generalized convulsions. Seizures last from ten seconds to two minutes but are rarely more than thirty seconds. The patient may experience up to one hundred attacks a day. Usually the person has a premonition of the attack through unusual sensations of light, sound, and taste. After the attack, the patient continues activities as if nothing has happened. Seizures are most prevalent during the first ten years of life; 50% of children with absence seizures have tonic-clonic activity as they grow older.
- **Myoclonic** This type occurs with sudden, massive, and brief muscle jerks, which may throw the patient down, or nonmassive, quick jerks of the arm, hand, leg, or foot. Consciousness is not lost, and this seizure type can occur during sleep.
- **Atonic** This type begins with sudden loss of both muscle tone and consciousness. The patient may collapse, the head may drop, and the jaw may slacken. An arm or leg may go limp. The seizure lasts a few seconds to a minute, and then the patient can stand and walk again.

STATUS EPILEPTICUS *Status epilepticus* is a serious disorder that comprises continuous tonic-clonic convulsions, with or without a return to consciousness, lasting at least thirty minutes. It is characterized by high fever and lack of oxygen severe enough to cause brain damage or death. Of the patients who have convulsive *status epilepticus*, 10% die regardless of treatment, often as a complication of sudden drug withdrawal. Therapy is aimed at stopping the convulsions and preventing brain damage. **Valium (diazepam)** is the drug of choice; it takes thirty to sixty seconds for the effects to become apparent. If this does not work, then **Dilantin (phenytoin)** or barbiturates are administered. If antiepileptic therapy does not work and the seizure continues for more than sixty minutes, intubation and general anesthetics are used as a last resort.

Antiepileptic Drug Therapy

Epilepsy can have a profound effect on one's health, quality of life, and ability to function. The optimum antiepileptic therapy would be complete seizure control without compromising the patient's quality of life. Thus, there are two goals of therapy with anticonvulsants. The first goal is to control seizures or to reduce their frequency so the patient can live an essentially normal life. The second goal is to prevent emotional and behavioral changes that may result from the seizures.

Important in the development of antiepileptics is knowledge of the mechanism of neuron activity. In epilepsy, the neuron activity occurs in three stages.

1. polarized (resting)
2. depolarized (firing)
3. repolarized (return to resting)

The entrance of sodium and calcium into the cell causes polarization and depolarization. When sufficient ions accumulate, an electrical charge is transmitted to axon terminal bulbs, which release neurotransmitters. If this happens excessively, neurons fire uncontrollably, causing a seizure. If a drug can block this firing by raising the threshold of depolarization, it can control seizures.

The most important concept in treating epilepsy is to begin with a single drug (monotherapy) and increase the dosage. Once an optimal dosage has been determined, it is essential that the plasma concentration remain stable to ensure seizure control and minimize the risk of side effects. Abrupt discontinuation should be avoided because of the risk of triggering *status epilepticus.* The newer drugs are seizure-specific; that is, their pharmacologic action is directed toward controlling a certain type of seizure activity.

Except in life-threatening situations, single-drug therapy should be initiated at a low dosage (one fourth to one third of the usual daily dosage). The dosage is then increased gradually over three or four weeks until seizures are controlled or adverse effects occur.

Polytherapy should be considered for patients who do not respond to monotherapy. The need for therapy should be evaluated periodically. Some patients can discontinue therapy if they have been seizure-free for several years. To discontinue an antiepileptic drug, the dosage should be decreased gradually over two to six months to prevent withdrawal seizures. The potential for drug interactions during antiepileptic therapy is high.

Antiepileptic drugs interact with each other and with other drugs through two major mechanisms. They can induct or inhibit the hepatic microsomal enzymes responsible for drug metabolism. They can also cause drug displacement from plasma protein.

One possible reason for lack of response to antiepileptic drug therapy is use of an agent inappropriate for the seizure type. In the past, most patients with epilepsy were treated with phenytoin, phenobarbital, or both. Clinicians now recognize that different seizure types require different antiepileptic agents. A drug that controls one seizure type may exacerbate another type. Monotherapy is preferred to multiple-drug therapy because it costs less and causes fewer adverse effects, drug interactions, and compliance problems. Table 9.1 presents the most-commonly used anticonvulsants.

Table 9.1	Most-Commonly Used Anticonvulsants for Partial and Generalized Seizures	
Generic Name	**Brand Name**	**Dosage Form**
carbamazepine	Tegretol	tablet, chewable, suspension
	Epitol	tablet
clonazepam	Klonopin	capsule
divalproex	Depakote	tablet, capsule
ethosuximide	Zarontin	capsule, syrup
fosphenytoin	Cerebyx	IV
gabapentin	Neurontin	capsule
lamotrigine	Lamictal	tablet
levetiracetam	Keppra	tablet
oxcarbazepine	Trileptal	tablet
phenobarbital	Barbita, Luminal, Solfoton	tablet, capsule, solution, IM, IV
phenytoin	Dilantin	tablet, capsule, suspension, IV
primidone	Mysoline	tablet, suspension
topiramate	Topamax	tablet
valproic acid	Depakene	capsule, syrup
zonisamide	Zonegran	capsule

Of epilepsy patients, 30% are poorly controlled with medication and 30% do not comply with therapy because of some of the drug's side effects. The most common side effects are sedation and loss of cognitive processes (i.e., mental perception, memory, judgment).

Carbamazepine, phenytoin, Depakote, and Depakene act on sodium channels to stabilize the neuronal membrane and may decrease the release of excitatory neurotransmitters. Barbiturates and benzodiazepines enhance the inhibitory effect of GABA. The mechanism of gabapentin is unknown. However, it does not interact with GABA receptors.

The therapeutic regimens indicated for the various types of seizures are listed in Table 9.2.

Sometimes two drugs are given together to induce one or the other or to limit the side effects. These drugs all have relatively narrow therapeutic ranges. In some patients, even minor changes in bioavailability can compromise control or result in toxicity. Maintaining a consistent rate and extent of absorption, and thus stable plasma concentrations, is important. Factors that can alter either the rate or the extent of absorption include storage conditions, the drug's physiochemical characteristics, the dosage form, and the patient's physical condition. Pharmacokinetic interactions result from some alteration of absorption, protein binding, metabolism, or elimination.

Zarontin (ethosuximide) is the drug of choice for absence seizures. It reduces calcium transport and increases the seizure threshold. Because of its long half-life, it can usually be given once daily to achieve therapeutic plasma concentrations. The patient should be told to take the dose with food and to not discontinue it abruptly. The drug may cause drowsiness and impair judgment. Patients should have a complete blood count (CBC) every four months during therapy. The side effects are drowsiness, headache, dizziness, nausea, and vomiting.

Depakene (valproic acid) and **Depakote (divalproex)** are two agents to increase the availability of GABA and are indicated for managing simple and complex absence seizures, mixed seizure types, and myoclonic and generalized tonic-clonic seizures. They may also be effective in partial seizures and infantile spasms. The patient should take the dose with water (not with a carbonated drink)

| Table 9.2 | **Therapeutic Regimens for Seizures** |

Seizure Type	Anticonvulsant		
	First Line	**Second Line**	**Third Line**
partial seizure (simple or complex)	carbamazepine or phenytoin	gabapentin or lamotrigine	phenobarbital, primidone, or valproic acid
absence (petite mal)	ethosuximide or valproic acid	clonazepam	
atonic, atypical absence, and myoclonic	valproic acid	clonazepam	
tonic-clonic, tonic, and clonic	carbamazepine, phenytoin, or valproic acid	phenobarbital or primidone	
status epileptius	phenytoin IV diazepan IV lovazepan IV		

and should not chew, break, or crush the tablets or capsules. Patients should be warned to not use aspirin or aspirin products, as these could lead to *serious* valproic acid toxicity. Routine hepatic and hematologic tests are indicated during therapy. Patients should report severe or persistent sore throat, fever, fatigue, bleeding, or bruising. Side effects include drowsiness and impaired judgment or coordination.

Dilantin (phenytoin) is used to manage generalized tonic-clonic, simple-partial, and complex-partial seizures and to prevent seizures after head trauma and neurosurgery. It works in the motor cortex by promoting sodium ion outflow from cells, thus stabilizing the membrane threshold. It is useful for all types of seizures except absence. In some patients, small changes in dose result in large changes in serum concentration. Side effects may or may not be related to dose and are reversible when the dose is reduced. Table 9.3 lists phenytoin's dose-related and non dose-related side effects.

Phenytoin-induced megaloblastic anemia with folic acid deficiency occurs in less than 1% of patients. Prophylactic folic acid supplementation is unnecessary and may alter phenytoin metabolism. Patients should receive routine hepatic and hematologic tests. Phenytoin must be discontinued if even a mild rash appears. The symptoms usually occur within the first eight weeks of therapy and include hepatitis, lymphadenopathy, and hematologic alterations. The rash can progress to Stevens-Johnson syndrome.

Antacid and phenytoin doses should be spaced two to three hours apart. Phenytoin is a potent inducer of hepatic microsomal enzymes and binds avidly to plasma proteins. It interacts with many other drugs. A few interactions are listed in Table 9.4.

Phenytoin adsorbs to nasogastric tubes and must be thoroughly flushed through the tube. In the liquid form, there is a noticeable difference in the concentration of drug from the top of the bottle to the bottom. The drug concentration is much higher when the dose comes from the bottom of the bottle. The bottle should be well shaken before each dose; it can also be stored upside down to help counteract this difference.

Table 9.3	Phenytoin Side Effects
	Side Effects
Dose-Related	ataxia diplopia dizziness drowsiness encephalopathy involuntary movements (at doses > 30 mcg/mL)
Non Dose-Related	gingival hyperplasia peripheral neuropathy vitamin deficiencies

Table 9.4	Phenytoin Interactions		
	alcohol carbamazepine cimetidine clonazepam corticosteroids	cyclosporine heparin oral contraceptives fluoxetine rifampin	theophylline tolbutamide valproate warfarin

Phenytoin can only be mixed in normal saline and should never be infused faster than 50 mg/min. It is one of the few drugs that might be mixed on the floor because it precipitates out so quickly. IV phenytoin should be marked as a "high alert" drug in a hospital setting because of the many problems it presents.

Cerebyx (fosphenytoin) is used instead of IV Dilantin. It is a prodrug (precursor or inactive form) that is rapidly converted to phenytoin after administration. It has the advantage of being water soluble and, therefore, better tolerated. This means fewer infusion reactions (pain, burning, or tissue damage) and more reliable treatment. It does have an unusual side effect of brief, intense itching, usually in the groin, which might be a reaction to the phosphate in the injection, but it is not an allergic response.

Luminal (phenobarbital) is used for generalized tonic-clonic and partial seizures because it interferes with transmission of impulses from the thalamus to the cortex of the brain. Use of alcohol and other CNS depressants should be avoided. The drug should not be stopped abruptly. Phenobarbital is a C-IV agent because it has abuse potential. It can cause drowsiness and paradoxical hyperexcitability in children and the elderly. Periodic blood tests are required.

When filling a prescription for phenobarbital, the pharmacy technician should always check the patient's profile in the computer for other drugs being prescribed. Phenobarbital has several interactions with other drugs, some of which are listed in Table 9.5. If the patient has a rash or exhibits excessive drowsiness, ataxia, dysphagia, slurred speech, and confusion while taking this drug, the physician should be notified immediately.

Mysoline (primidone) is indicated in generalized tonic-clonic and complex-partial seizures. The liver metabolizes the drug to phenobarbital, so the side effect profile and effects profile are similar to those of phenobarbital. Because megaloblastic anemia is a rare side effect of primidone, annual CBCs are recommended.

Tegretol and **Epitol (carbamazepine)** are used in the prophylaxis of generalized tonic-clonic, partial (especially complex-partial), and mixed partial or generalized seizure disorders. They are also used to treat bipolar disorders. The antiepileptic effect may be related to its effects on sodium channels to limit sustained, repetitive firing and alter synaptic transmission. Blood monitoring is important; since carbamazepine induces its own metabolism, the plasma concentration may be lower than expected. The patient should report bleeding, bruising, jaundice, abdominal pain, pale stools, mental disturbances, fever, chills, sore throat, or mouth ulcers. The drug may also cause drowsiness. Like all the other anticonvulsants, carbamazepine has many interactions with other drugs, and these are listed in Table 9.6.

Carbamazepine's side effects can be serious, the most serious being aplastic anemia, but this is rare. A rash may occur, but it does not necessarily mean the drug must be discontinued. The drug should be taken with food to offset GI disturbances. The most serious adverse reaction is fatal hepatotoxicity. The patient should receive hepatic and hematologic tests for the first six months.

Neurontin (gabapentin) is used as adjunctive therapy (drugs added to existing therapy) for drug-refractory (not responsive to treatment) partial and generalized

Warning
Cerebyx looks and sounds like Celexa and Celebrex; be careful in dispensing.

Table 9.5	**Phenobarbital Interactions**	
benzodiazepines	doxycycline	quinidine
beta blockers	griseofulvin	theophylline
CNS depressants	haloperidol	tricyclic antidepressants
corticosteroids	oral contraceptives	warfarin
cyclosporine	phenothiazines	

Table 9.6	Carbamazepine Interactions	
benzodiazepines	ethosuximide	thyroid preparations
cimetidine	isoniazid	tricyclic antidepressants
corticosteroids	MAOIs	valproic acid
cyclosporine	oral contraceptives	verapamil
diltiazem	phenytoin	warfarin
doxycycline	propoxyphene	
erythromycin	theophylline	

Warning

Neurontin and Noroxin could be differentiated by dose. Neurontin is usually 100 mg and Noroxin is 400 mg.

Warning

Lamictal, Lamisil, and Lomotil could be easily mistaken for each other.

Warning

Boxed warnings are special warnings about a drug highlighted in a box in the FDA-approved product information. A black boxed warning is the most serious.

seizures, secondary to the initial seizure in adults with epilepsy. However, it is not effective for absence seizures. It was designed to mimic the neurotransmitter GABA, but studies have shown that it must have another mechanism of action. It does not modify plasma concentrations of standard anticonvulsant medication as do other anticonvulsant drugs. Side effects are somnolence, dizziness, ataxia, fatigue, nystagmus, tremors, and double vision. There are no reported significant drug interactions. Renal function should be monitored.

Gabapentin is being prescribed for neuropathic pain, a stinging and burning pain resulting from nerve damage, such as the type of pain seen in patients with diabetic neuropathy or post-herpetic neuralgia. This pain is treated first with tricyclic antidepressants. If that does not work, the next step is anticonvulsants. Gabapentin seems to work well for some patients, even those with severe and refractory pain. It is also less sedating than the other agents.

The only indication for **Klonopin (clonazepam)**, a C-IV benzodiazepine, is prophylaxis of seizures. It suppresses the spike-and-wave discharge in absence seizures by depressing nerve transmission in the motor cortex. The patient should be told to avoid alcohol and other CNS depressants and to not discontinue the drug abruptly. Physical or psychological dependence may result from its use.

Lamictal (lamotrigine) provides add-on therapy for adults with partial seizures, with or without generalized secondary seizures. The drug works by blocking sodium channels, thereby stabilizing neuronal membranes. Lamotrigine does not affect serum concentrations of phenobarbital, phenytoin, or primidone, but it may affect the pharmacokinetics or pharmacodynamics of carbamazepine and valproate. The drug has a new boxed warning in the FDA-approved product information about fatal rashes. The pharmacist should tell patients to call the physician immediately if a rash appears, but should not tell them to discontinue the drug.

Topamax (topiramate) is for treating partial onset seizures in adults. Although its mechanism of action is not well understood, the most common theories propose that topiramate blocks sodium channels and subsequently enhances the activity of GABA and antagonizes glutamine receptors. It is add-on therapy to carbamazepine or phenytoin. It works well but causes significant cognitive effects (e.g., slowed thinking, slowed speech, and difficulty concentrating). Therapy should start with a low dose and be titrated slowly over eight weeks. Topiramate can increase phenytoin levels. It is a weak carbonic anhydrase inhibitor, so it increases the risk of kidney stones. Patients should drink plenty of water.

Trileptal (oxcarbazepine) blocks voltage sensitive sodium channels and thereby stabilizes hyperexcited neuronal membranes. This drug is most frequently used as an adjunct to other therapies. However, for partial seizure, oxcarbazepine can be used as monotherapy. Female patients taking oxcarbazepine must be warned that this drug decreases the effectiveness of birth control pills. Patients should also be warned about the potentially debilitating drowsiness associated with oxcarbazepine therapy.

Keppra (levetiracetam) is an adjunctive therapy for partial seizures. Keppra's mechanism of action is unknown. This drug also causes drowsiness.

Zonegran (zonisamide) is a sulfonamide with anticonvulsant activity. Patients must be warned about the potentially serious sulfonamide reactions and the pharmacy technician should check for sulfa allergies when dispensing this drug. Patients should also be instructed to report any skin rashes and drink six to eight glasses of water a day to reduce the risks of kidney stones.

ANTI-PARKINSON AGENTS

Parkinson's disease affects about one in one hundred persons over age sixty. About 115 million Americans have the disease. With the elderly increasing in number, expect to see more and more cases of this debilitating disease.

Parkinson's Disease

The extrapyramidal system is a complex functional unit of the CNS involved in the control of motor activities. Parkinson's disease is the most common of the extrapyramidal diseases, a group of disorders resulting from pathologic alterations of the basal ganglia. A distinguishing feature is the presence of Lewy bodies, hyaline-like masses of cytoplasmic proteins consisting of a dense core and a peripheral filamentous halo. As Parkinson's disease progresses, the number of Lewy bodies increases.

Voluntary movement requires complex neurochemical messaging in the brain. Nerve impulses travel, via electrical impulses and neurotransmitters, from the cerebral cortex to the basal ganglia and back to the cerebral cortex via the thalamus. Transmission of information about the initiation of movement, muscle tone, and posture is affected by the balance of neurotransmitters in the basal ganglia. Normal movement requires that the two primary neurotransmitters—dopamine, an inhibitor, and acetylcholine (ACh), a stimulator—be in balance.

In a healthy person, dopaminergic neurons in the substantia nigra release an amount of dopamine sufficient to control the stimulating effect of ACh on large motor and fine muscle movements. In parkinsonism, however, there is progressive destruction of dopaminergic neurons in the nigrostriatal pathway, so an insufficient amount of dopamine is produced to counterbalance ACh production. This results in a predominance of cholinergic neuronal activity.

Parkinson's disease occurs as a result of pathologic alterations in the extrapyramidal system, a complex functional unit of the CNS involved in controlling motor activities. The extrapyramidal system is composed of the basal nuclei, symmetric, subcortical masses of gray matter embedded in the lower portions of the cerebral hemisphere. The disease is characterized by muscular difficulties and postural abnormalities. See Figure 9.1 for an illustration of the location of the basal nuclei. Three characteristic signs of Parkinson's disease are resting tremor, rigidity, and akinesia. These may manifest by poor posture control, shuffling gait, and loss of overall muscle control (e.g., flexed stance, difficulty in turning, hurried gait, and flat emotional affect).

Parkinson's Disease Drug Therapy

The interaction between two neurotransmitters, ACh and dopamine, controls normal function of the basal ganglia. Degeneration of neurons containing dopamine within the CNS creates a deficiency; the results are a dominance of ACh activity that produces excessive motor nerve stimulation. Drug therapy is aimed at objective symptomatic relief; it does not, however, alter the underlying disease process.

Figure 9.1

Cutaway View of the Brain

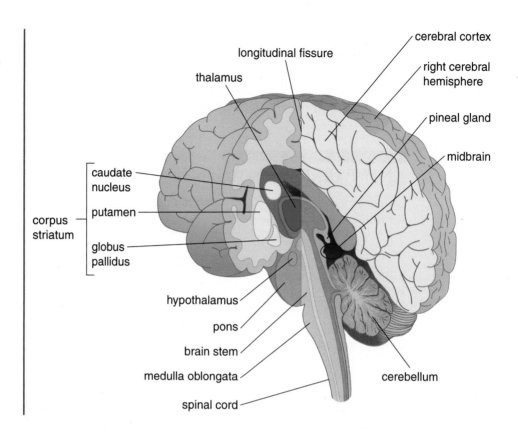

Temporary or prolonged remission allows the patient to live a productive life. Table 9.7 presents the most-commonly used agents for patients with Parkinson's disease.

A problem in the treatment of parkinsonism is the side effects of the drugs. Patients have to tolerate some side effects. Drugs with numerous problems may necessitate constant change in the medication. Often, emotional and psychological support is needed.

Drug therapy has improved greatly the functional ability and clinical status of the patients. The search continues for new agents to prolong the length of effective treatment or reverse the disease.

Table 9.7   Most-Commonly Used Anti-Parkinson Agents

Generic Name	Brand Name	Dosage Form
amantadine	Symmetrel	capsule
benztropine	Cogentin	tablet, IM, IV
bromocriptine	Parlodel	tablet, capsule
entacapone	Comtan	tablet
levodopa	Dopar	capsule
	Larodopa	tablet
levodopa-carbidopa	Sinemet	tablet
pergolide	Permax	tablet
pramipexole	Mirapex	tablet
ropinirole	Requip	tablet
selegiline	Eldepryl	capsule
tolcapone	Tasmar	tablet
trihexyphenidyl	Artane	capsule, elixir, tablet

Table 9.8	Additional Classifications of Anti-Parkinson Agents	

Generic Name	Brand Name	Additional Classification
amantadine	Symmetrel	antiviral
benztropine	Cogentin	antidyskinetic
bromocriptine	Parlodel	ergot alkaloid
selegiline	Eldepryl	MAOI selective MOAB inhibitor

Some drugs used to treat parkinsonism also fit into other drug classifications. Table 9.8 lists these drugs and their additional classifications.

Dopar and **Larodopa (levodopa)**, precursors of dopamine, cross the blood-brain barrier and are metabolized into dopamine in the brain. Dopamine does not cross the blood-brain barrier. Levodopa is converted into dopamine by the peripheral tissues, so the brain does not receive the full dose. This drug has very undesirable effects. The dosage is limited because of the potential for nausea, vomiting, and cardiac arrhythmia. There is also the on-off phenomenon which occurs in as many as two-thirds of Parkinson patients after about five years of therapy. It is a wide fluctuation of functional states, ranging from a hyperkinetic to a hypokinetic state, potentially occurring several times a day. The hyperkinetic state is characterized by dyskinesias and good functional status; the hypokinetic state is characterized by akinesia "freezing" episodes and painful dystonic spasms. These fluctuations are associated primarily with the CNS availability of levodopa at post-synaptic dopamine receptors. Patients may be well controlled on levodopa for several years, and then suddenly they assume a state of akinesia, masked facies (a lack of emotional reflection that presents as a stare with a relentless, unblinking look), and stooped posturing. The drug may just as suddenly start working again. It also causes neuropsychiatric disorders, dementia, loss of memory, hallucinations, and postural hypotension (reduced blood pressure due to inhibition of neurons responsible for vasoconstriction). Levodopa should be carefully titrated to provide optimal control at minimal doses so that the on-off phenomenon is delayed as long as possible.

Sinemet (levodopa-carbidopa) is probably the most-commonly used drug in parkinsonism. The carbidopa prevents peripheral conversion and less dopaminergic side effects. It does not affect the CNS metabolism of levodopa, and lower doses of levodopa can be used as brain concentrations of dopamine increase. There is a smoother, more rapid induction into therapy with this drug.

Parlodel (bromocriptine), an ergot alkaloid with dopaminergic properties, inhibits prolactin secretion (and is also used to dry up milk in breast-feeding mothers). It improves symptoms of Parkinson's disease by directly stimulating dopamine receptors in the corpus striatum. It is usually used with levodopa or Sinemet. The drug should be taken with food or milk. The patient should limit use of alcohol and avoid exposure to cold. Blood pressure should be closely monitored. Drowsiness, nausea, and hypotension are the most common side effects.

Symmetrel (amantadine) is useful to treat parkinsonism and as prophylaxis and treatment for influenza, a viral infection. Its anti-Parkinson activity is a result of blocking the reuptake of dopamine into presynaptic neurons and causing direct stimulation of postsynaptic receptors. The second dose of the day should be taken in the early afternoon to decrease the incidence of insomnia. Abrupt discontinuation of therapy should be avoided.

Eldepryl (selegiline) is a potent MAO type B inhibitor found primarily in the brain. It plays a major role in the metabolism of dopamine and may increase dopaminergic activity by interfering with dopamine reuptake at the synapse. The daily dose should not exceed 10 mg.

Cogentin (benztropine) blocks central cholinergic receptors, helping to balance cholinergic activity in the basal ganglia. Indications for the use of this drug are acute dystonic reactions, parkinsonism, and drug-induced extrapyramidal reactions. It may also prolong dopamine's effects by blocking dopamine reuptake and storage at central receptor sites. This drug should be administered after meals to prevent GI irritation. Constipation is the primary side effect. It should not be discontinued abruptly.

Permax (pergolide) is an ergot alkaloid similar to bromocriptine but more potent and longer-acting. This drug stimulates dopamine$_1$ and dopamine$_2$ receptor sites and is used as adjunctive treatment to Sinemet for Parkinson's disease. Pergolide must be taken with food or milk. The primary side effects are hypotension (the patient should rise slowly from sitting or lying positions), insomnia, abnormal vision, and diarrhea. Any confusion or change in mental status should be reported to the physician.

Artane (trihexyphenidyl) is an adjunctive treatment of Parkinson's. It is also used in treatment of drug-induced extrapyramidal symptoms (EPS) and acute dystonic reactions. It is thought to block excess ACh. It should be taken with food and alcohol should be avoided. It may cause excessive dryness of the mouth.

Mirapex (pramipexole) is a dopamine agonist, which is more selective for dopamine$_2$ receptors but has also been shown to bind to dopamine$_3$ and dopamine$_4$ receptors. This drug works as well as other anti-Parkinson's drugs but has fewer side effects. Unlike Permax and Parlodel, Mirapex is not an ergot derivative. Mirapex should be prescribed early in the disease either as a monotherapy or in combination with Sinemet. It should be taken with food to reduce nausea.

Requip (ropinirole), like Mirapex, has a high in vitro specificity activity at the dopamine$_2$ and dopamine$_3$ receptors, binding with higher affinity of the dopamine$_3$ receptors. The precise mechanism of action is unknown. It can be taken without regard to food. Hypotension, especially at the beginning of therapy or dose escalation can cause severe dizziness, especially with a change in position.

Tasmar (tolcapone) is the first of a new class of anti-Parkinson's agents known as COMT (catechol-o-methyl transferase) inhibitors. The inhibitition of COMT, an enzyme that metabolizes levodopa in the body, allows greater levels of levodopa to reach the brain, thereby extending the drug's beneficial life. The COMT inhibitors have no clinical effect unless they are combined with levodopa. Talcapone was approved by the FDA in 1998 but has since been linked to three fatal liver injuries. As a result the medication now carries a warning label recommending its use be limited to people who do not respond to or are not appropriate candidates for other available treatments. Tolcapone has been shown to increase patient "on-time" by an average of two to three hours per day. The drug should be discontinued if the patient does not demonstrate any improvement within three weeks.

Comtan (entacapone) is the second COMT inhibitor to be approved by the FDA. Whereas tolcapone penetrates the CNS, entacapone acts peripherally. Thus, entacapone is expected to be less toxic than tolcapone. Entacapone is indicated for patients who are experiencing a deteriorating response to levodopa in the earlier stages of motor fluctuations. This drug can be taken without regard to food.

OTHER CNS DISORDERS

Several other neurologic disorders share symptoms and signs with the convulsive disorders and Parkinson's disease. They include myasthenia gravis, attention-deficit hyperactivity disorder and attention-deficit disorder, Amyotrophic Lateral Sclerosis (ALS), Multiple Sclerosis (MS), and Alzheimer's disease.

Myasthenia Gravis

Myasthenia gravis is a disorder of the neuromuscular junction resulting from autoimmune damage to the nicotine cholinergic receptors. The ACh receptors are destroyed at the motor end plate (Figure 9.2). The disorder is characterized by weakness and fatigability, especially of the skeletal muscles, due to the reduction in number of ACh receptors at the myoneural junction. The weakness is typically worse after exercise and better after rest, but may be constant. Presenting signs include ptosis (paralytic drooping of the upper eyelid), diplopia, dysarthria, dysphagia, extremity weakness, and respiratory difficulty. The clinical course is variable and includes spontaneous remissions and exacerbations.

Acetylcholinesterase drugs can produce clinical improvement in all forms. They allow ACh to last longer and may be used with corticosteroids. This does not inhibit or reverse the basic immunologic flaw. The ACh remaining in the junction sites interacts with ACh receptors for longer periods of time. Table 9.9 lists the most-commonly used drugs for myasthenia gravis.

Tensilon (edrophonium) is used to diagnose myasthenia gravis. It often produces marked improvement of patients' strength. The response lasts five minutes.

Figure 9.2

Motor End Plate
The interface between the nervous system and the muscular system is the neuromuscular junction.

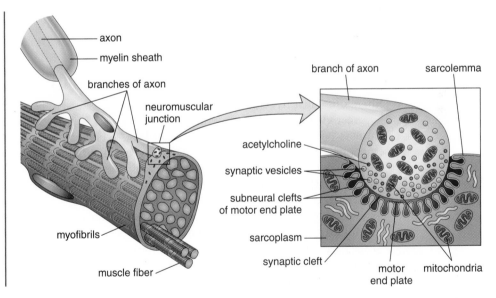

Table 9.9	Most-Commonly Used Agents for Myasthenia Gravis

Generic Name	Brand Name	Dosage Form
azathioprine	Imuran	tablet, IV
cyclophosphamide	Cytoxan	tablet, IV
edrophonium	Tensilon	IV
neostigmine	Prostigmin	tablet, IM, IV, SC
pyridostigmine	Mestinon	tablet, syrup, IM, IV

Prostigmin (neostigmine) and **Mestinon (pyridostigmine)** are used to treat myasthenia gravis or to reverse nondepolarizing muscle relaxants. They block ACh hydrolysis by cholinesterase, resulting in ACh accumulation at cholinergic synapses, increasing stimulation of cholinergic receptors at the myoneural junction. They interact with procainamide, quinidine, corticosteroids, succinylcholine, and magnesium. The drugs should be taken with food or milk. It is equally important to take them exactly as directed and at the same time each day.

These oral, IM, and IV drugs inhibit the destruction of ACh by acetylcholinesterase, which facilitates transmission of impulses across the myoneural junction. Side effects are generally due to exaggerated pharmacologic effects. The most common side effects are salivation and muscle fasciculation. The physician should be notified of any nausea, vomiting, muscle weakness, severe abdominal pain, or difficulty in breathing.

Chemotherapeutic agents are sometimes used in treating myasthenia gravis. The side effects of these immunosuppressive drugs are leukopenia, pancytopenia, infection, GI irritation, and abnormal liver function tests.

Imuran (azathioprine) suppresses cell-mediated hypersensitivity, alters antibody production, and reverses neuromuscular blockade. It is taken with food to avoid nausea.

Cytoxan (cyclophosphamide), an alkylating agent, prevents cell division by cross-linking deoxyribonucleic acid (DNA) strands. Guidelines for preparing and disposing of chemotherapeutic agents should be followed. Administration with cold foods, such as ice cream, should improve the oral dose. Fluids should be taken liberally (3 liters per day). Cystitis is a frequently occurring side effect, even months after therapy has been discontinued. Uric acid, CBCs, and renal and hepatic functions should be monitored. Alopecia is a side effect, as well as nausea, vomiting, and bone marrow depression. The side effect profile is typical of any chemotherapeutic drug.

Attention-Deficit Hyperactivity Disorder and Attention-Deficit Disorder

Attention-deficit hyperactivity disorder (ADHD) is assessed by three characteristics: hyperactivity, impulsivity, and distractibility. ADHD is characterized by purposeless, chronic, pervasive, driven behavior that blocks a child from participating in social, emotional, and academic learning. On the other hand, attention-deficit disorder (ADD) has less hyperactivity. The ADD child is more lethargic and easily distracted than an ADHD or a child without these disorders. Attention-deficit hyperactivity and attention-deficit disorders are more common in boys than girls. Although ADHD is thought of as a disease of childhood, some symptoms can persist into adult life. Several drugs are used primarily for this disorder, and they are listed in Table 9.10.

Table 9.10	**Most-Commonly Used Agents for Attention-Deficit Disorders**	
Generic Name	**Brand Name**	**Dosage Form**
amphetamine-dextroamphetamine	Adderall	tablet
clonidine	Catapres	tablet
	Catapres-TTS	transdermal system
desipramine	Norpramin	capsule, tablet
imipramine	Tofranil	tablet, capsule, IM
methylphenidate	Ritalin	tablet
nortriptyline	Aventyl, Pamelor	capsule, oral solution
pemoline	Cylert	tablet, chewable

Ritalin (methylphenidate), a C-II agent, is the drug of choice to treat attention-deficit disorders and narcolepsy. It often improves concentration by increasing the levels of neurotransmitters in the brain. It should be used as an adjunct to psychosocial measures. Like amphetamine, it has a paradoxical calming effect in hyperactive children. A CBC differential (number of types of cells) and platelet count should be monitored during long-term therapy. Intermittent drug-free periods when stress is less (such as during weekends and vacations) may help prevent development of tolerance and permit decreased dosage when the drug is resumed. Caffeine may decrease this drug's efficacy, so the patient should avoid coffee, tea, and colas. The patient should get plenty of rest. The drug does have abuse potential.

Cylert (pemoline), a C-IV agent, is an alternative to methylphenidate. It does not seem to work as well but is less likely to be abused. It can cause serious liver toxicity. The manufacturer has added a boxed warning to the product information that liver failure can come on suddenly and may not be detected with periodic screening.

Tofranil (imipramine) is a tricyclic antidepressant. It is sometimes used for ADD, ADHD, and is also used to treat bedwetting in children.

Norpramin (desipramine) and **Aventyl** and **Pamelor (nortriptyline)** are also TCAs used to treat these disorders.

Catapres and **Catapres-TTS (clonidine)** are helpful in controlling aggression. These drugs stimulate alpha adrenergic receptors in the brain stem and thereby reduce sympathetic nervous system overflow. They reduce hyperactivity and improve sleep. For Catapres, the treatment should start with a low dose of the drug, taken before bedtime.

Adderall (amphetamine-dextroamphetamine), a C-II agent, is an alternative to other stimulants. Its effects can last about six hours, long enough to get some children through the school day. The primary side effect is depression as the drug wears off. After six hours, some children become depressed.

Amyotrophic Lateral Sclerosis (ALS)

Amyotrophic lateral sclerosis (ALS), also known as Lou Gehrig's disease, is a progressive degenerative disease of the nerves that leads to muscle weakness, paralysis, and eventually death. It is thought to be caused by excessive levels of glutamate, an excitatory neurotransmitter that causes nerve damage.

Until recently there were no drugs to treat this syndrome. **Rilutek (riluzole)** is the first drug approved for ALS. It inhibits the release of glutamate, inactivates sodium channels, and interfers with intracellular events following transmitter binding at excitatory receptors. Riluzole has been shown to improve survival by approximately three months in some patients.

Multiple Sclerosis (MS)

Multiple sclerosis (MS) is considered to be an autoimmune disease in which the myelin sheaths around nerves degenerate. The patient loses use of the muscles, and often eyesight is affected. In the later stages of the disease, there is severe trembling. Some drugs can slow the progression of the disease, but there is no cure. Table 9.11 lists the agents most-commonly used to treat MS.

Betaseron is for use in ambulatory patients with relapsing, remitting MS. It is given every other day. Most patients report flulike symptoms, and to avoid these, prophylaxis with acetaminophen is indicated. A photosensitivity reaction may occur.

Avonex is an interferon but chemically different from Betaseron. It reduces the frequency of attacks in patients with the relapsing-remitting form of MS. It also delays disability (the only drug that has been able to do this). It is given once a

Table 9.11   Most-Commonly Used Agents for Multiple Sclerosis

Generic Name	Brand Name	Dosage Form
glatiramer acetate	Copaxone	injection, SC
interferon beta-1a	Avonex	single-dose vial, SC
interferon beta-1b	Betaseron	injection, SC
tizanidine	Zanaflex	tablet

week and has fewer side effects. The cost is about the same as for Betaseron. The drug should not be exposed to high temperatures or freezing.

Copaxone (glatiramer acetate) seems to block the autoimmune reaction against myelin that leads to nerve damage. It decreases the frequency of relapses, but it has not been shown to slow disease progress. It is given every day by subcutaneous injection. It may cause local injection-site reactions and brief flushing, chest pain, and shortness of breath; these are bothersome but benign. The drug must be stored frozen.

Zanaflex (tizanidine) is indicated to reduce muscle spasticity in MS and spinal cord injuries. This drug works via the inhibition of presynaptic motor neurons. Zanaflex is the first new oral drug approved for spasticity since Lioresal (baclofen). It is structurally similar to clonidine and has similar side effects (dry mouth, sedation, dizziness, and hypotension).

Lioresal (baclofen) is a skeletal muscle relaxant used to treat MS, spinal cord lesions, intractable hiccups, and bladder spasticity. It inhibits transmission of reflexes at the spinal cord level with resultant relief of muscle spasticity. Onset requires three to four days. It should be taken with food and may cause drowsiness.

Alzheimer's Disease

Alzheimer's disease is a form of dementia. This disease was first described by German psychiatrist, Alois Alzheimer in 1907. It is a degenerative disorder of the brain that leads to progressive dementia (loss of memory, intellect, judgment, orientation, and speech) and changes in personality and behavior. In the early stages of the disease, the patient complains of memory deficit, forgetfulness, and/or misplacement of ordinary items. Depression is a part of the disease profile. As the disease progresses, complex tasks become impossible (for example, managing personal finances), concentration becomes poor, and in the final stages there is complete incapacitation, disorientation, and failure to thrive. There are no agents that will reverse the cognitive abnormalities. The depression associated with the disease is often treated with antidepressants determined by existing symptoms and adverse drug reaction profiles. Amitriptyline should be avoided in these patients due to its high anticholinergic profile. Agitation and sleep disturbances should be treated with short-acting benzodiazepines. Table 9.12 lists the drugs most commonly used to treat Alzheimer's disease.

Table 9.12   Most-Commonly Used Agents for Alzheimer's

Generic Name	Brand Name	Dosage Form
donepezil	Aricept	tablet
gingko	(any)	tablet
tacrine	Cognex	tablet

Cognex (tacrine) is a cholinesterase inhibitor. The most common side effect is an increase in liver function tests. It is metabolized through cytochrome P-450 so it interacts with other drugs that are metabolized through that system. It must be taken four times a day on an empty stomach.

Warning
Aricept and AcipHex labels are nearly identical.

Aricept (donepezil) is similar to Cognex. Both cause improvements in memory and alertness, but Aricept is more selective for the cholinesterase that is in the CNS. This means less nausea, vomiting, and diarrhea. Also, liver function tests are not necessary. Aricept is also more convenient. Unlike Cognex, Aricept is given only once a day at bedtime.

Gingko, an herb, has shown good results in improving cognitive function and social behavior in Alzheimer's patients. Use the concentrated gingko tablets. They have antioxidant and anti-inflammatory effects. Gingko improves blood flow and inhibits platelet aggregation. It is much less expensive than the other drugs and, of course, is an OTC drug. It takes six to twelve weeks to see improvement.

Chapter Summary

Epilepsy

- Epilepsy is a common neurologic disorder defined as paroxysmal, recurring seizures. It involves disturbances of neuronal electrical activity that interfere with normal brain function.
- Two major classifications of seizures are generalized and partial.
- The objective of antiepileptic drug therapy is to eliminate seizures without compromising the patient's quality of life because of adverse effects.
- All anticonvulsants have very narrow dose/therapeutic ranges. A slight dose change can result in loss of seizure control or toxicity.
- Different seizure types require different drugs.
- The first-line drug for simple or complex seizures is carbamazepine or phenytoin; for absence seizures it is ethosuximide or valproate; for atonic, absence, myoclonic, and atypical seizures it is valproate; for tonic-clonic and tonic and clonic seizures it is carbamazepine or phenytoin or valproate.
- Boxed warnings are special warnings about a drug highlighted in a box in the FDA-approved product information.

Anti-Parkinson Agents

- For normal movements to be performed, the two primary neurotransmitters—dopamine (an inhibitor) and acetylcholine (a stimulator)—must be in balance. In parkinsonism these transmitters are not in balance.
- Dopamine will not cross the blood-brain barrier, so it must be combined with drugs that will.
- Sinemet, a levodopa-carbidopa preparation, is probably the most-commonly used drug in parkinsonism.
- Parlodel is used to treat parkinsonism; it is also used to dry up breast milk in a nursing mother.
- Eldepryl is an MAOI used in treating parkinsonism.

Other CNS Disorders

- Acetylcholinesterase drugs can produce clinical improvement in all forms of myasthenia gravis.
- Ritalin is the drug of choice to treat attention-deficit disorders.
- Ritalin is a CNS stimulant and C-II controlled substance used primarily for attention deficit disorders in children and narcolepsy in adults.
- Rilutek (riluzole) is the first drug approved for amyotrophic lateral sclerosis (Lou Gehrig's disease). It inhibits the release of glutamate and seems to improve survival by about three months.
- Among the drugs used to treat multiple sclerosis are two chemically different interferons.
- Copaxone is an MS drug that must be kept frozen.
- Zanaflex is the first oral drug approved for spasticity since Lioresal.
- Alzheimer's is a progressive form of dementia.
- Cognex and Aricept are used to treat Alzheimer's; Aricept has fewer side effects.
- Gingko has shown good results in improving cognitive function and social behavior in Alzheimer's patients.

Drug Summary

The following drugs were discussed in this chapter. Each generic drug name is followed in parentheses by one or more brand names. An asterisk (*) indicates drugs frequently written using *either* brand *or* generic name. These need to be memorized.

Anticonvulsants
carbamazepine (Tegretol, Epitol)*
clonazepam (Klonopin)*
divalproex (Depakote)
ethosuximide (Zarontin)*
fosphenytoin (Cerebyx)
gabapentin (Neurontin)
lamotrigine (Lamictal)
levetiracetam (Keppra)
oxcarbazepine (Trileptal)
phenobarbital (Solfoton, Bellatal, Luminal)*
phenytoin (Dilantin)*
primidone (Mysoline)*
topiramate (Topamax)
valproic acid (Depakene)*
zonisamide (Zonegran)

Anti-Parkinson Agents
amantadine (Symmetrel)*
benztropine (Cogentin)*
bromocriptine (Parlodel)*
entacapone (Comtan)
levodopa (Dopar, Larodopa)
levodopa-carbidopa (Sinemet)*
pergolide (Permax)
pramipexole (Mirapex)
ropinirole (Requip)
selegiline (Eldepryl)
tolcapone (Tasmar)
trihexyphenidyl (Artane)

Myasthenia Gravis
azathioprine (Imuran)
cyclophosphamide (Cytoxan)
edrophonium (Tensilon)
neostigmine (Prostigmin)
pyridostigmine (Mestinon)

Attention-Deficit Disorders
amphetamine-dextroamphetamine (Adderall)
clonidine (Catapres, Catapres-TTS)
desipramine (Norpramin)
imipramine (Tofranil)*
methylphenidate (Ritalin)*
nortriptyline (Aventyl, Pamelor)
pemoline (Cylert)

Amyotrophic Lateral Sclerosis (ALS)
riluzole (Rilutek)

Multiple Sclerosis (MS)
baclofen (Lioresal)
glatiramer acetate (Copaxone)
interferon beta-1a (Avonex)
interferon beta-1b (Betaseron)
tizanidine (Zanaflex)

Alzheimer's Disease
donepezil (Aricept)
gingko (any)
tacrine (Cognex)

Chapter Review

Pharmaceuticals and Body Functions

Select the best answer from the choices given.

1. Seizures can be caused by
   a. epilepsy.
   b. alcohol withdrawal.
   c. infection.
   d. All of the above

2. The two major classifications of seizures are
   a. generalized and partial.
   b. simple-partial and complex-partial.
   c. tonic-clonic and atonic.
   d. absence and myoclonic.

3. Goals of epilepsy therapy are
   a. to control seizures or reduce their frequency to the extent that the patient can live essentially a normal life.
   b. to prevent emotional and behavioral changes.
   c. a and b.
   d. None of the above

4. Which is the drug of choice for absence seizures?
   a. Dilantin
   b. Depakote
   c. Depakene
   d. Zarontin

5. Which drug has a new boxed warning about fatal rashes?
   a. Cerebyx
   b. Klonopin
   c. Lamictal
   d. Neurontin

6. Which liquid drug should be well shaken before administering?
   a. Phenytoin
   b. Primidone
   c. Carbamazepine
   d. Phenobarbital

7. Which anticonvulsant is a scheduled drug?
   a. Phenytoin
   b. Primidone
   c. Carbamazepine
   d. Phenobarbital

8. Which drug is metabolized to phenobarbital?
   a. Carbamazepine
   b. Primidone
   c. Phenytoin
   d. Valproic acid

9. Which anticonvulsants are used to treat bipolar disorders?
   a. Carbamazepine and valproic acid
   b. Phenytoin and ethosuximide
   c. Phenobarbital and gabapentin
   d. Clonazepam and Klonopin

10. The only approved indication for Klonopin is
    a. migraine headaches.
    b. anxiety.
    c. seizures.
    d. None of the above

The following statements are true or false. If the answer is false, rewrite the statement so it is true.

_____ 1. The drug of choice for convulsive *status epilepticus* is Klonopin.

_____ 2. Dopamine crosses the blood-brain barrier.

_____ 3. Sinemet is an antiparkinson drug that has an "on-off" phenomenon.

_____ 4. The most-commonly used drug in parkinsonism is levodopa.

_____ 5. Amantadine can be used for prophylaxis and treatment of flu.

_____ 6. Parlodel can be used to dry up milk in a nursing mother.

_____ 7. Cylert is the drug of choice in treating attention-deficit hyperactivity disorder.

_____ 8. Copaxone must be kept frozen.

_____ 9. Cylert has been the causative factor of some liver toxicity.

_____ 10. Attention-deficit hyperactivity disorder has been characterized by hyper-activity, distractibility, and impulsivity.

Diseases and Drug Therapies

1. List five causes of seizures.
2. List the three stages of neuron activity in epilepsy.
3. What is the big advantage of Lamictal in the treatment of seizures?
4. What are the uses of Parlodel?

Dispensing Medications

The following prescriptions are brought in. Identify a possible disease state that is being treated.

1. 25-year-old woman: Parlodel
2. 10-year-old boy: Zarontin
3. 50-year-old man: Parlodel
4. 50-year-old man: Sinemet
5. 20-year-old man: Symmetrel
6. 50-year-old man: Permax
7. 50-year-old man: Ritalin
8. 10-year-old boy: Ritalin
9. 35-year-old man: Rilutek
10. 25-year-old woman: Betaseron

Internet Research

Use the Internet to complete the following assignments.

1. Locate information related to ongoing clinical trials aimed at the development of new treatments for Parkinson's disease. Create a table listing at least five experimental therapies. Indicate the phase (one through three) of testing presently underway and where (institution and country) the trials are taking place. List your Internet sources.
2. Identify three Internet sites that offer guidance related to the management of epilepsy. Which of these sites would you recommend most highly to a patient and why?

Respiratory, GI, Renal, and Cardiac Drugs

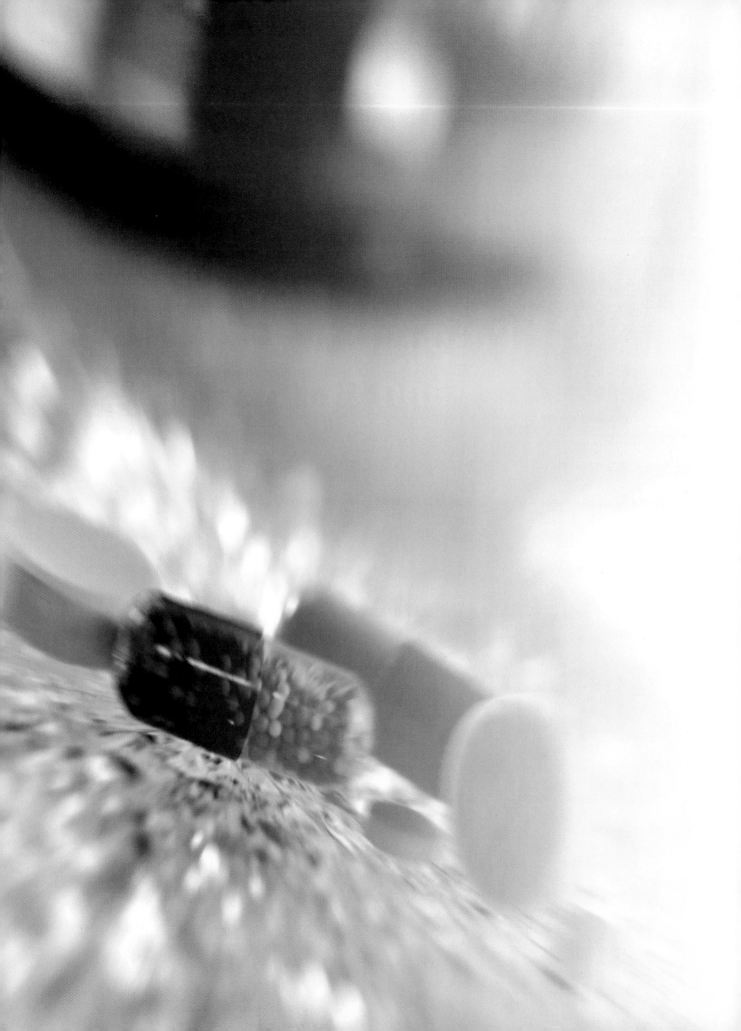

Respiratory Drugs

Learning Objectives

◇ Differentiate the pulmonary diseases.

◇ Learn the pathophysiology and treatment of asthma.

◇ Define the goals of asthma treatment.

◇ Discuss the pathophysiology and treatment of emphysema and chronic bronchitis.

◇ Learn how pneumonia, cystic fibrosis, and respiratory distress syndrome fit into this category of diseases.

◇ Be aware of the reemergence of tuberculosis and of treatment for this disease.

◇ Outline smoking cessation plans and supportive therapy.

Chronic obstructive pulmonary disease (COPD) encompasses two major diseases: emphysema and chronic bronchitis. COPD is irreversible. Asthma, a reversible syndrome, obstructs inspiration, whereas emphysema and chronic bronchitis obstruct expiration. Related diseases, also obstructive, are pneumonia and other respiratory tract infections, cystic fibrosis, respiratory distress syndrome, and tuberculosis. Closely linked to many of these diseases is smoking; many innovative drugs are available to help the smoker quit.

ASTHMA

Asthma is a lung disease precipitated by specific triggering events that have relative degrees of importance from patient to patient. It is a reversible airway obstruction with intermittent attacks. Studies strongly support the concept of genetic predisposition to developing asthma. An allergic component is present in 35% to 55% of patients. The allergens that provoke asthma are airborne and evoke the response through classic allergic pathways.

Asthma differs from normal pulmonary defense mechanisms in its severity of bronchospasm and apparent failure of normal dilator systems, excessive production of mucus that plugs airways, and the presence of sometimes severe long-term inflammatory reactions that may lead to patchy shedding of the small airways' lining. The asthmatic lung is more sensitive and responds to lower doses of allergen challenge than the normal lung.

Asthma is a disease in which inflammation (irritation in the lungs) causes the patient's airways to tighten. Asthma is most commonly classified as either allergic, exercise-induced, or nonallergic. Asthma has the following characteristics: reversible small airway obstruction, progressive airway inflammation, and increased airway responsiveness to a variety of endogenous and exogenous stimuli. These characteristics translate into recurrent episodes of wheezing, dyspnea, and cough that have both acute and chronic manifestations in most patients.

The Asthmatic Response

Mast cells mediate a variety of cells and events in the inflammatory process. These cells are activated by immunoglobulin E (IgE), air inhalation during exercise, cold weather, and allergens. This leads to airway obstruction caused by smooth-muscle contractions, increased secretion of mucus, and increased vascular permeability (see Figure 10.1).

An asthma attack consists of two phases or responses. The first response is often triggered by an antigen antibody reaction and is characterized by degranulation of the mast cells, which releases histamine and other mediators, resulting in immediate bronchospasm (constriction of bronchial smooth muscle) and increased production of mucus, which often forms plugs in the small airways with plasma leaking into tissue. This results in the release of mediators: histamines, eosinophils, chemotactic factor, platelet-activating factor, bradykinin, prostaglandins, and leukotrienes. The second response is bronchoconstriction with delayed, sustained reactions including epithelial damage that make the airway more sensitive to further challenge, even weeks after exposure. The late response causes self-sustaining inflammation.

The most useful measure to assess severity and follow the course of asthma on a regular basis is the peak expiratory flow rate (PEFR), the maximum flow rate generated during a forced expiratory maneuver, measured in liters per minute. A measurement below 50% indicates a medical alert; immediate treatment with a bronchodilator and anti-inflammatory agent is needed, and the physician should be notified.

Goals of Asthma Care and Management of the Disease

For the patient, the goals of asthma care are to

◇ sleep well every night
◇ be able to go to work or school every day

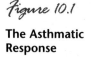

The Asthmatic Response

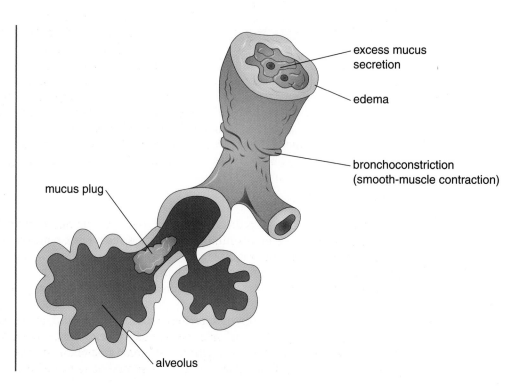

excess mucus secretion

edema

bronchoconstriction (smooth-muscle contraction)

mucus plug

alveolus

- be free from wheezing all day
- have good control of coughing
- be able to continue with activities and exercise
- tolerate medicines well

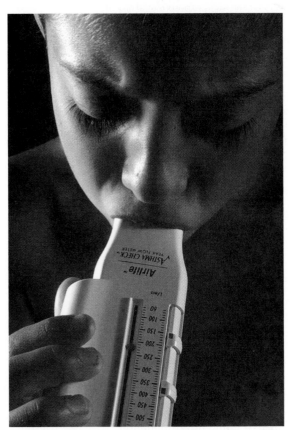

A peak flow meter is a valuable tool for asthma patients to use to measure and manage symptoms.

As part of good asthma care, the asthmatic patient must learn to manage the disease and its complications and to limit the amount of exposure to irritants that will cause airway inflammation. The patient will need to learn which things trigger asthma attacks and how to control those trigger factors. For example, the asthmatic patient should avoid contact with smoke as much as possible because smoke definitely harms patients with asthma. Also, because most asthmatics are allergic to dust mites, patients should follow simple dust mite control steps, including washing sheets and mattress pads at least once a week in hot (130° F or hotter) water. Asthma patients should obtain a yearly flu vaccination.

Symptoms alone are not always the best measure of respiratory status. For this reason, patients must learn to use a peak flow meter. The peak flow meter should be used twice a day and the results should be recorded in a diary as an aid to better management. Often, simply adjusting the asthma medications on the basis of the peak flow meter readings helps effectively manage asthma.

It is imperative that asthmatics and caregivers be aware of the signs and symptoms of *status asthmaticus*, which is a potentially life-threatening condition. An episode of *status asthmaticus* begins as any other asthma attack but, unlike an ordinary attack, it will not respond to normal management. The patient suffering from such an episode will experience increasing difficulty in breathing and will exhibit blue lips and nail beds. Finally, the patient may potentially lose consciousness. *Status asthmaticus* clearly constitutes a medical emergency and the patient should receive prompt attention. This may involve a visit to the emergency room.

Asthma Drug Therapy

The mainstay of asthma management is drug therapy. The appropriate drug therapy is defined by the persistence of the asthma attacks the patient suffers. The phases of the disease begin with intermittent attacks, followed by mild to severe, persistent symptoms. Treatment should start at the step most appropriate to the condition's initial severity. Table 10.1 lists the drug therapy for each step in the progression of the disease.

A rescue course of corticosteroids may be needed at any time and any step. If control is not achieved, the patient's medication technique and compliance, and then avoidance of allergens or other trigger factors (environmental control) should be reviewed. If these are all adequate, treatment should be reviewed every three to six

Table 10.1	Stepwise Approach to Asthma Therapy

Step 1. Intermittent Attacks
- Short-acting oral or inhaled β₂ agonist as needed for symptom control, but less than once a week. (Examples of short-acting inhaled β₂ agonists include albuterol, bitolterol, isoetharine, isoproterenol, metaproterenol, and pirbuterol.)
- Inhaled β₂ agonist or cromolyn sodium before exercise or exposure to allergen.
- Move patient to Step 2 when more than one canister a month is needed.
- Daily medications: none.

Step 2. Mild, Persistent Disease
- Short-acting oral or inhaled β₂ agonist as needed for symptom control, not to exceed three to four times in one day.
- Daily medications: inhaled corticosteroid *or* mast cell stabalizer *or* sustained-release (SR) β₂ agonist; may add long-acting bronchodilator (especially for nighttime symptoms). Examples of long-acting inhaled β₂ agonists include salmeterol and terbutaline.
- Leukotriene modifiers are second-line agents for this stage as well as theophylline for resistant cases.

Step 3. Moderate, Persistent Disease
- Short-acting oral or inhaled β₂ agonist as needed for symptom control, not to exceed three to four times in one day.
- Daily medications: inhaled corticosteroid *and* long-acting bronchodilator, especially for nighttime symptoms, *and either* an SR long-acting β₂ agonist *or* a long-acting oral β₂ agonist. For some patients, adding Serevent works better than doubling the inhaled corticosteroid.

Step 4. Severe, Persistent Disease
- Short-acting oral or inhaled β₂ agonist as needed for symptom control.
- Daily medications: inhaled corticosteroid *and* long-acting bronchodilator, *and either* an SR long-acting β₂ agonist *and/or* a long-acting oral β₂ agonist and oral corticosteroid long term.

months. If control is sustained for at least three months, a gradual stepwise reduction in treatment may be possible.

For exercise-induced asthma the best treatment is inhalation of terbutaline or albuterol, which provides protection for two hours after inhalation.

Beta blockers are contraindicated in asthmatics because they constrict the bronchial tubes. They should avoid antihistamines in an acute attack. Many asthmatics are sensitive to aspirin and other drugs such as NSAIDs, penicillins, cephalosporins, and sulfas.

By far, the predominant use of inhaled medications is for the treatment of asthma. In treating asthma, one of the most common methods of administering medication is by nebulizer, which uses a stream of air flowing past a liquid to create a fine mist. The nebulizer utilizes a compressor which propels air past a solution containing the medication, causing a fine mist. While breathing normally, the patient inhales the mist through a mouthpiece or mask. The drug thus has a higher likelihood of being deposited further into the lungs. It is a very effective delivery system, especially for young children. If not properly cared for, home nebulizers can be a source of bronchitis and infections. Therefore, nebulizers should be cleaned daily. Contaminated saline can create a problem for the patient.

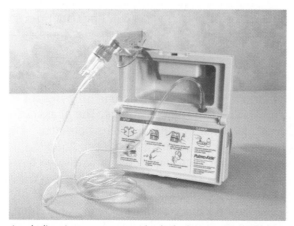

A nebulizer is a common method of administering asthma medication. It is especially effective for children.

The other important method of administering asthma medications is by a metered dose inhaler (MDI)—sometimes called a "puffer"—that contains medication and compressed gas. The MDI delivers a specific amount of medication with each actuation. In both methods, the idea is to suspend the medication in particles or droplets fine enough to penetrate to the deepest parts of the lungs.

The metered dose inhaler is sometimes ordered to be used with a spacer. A spacer is recommended to decrease the amount of spray deposited on the back of the throat and swallowed. The spacer chamber holds the drug mist until the patient is ready to breathe. It also allows the patient to breathe the mist in at a slower, more effective rate, depositing the drug further in the lungs. It can reduce side effects by more effectively delivering the drug to the lower portions of the lungs and leaving fewer particles in the oropharynx to be absorbed. It is extremely useful for children and the elderly who have a hard time coordinating an inhaler.

Patients should always use the lowest effective dose. Serevent should be added to inhaled corticosteroid if needed to decrease the steroid dose needed for control. Table 10.2 lists the most-commonly used agents for asthma.

Long-term control medications are cromolyn, nedocromil, inhaled steroids, theophylline, long-acting β_2 agonists, and leukotriene antagonists. Quick relief medications for reversal of acute exacerbations include short-acting β_2 agonists, systemic corticosteroids, and ipratropium. Some physicians may begin patients at a higher step to gain control and then reduce therapy to the minimum required for control. There is evidence supporting a more aggressive initial approach.

If a spacer is added to the metered dose inhaler, the medication will penetrate deeper into the tissue of the lungs than if the metered dose inhaler was used without a spacer.

BRONCHODILATORS Adrenalin (epinephrine) is the drug of choice for acute attacks. It is given subcutaneously immediately. Many asthmatics carry an EpiPen. Epinephrine acts as a bronchodilator through β_2 receptos, relaxing smooth muscles and relief of bronchospasm. The OTC aerosols, Primatene Mist and Bronkaid Mist, should not be used more than eight times a day.

Side effects of epinephrine need to be monitored. The alpha agonist actions of the drug increases blood pressure, which increases risk of angina, aortic rupture, and cerebral hemorrhage due to vasoconstriction. The β_1 agonist action causes palpitation, tachycardia, and arrhythmias. The β_2 agonist action causes CNS stimulation (nervousness, tremor, anxiety, nausea, vomiting) and relaxation of uterine muscles. The β_2 agonists may also have a dry mouth side effect.

The pharmacy technician should be alert to the potential for patient over-dependence on short-acting β_2 agonists. If the patient is using more than one canister a month, the prescribing physician should be notified by the pharmacist. Such over-dependence is generally a sign that the patient's asthma is not being adequately controlled and that the physician needs to consider alternative treatment regimens.

Proventil, **Proventil HFA**, and **Ventolin (albuterol)** are bronchodilators used in cases of airway obstruction, such as asthma or chronic obstructive pulmonary disease

Table 10.2   Most-Commonly Used Agents for Asthma

Generic Name	Brand Name	Dosage Form
Bronchodilators		
albuterol*	Proventil, Ventolin	aerosol, capsule, solution, syrup, tablet
	Proventil HFA	inhaler
	Volmax	tablet
bitolterol	Tornalate	inhaler, inhalation solution
epinephrine	Adrenalin	SC, IM, IV
	Primatene Mist,	aerosol
	Bronkaid Mist	
ipratropium bromide*	Atrovent	inhaler, nasal spray
ipratropium-albuterol	Combivent	aerosol
isoetharine*	Bronkosol	inhaler
isoproterenol*	Isuprel	tablet, inhaler, IV
levalbuterol	Xopenex	solution
metaproterenol*	Alupent	tablet, syrup, inhaler
pirbuterol	Maxair	inhaler
salmeterol	Serevent	inhaler, inhalant disks
terbutaline*	Brethaire	tablet, inhaler, IV
Xanthine Derivatives		
aminophylline	Truphylline	tablet, liquid, IM, IV
theophylline*	Theo-dur	capsule, tablet, solution
	Slo-Phyllin	tablet, syrup, IV
Leukotriene Inhibitors		
montelukast	Singulair	tablet
zafirlukast	Accolate	tablet
zileuton	Zyflo	tablet
Corticosteroids, Oral		
dexamethasone	Decadron	tablet, elixir
hydrocortisone	Solu-Cortef	tablet, suspension
methylprednisolone	Solu-Medrol	tablet
prednisolone	Pediapred	solution
prednisone	Deltasone	tablet, syrup
Corticosteroids, Inhalant		
beclomethasone	Beclovent, Vanceril	inhaler
	Vancenase	nasal spray
budesonide	Rhinocort	inhaler
	Pulmicort Turbuhaler	inhaler
	Pulmicort Respules	capsule
dexamethasone	Decadron	inhaler
flunisolide	AeroBid	inhaler
fluticasone	Flovent	inhaler
	Flonase	nasal spray
triamcinolone	Azmacort	inhaler
Mast Cell Stabilizers		
cromolyn sodium	Intal	inhaler, nebulizer solution
	Nasalcrom	solution
nedocromil	Tilade	inhaler

* These products come in forms other than inhalants, such as liquids for use in nebulizers, syrups, and injections. Pharmacists and pharmacy technicians should always carefully read the prescription and choose the correct dosage form.

(COPD). They relax bronchial smooth muscle by action on pulmonary β_2 receptors with little effect on heart rate. Albuterol is administered by inhalation or orally for relief of bronchospasms. Duration is three to six hours. Proventil HFA is an inhaler without chlorofluorocarbons. Volmax is an albuterol supplied as an extended-release tablet. These drugs are associated with side effects of tremor and nervousness.

Tornalate (bitolterol) is used to prevent and treat bronchial asthma. It selectively stimulates β_2-adrenergic receptors in the lung, relaxing bronchial smooth muscle; it has minor β_1 activity. Duration ranges from three to six hours.

Xopenex (levalbuterol) is the R isomer of albuterol. It is the active component of the drug. It can be given at lower doses. The side effects of tremor and nervousness are thought to be caused by the S isomer. This drug is more effective than the S isomer with fewer side effects.

Bronkosol (isoetharine) is a bronchodilator for bronchial asthma and for reversible bronchospasm occurring with bronchitis and emphysema. It relaxes bronchial smooth muscle by action on β_2 receptors. Normally it is used only by inhalation for the treatment of acute episodes of bronchoconstriction, but it can be used around-the-clock to promote less variation in serum levels.

Isuprel (isoproterenol) is indicated for treating reversible airway obstruction, as in asthma or COPD. It stimulates β_1 and β_2 receptors, resulting in relaxation of bronchial, GI, and uterine smooth muscle, increased heart rate and contractility, and vasodilation of peripheral vasculature. It may be used up to five times a day with no more than two inhalations at one time with one to five minutes between inhalations, and no more than six inhalations should be administered in one hour.

Alupent (metaproterenol) is a bronchodilator for reversible airway obstruction, such as asthma or COPD. It has a rapid onset of action within minutes, peak effect in one hour, with prolonged effect (four hours) and acts primarily on β_2 receptors, with little or no effect on heart rate.

Maxair (pirbuterol) is a short-acting bronchodilator used to prevent and treat reversible bronchospasm, especially asthma. It is a selective β_2 agonist with four to six hours duration of action. The patient should not exceed the recommended dose of twelve inhalations per day. Allow at least two minutes between inhalations and at least five minutes before using inhaled steroids.

Serevent (salmeterol) is indicated for maintenance therapy of asthma. It is a β_2 agonist with long duration of action and onset of action in thirty to sixty minutes. It is taken twice a day. It should be reserved for patients with more serious asthma or those already receiving anti-inflammatory therapy. Its long duration of action makes it particularly useful for nocturnal symptoms of asthma. It should not be used to treat rescue situations. Deaths have been implicated with the improper use of this drug.

Brethaire (terbutaline) is a long-acting bronchodilator for reversible airway obstruction and bronchial asthma. It can be used parenterally for *status asthmaticus*. Excessive use may lead to paradoxical bronchoconstriction. If this occurs, discontinue immediately. It is a β_2 agonist. (Terbutaline is also used in obstetrics as a premature labor inhibitor due to its relaxation of uterine muscle.)

Atrovent (ipratropium bromide) blocks the action of acetylcholine at parasympathetic sites in bronchial smooth muscle, causing bronchodilation. It is derived from atropine and is not for acute management, but for prevention. It is short-acting and is not absorbed into general circulation when it is inhaled, so it does not cause arrhythmias.

XANTHINE DERIVATIVES **Theo-dur** and **Slo-Phyllin (theophylline)** are phosphodiesterase inhibitors that reverse early bronchospasm associated with antigens or irritants. **Truphylline (aminophylline)** is the more soluble ethylenediamine solution of theophylline. Theophylline improves the contractility of the fatigued diaphragm. They are used only in lung disease unresponsive to other drugs. Blood levels are maintained from 8 mcg/mL to 20 mcg/mL. Theophylline has many interactions, and blood levels can become elevated quickly. It is used as a bronchodilator in reversible airway obstruction due to asthma, chronic bronchitis, and emphysema. Theophylline can also be used for neonatal apnea and bradycardia.

LEUKOTRIENE INHIBITORS Leukotrienes are metabolized from arachidonic acid, which is also responsible for forming prostaglandins. Leukotrienes increase edema, mucus, and vascular permeability and are 100 to 1,000 times more potent than histamine for these effects. Blocking receptors also blocks tissue inflammatory responses.

Accolate (zafirlukast) antagonizes leukotriene receptors, thus reducing edema, mucus, and vascular permeability. It is intended for prophylaxis and long-term treatment in patients twelve years of age or older. Side effects are headache, rhinitis, and cough. Good results are being reported with few side effects.

Zyflo (zileuton) is a leukotriene inhibitor that has strong warnings about liver toxicity. It can also double theophylline levels if the patient is taking that drug. While Accolate is a leukotriene receptor blocker, Zyflo reduces the production of leukotrienes.

Singulair (montelukast), like accolate, is a leukotriene receptor antagonist. This drug is indicated for the prophlaxis and chronic treatment of asthma. Singulair has been shown to decrease daytime asthma as well as nocturnal awakenings due to asthma attacks. It can also decrease the need for β-adrenergic agonists. It should not be used to treat acute attacks. Unlike the other leukotriene modifiers which can only be prescribed for adults or children over the age of twelve, Singulair has been approved for use in children over the age of six. Singulair also has the benefit of a once daily dosage, as opposed to the other leukotriene inhibitors which must be dosed two to four times a day. A headache is the most common side effect associated with Singulair.

CORTICOSTEROIDS Corticosteroids stimulate adenylate cylase and inhibit inflammatory cells. These drugs inhibit the late-phase inflammatory reaction but have no effect on immediate hypersensitivity. Corticosteroids are reserved for more difficult cases and may be prescribed on an alternate-day basis or as a tapering dose when short-term therapy is indicated. Inhaled corticosteroids may be successful when other drugs are not. The primary side effects of these drugs if inhaled are oral candidiasis, irritation and burning of the nasal mucosa, hoarseness, and dry mouth. This irritation can sometimes lead to episodes of coughing. If corticosteroids are taken orally for a long period in a dosage exceeding 10 mg/day, they can cause growth of facial hair in females, breast development in males, "buffalo hump," "moon face," edema, weight gain, and easy bruising. A short-term course of high-dose corticosteroid will not cause these side effects. The patient should always be advised to rinse the mouth thoroughly with water after using a corticosteroid inhaler.

Large doses of inhaled corticosteroids have been associated with slowed growth in children. However, uncontrolled asthma can also slow growth. As such, the potential risks of corticosteriods are often outweighed by the benefits in this patient population. As noted in the descriptions below, a number of corticosteroids have been approved for use in pediatric patients over the age of six years.

Problems with corticosteroids are improper technique when using a metered-dose inhaler and patients' fears of the drugs due to the potential side effects. Too many asthmatics still are not using inhaled corticosteroids.

Flovent (fluticasone) is the same drug as that in the nasal spray Flonase. Flovent comes in three strengths. The lowest is for mild asthma and the highest is to wean patients off oral corticosteroids. It should be used twice daily and may take up to one to two weeks to reach maximum benefit. Other steroids are **Deltasone (prednisone), Solu-Cortef (hydrocortisone), Solu-Medrol (methylprednisolone), Decadron (dexamethasone), Pediapred (prednisolone), Beclovent (beclomethasone), Azmacort (triamcinolone)**, and **AeroBid (flunisolide)**.

Warning
Prednisone, Prilosec, and primidone could each be easily misread for the other.

The **Pulmicort Turbuhaler (budesonide)** formulation of budesonide uses a novel, dry powder, propellant-free inhalant which is breath-activated. This formulation requires less hand-lung coordination than other forms. As a result, it is easier to use. Moreover, the turbuhaler only needs to be primed prior to the initial uses rather than before each dose as with other corticosteroid inhalers. Pulmicort is associated with a lower frequency of coughing episodes relative to other inhaled corticosteroids. This drug can be prescribed to patients six years of age and older. As with other drugs in this class, patients should be instructed to rinse their mouth after each dose. Inadequate response to Pulmicort is often the result of an improper inhalation technique. The pharmacist can help correct this problem by providing appropriate instructions to the patient.

Pulmicort Respules (budesonide) is the first corticosteroid formulated for use in home nebulizers. This formulation has made possible the treatment of children as young as twelve months of age.

MAST CELL STABILIZERS **Intal** and **Nasalcrom (cromolyn sodium)** work topically in the airways. They are prophylactic drugs with no benefit for acute reactions. Cromolyn stabilizes mast cell membranes. It directly inhibits other inflammatory cells. The airways must be open before administration, so a bronchodilator is often given first. Cromolyn has an unpleasant taste after inhalation and side effects of hoarseness, dry mouth, and stuffy nose. This is a very effective drug, but patient compliance is a big problem. It is dosed four times a day, and most patients have difficulty fitting the four doses into their day's routine. The drug has many dosage forms, so care must be taken to select the correct one.

Tilade (nedocromil) is an anti-inflammatory that inhibits release and activation of mediators (histamines, leukotrienes, prostaglandins, and mast cells) associated with asthma. It is used for maintenance therapy in patients with mild to moderate asthma. It inhibits early and late bronchoconstrictive response to inhaled antigens, exercise, cold air, fog, and sulfur dioxide. The few side effects, including arthritis, rash, and tremors, are rare.

EMPHYSEMA AND CHRONIC BRONCHITIS

Emphysema and chronic bronchitis obstruct airflow on expiration. They sometimes occur together, and their pharmacologic therapy is similar.

Emphysema is characterized by destruction of the tiny alveoli, walls, or air sacs of the lungs. Typically, air spaces distal to the terminal bronchioles are enlarged. Patients have tachypnea, which gives them a flushed appearance. Major risk factors are cigarette smoking (which destroys the walls of the lungs), occupational exposure, air pollution, and genetic factors.

Chronic bronchitis is a result of several contributing factors. The most prominent of these include cigarette smoke; exposure to occupational dusts, fumes, and environmental pollution; and bacterial infection. This disease is characterized by a cough that produces purulent, green, or blood-streaked sputum. Most persons have a morning cough that is a result of irritation to the lungs. Studies of lungs from smoking and nonsmoking subjects clearly demonstrate that those who smoke cigarettes have bronchial inflammation and substantially increased numbers of alveolar macrophages.

Bronchitis is a condition due to destruction of the lungs' defense mechanisms. In chronic bronchitis, excessive production of tracheobronchial mucus is sufficient to cause cough with expectoration of at least 30 mL of sputum per twenty-four hours for three months of the year for more than two consecutive years. Patients are usually overweight, have a barrel chest, and tend to retain carbon dioxide. Acute bronchitis runs a brief course and is corrected by the body, often with the aid of antibiotics and generally does not return.

To understand the treatment for emphysema and chronic bronchitis, you must also understand the lungs' natural defense system. When this system is functioning properly, the host defenses of the respiratory tract provide good protection against pathogen invasion and remove potentially infectious agents from the lungs. The lungs are normally sterile below the first branch. It is when organisms breech this region that infection and inflammation are initiated.

The body's defenses include a number of different types of cells.

- ◇ Ciliary carpet, minute hairlike processes that beat rhythmically to move fluid or mucus over the surface.
- ◇ Goblet cells occur in increased numbers due to smoking.
- ◇ Clara cells are unciliated cells at the branching of the alveolar duct from the bronchioles.
- ◇ Epithelial cells produce a protein-rich exudate in the small bronchi and bronchioles.
- ◇ Type I pneumocytes in the alveolar membranes act as the phagocytes of the lung.
- ◇ Type II pneumocytes synthesize and secrete surfactant.
- ◇ Phagocytic cells clear trash and organisms from the lung.

The pharmacologic management of emphysema and bronchitis is still largely empirical, with methylxanthines, corticosteroids, β agonists, and ipratropium bromide forming the foundation of therapy. Oxygen administration and physiotherapy play an important role in treating lung diseases.

In both emphysema and chronic bronchitis, antibiotic therapy is sometimes needed if sputum changes from yellow to green, fever is present, or both.

Expectorants are sometimes used to stimulate respiratory secretions and counter dryness, which stimulates irritation and coughing. Drinking lots of water helps to break up mucus and enable the patient to cough up secretions. Water is the expectorant of choice.

A highly controversial aspect of treatment is the use of mucolytics, such as **Mucomyst (acetylcysteine)**, which break apart glycoproteins, thus reducing viscosity

Figure 10.2

Cellular Makeup of an Alveolus and Capillary Supply

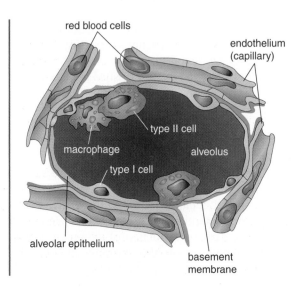

and promoting easier movement and removal of secretions. Another mucolytic enzyme, **Pulmozyme (dornase alfa)**, is sometimes used in cystic fibrosis.

Influenza and pneumococcal vaccinations are recommended for patients with chronic obstructive pulmonary disease.

OTHER LUNG DISEASES

Pneumonia

Pneumonia is a common lung infection occurring in persons of all ages and is caused by microorganisms gaining access to the lower respiratory tract by three routes.

- ◇ They are inhaled as aerosolized particles.
- ◇ They enter through the bloodstream.
- ◇ They are aspirated in oropharyngeal contents.

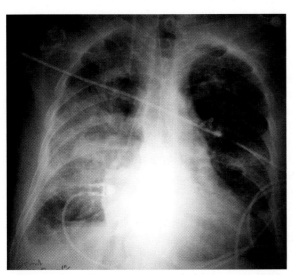

This x-ray shows that the patient's right lung contains fluid due to pneumonia.

Aspiration (inhalation of fluids from the mouth and throat) is a common occurrence in both healthy and ill persons during sleep. It is the major mechanism by which pulmonary pathogens gain access to the normally sterile lower airways and alveoli. Pneumonia is treated with antibiotics, depending on the causative organism.

Cystic Fibrosis (CF)

Cystic fibrosis (CF) is a disease that involves the gastrointestinal and pulmonary systems. It is fatal, but some patients survive into early adulthood. The morbidity and mortality of the disease are associated with disorders in the pulmonary system. The GI involvement is due to increased viscosity of secreted mucus and a relative deficiency of pancreatic digestive enzymes.

Hypoxia with resultant cyanosis and digital clubbing are common. A patient's respiratory status follows a cyclic pattern, from a state of relative well-being to one of acute pulmonary deterioration. Management of the pulmonary aspect of this disease can be broken down into two areas: respiratory therapy and antibiotic therapy.

The cornerstone of respiratory therapy is percussion, a tapping movement to induce cough and expectoration of sputum from the lungs, which is often preceded by nebulizer therapy during which nebulized sterile water or normal saline is breathed to liquefy pulmonary secretions.

Mucomyst or bronchodilators may be added to the nebulizer solution to prevent bronchospasm and further liquefy the secretions. Mucomyst has a very unpleasant taste and odor, and many patients prefer not to use it. Normal asthmatic bronchodilators are appropriate for cystic fibrosis. Theophylline may be of benefit; however, theophylline clearance in CF patients may differ from that in asthmatics, and clearance and dosage should be carefully monitored. Table 10.3 lists the most-commonly used agents for CF.

Pulmozyme (dornase alfa) selectively breaks down DNA that is released by degenerating leukocytes. The leukocytes collect in response to infection. By destroying DNA in the mucus, dornase alfa helps reduce secretion viscosity.

Most CF patients are at high risk for complications from influenza, so influenza vaccine should be given yearly. Most clinicians treat pulmonary exacerbations with antibiotics, although this may be controversial.

Respiratory Distress Syndrome (RDS)

Respiratory distress syndrome (RDS) occurs in newborns during the first few hours of life. Its characteristics—acute asphyxia with hypoxia and acidosis—can inhibit pulmonary surfactant production. Two causative factors are prematurity and maternal diabetes. If RDS occurs, surfactant is administered. Table 10.4 lists the most-commonly used agents for RDS.

Survanta (beractant) is the drug of choice for RDS. It is a natural agent extracted from cattle lung and supplied as a suspension for intratracheal administration. It replaces deficient or ineffective endogenous lung surfactant in neonates and prevents the alveoli from collapsing during expiration by lowering the surface tension between the air and alveolar surfaces. It is used for prophylactic therapy in high-risk infants and rescue therapy within eight hours of birth.

Exosurf (colfosceril) is a lung surfactant which, by reducing surface tension in the lung, stabilizes the alveoli from collapsing in infants. Once reconstituted, the drug must be used immediately.

Infasurf (calfactant) replaces deficient endogenous lung surfactant and is indicated for neonates who are less than seventy-two hours of age. This drug seems to have a decreased incidence of air leaks and the infants require less oxygen. This drug should be stored in the refrigerator. The suspension settles and should be swirled gently but not shaken to redisperse the medication. It is not necessary to warm before administration. Unopened vials at room temperature may be returned to the refrigerator within twenty-four hours.

Respiratory Tract Infections

Respiratory tract infections are usually caused by viruses. The common cold is a mild self-limited viral infection. Symptoms are readily recognized by the patient and

Table 10.3	Most-Commonly Used Agents for Cystic Fibrosis	
Generic Name	**Brand Name**	**Dosage Form**
acetylcysteine	Mucomyst	solution
dornase alfa	Pulmozyme	solution, single-dose ampule

Table 10.4	Most-Commonly Used Agents for Respiratory Distress Syndrome	
Generic Name	**Brand Name**	**Dosage Form**
beractant	Survanta	suspension
calfactant	Infasurf	suspension
colfosceril	Exosurf	powder for injection

include mild malaise, rhinorrhea, sneezing, scratchy throat, and fever. Bacterial sinusitis and otitis are frequent complications necessitating antimicrobial therapy. Antibiotics and sometimes antivirals are used in treating these problems. However, viruses are the most common cause of infections to the respiratory system.

Tuberculosis (TB)

Mycobacterium tuberculosis most often affects the lung. Tuberculosis (TB) may spread in the body by traveling leukocytes and lymph. A follicle forms and is surrounded by epithelial cells. The mass may spread or liquefy, forming a cavity filled with fluid and teeming with organisms. The fluid may move in the direction of least resistance, spreading organisms and disease within the organ, thereby destroying more tissue (formation of a fibrosis). *M. tuberculosis* likes areas of high oxygen; lesions concentrate primarily in the lung, but also in bone and kidney tissue. TB is transmitted by respiratory droplets inhaled into the lungs of persons at risk. Suspended in the air, these droplets descend one to two inches per hour.

TB patients can be divided into two classes on the basis of disease and antibody production.

1. Exposed but no disease. These patients produce TB antibodies. Persons who test positive to the TB skin test nearly always test positive. This does not mean they have the disease.
2. Exposed and have active organisms. These patients may or may not produce antibodies. Only one in ten persons infected contract active disease over a lifetime; therefore, the risk to a healthy infected person is 10% over a lifetime. Significant signs and symptoms of the disease include weight loss, spitting blood, night sweats and night fever, chest pain, and malaise.

The agent in the TB test is purified protein derivative (PPD) from killed bacteria. This product is injected intradermally. Persons who have been exposed to or have the disease show a wheal-and-flare reaction within forty-eight hours at the injection site. A false-negative reaction may occur in persons recently exposed and in older persons who have delayed-type hypersensitivity. If the reading is positive, the patient is directed to have an x-ray taken to detect a lung shadow that may indicate active disease. TB is a disease that generally develops slowly; it may take twenty years to develop from the time of exposure. If the disease is arrested early (four to ten weeks after exposure), patients have a risk of reactivity for the remainder of their life. The highest incidence of infection occurs one to two years after exposure. The medical history of the patient should be watched for disease symptoms such as weight loss, fever, night sweats, malaise, and loss of appetite.

Patient compliance is a major problem in treating this disease. The length of therapy and the number of medications are problematic. Active disease should not be treated with a single agent. TB is seen primarily in alcoholics, the prison population, the immunocompromised, and the elderly. It should be included in the differential diagnosis of patients with fever of unknown origin, subacute meningitis, or chronic infection at any site.

The goals of TB therapy are to

◇ initiate treatment promptly
◇ convert the sputum culture to negative as soon as possible
◇ achieve cure without relapse
◇ prevent emergence of drug-resistant strains

Table 10.5 describes the most-commonly used agents for treating TB. The primary agents used are isoniazid, rifampin, ethambutol, streptomycin, and pyrazinamide. Isoniazid and rifampin are highly effective if used in combination. Streptomycin is recommended as a third drug, especially because it can be injected twice weekly to guarantee compliance. Combinations of drugs are necessary for treating TB but not for prophylaxis. The purpose of the combinations is to prevent the development of resistance to the drug. However, a new strain of *M. tuberculosis* that is very resistant to many currently used drugs and difficult to treat has now developed.

The treatment regimen for TB is different depending on the patient's symptoms. For patients with no symptoms, a positive purified protein derivative (PPD), and a positive x-ray, the disease is treated with a single agent, usually isoniazid (INH), 300 mg once daily for twelve months. For patients with the clinical disease, at least two agents to which the organism is susceptible will be administered. There are three options.

◇ **Option A** Give isoniazid and rifampin daily for eight weeks, followed by isoniazid and rifampin two to three times a week for sixteen weeks. If isoniazid resistance develops, add ethambutol or streptomycin. Treatment should extend for at least six months and then should be continued for three months beyond sputum culture conversion to negative.

◇ **Option B** Give isoniazid, rifampin, and pyrazinamide with streptomycin *or* ethambutol for two weeks, followed by the same drugs two to three times a week for six weeks; then isoniazid and rifampin two times a week for sixteen weeks.

◇ **Option C** Give isoniazid, rifampin, and pyrazinamide with ethambutol *or* streptomycin three times a week for six months.

The new strain of *M. tuberculosis* that has developed shows resistance to the usual drug regimens. The severe side effect profile and the length of time required for treatment of active TB create serious compliance problems. Patients being treated for active TB should avoid alcohol. They should also receive multiple drugs to reduce the chance for resistance to develop. Most patients receive the drug isoniazid. If resistance to isoniazid develops, rifampin is the drug of choice. When the disease exhibits resistance to both these agents, the following combinations are recommended: pyrazinamide plus Myambutol; pyrazinamide plus Cipro or Floxin.

Table 10.5	**Most-Commonly Used Agents for Tuberculosis**	
Generic Name	**Brand Name**	**Dosage Form**
capreomycin	Capastat	IM
ciprofloxacin	Cipro	IM, IV, ophthalmic, tablet
cycloserine	Seromycin	capsule
ethambutol	Myambutol	tablet
ethionamide	Trecator-SC	tablet
isoniazid (INH)	Laniazid	tablet, syrup
	Nydrazid	IM
	Rifamate	capsule
	Rifater	tablet
ofloxacin	Floxin	IV, ophthalmic, tablet
pyrazinamide	Tebrazid	tablet
rifampin	Rifadin	capsule, IV
	Rimactane	capsule
rifapentine	Priftin	tablet
streptomycin	(none)	IM, IV

Rifadin and **Rimactane (rifampin)** work through the inhibition of RNA synthesis. Side effects include the discoloration of urine, tears, and sweat. This discoloration can permanently stain soft contact lenses. Rifampin interferes with oral contraceptives and thus female patients taking this drug must be advised to seek alternative forms of birth control. Rifampin must be taken on an empty stomach.

Priftin (rifapentine) has a longer duration of action than rifampin and, therefore, has the advantage of a less frequent administration schedule, leading to improved patient compliance. Priftin is always used as an adjunctive therapy. This drug has the same side effect profile as rifampin. It must be taken with food.

SMOKING CESSATION

Cigarette smoke contains more than four thousand chemical compounds, including at least forty-three carcinogens. Nicotine, the physically addictive component of tobacco, is readily absorbed in the lungs from inhaled smoke. Nicotine from smokeless tobacco products, such as chewing tobacco and snuff, is absorbed across the oral or nasal mucosa, respectively.

Cigarette smokers lose about fifteen years of life. Leukemia and cancers of the mouth, pharynx, larynx, esophagus, pancreas, cervix, kidney, and bladder are associated with smoking. Evidence also links smoking with other cancers, such as ovarian, uterine, and prostate. Nicotine and polycyclic aromatic hydrocarbons in cigarette smoke induce the production of hepatic enzymes responsible for metabolizing caffeine, theophylline, imipramine, and other drugs. Smoking increases plasma cortisol and catecholamine concentrations, which affect treatment with adrenergic agonists and adrenergic-blocking agents.

Smoking increases the risk of heart disease, COPD, and stroke. The acute risks include shortness of breath, aggravation of asthma, impotence, infertility, and increased serum carbon monoxide concentration.

Environmental (second-hand) tobacco smoke poses a substantial health threat because it contains all the carcinogens and toxins present in cigarette smoke. Children living in a household with smokers have a higher risk of respiratory infection, asthma, and middle-ear infection than those who live with nonsmokers. Birth defects may be related to the mother's smoking during pregnancy.

The physical benefits of smoking cessation include a longer life and better health (i.e., decreased risk of lung, laryngeal, esophageal, oral, pancreatic, bladder, and cervical cancers; coronary heart disease; and other diseases aggravated by smoking). A few personal benefits from smoking cessation are listed in Table 10.6.

Table 10.6	Personal Benefits to Smoking Cessation

better performance in sports and sex
better-smelling home, car, clothing, and breath
economic savings
freedom from addiction
healthier babies
improved health
improved self-esteem
improved sense of taste and smell
no concern about exposing others to smoke
no worry about quitting
setting a good example for children and young adults

Nicotine is extensively metabolized in the liver and to a lesser extent in the kidneys and lungs. One major urinary metabolite, cotinine, has a longer half-life (fifteen to twenty hours) and a tenfold higher concentration than nicotine.

Nicotine is a ganglionic cholinergic-receptor agonist with complex, usually dose-related, pharmacologic effects. These effects include central and peripheral nervous system stimulation and depression, respiratory stimulation, skeletal muscle relaxation, catecholamine release by the adrenal medulla, peripheral vasoconstriction, and increases in blood pressure, heart rate, cardiac output, and oxygen consumption. Chronic nicotine ingestion leads to physical and psychological dependence. Smoking cessation results in withdrawal symptoms, usually within twenty-four hours. These symptoms are listed in Table 10.7.

Planning to Stop Smoking

Behavior-reinforcing properties of nicotine include relaxation, increased alertness, decreased fatigue, improved cognitive performance, and a "reward" effect (pleasure or euphoria). Increased alertness and cognitive performance result from stimulation of the cerebral cortex, which can occur at low doses. The reward effect, mediated by the limbic system, occurs at high doses.

The key to smoking cessation is total abstinence. Because drinking alcohol is strongly associated with relapse to tobacco use, smokers should reduce their alcohol consumption or abstain from drinking altogether during the quitting process. Individual or group counseling is highly recommended.

The steps in establishing a plan for quitting are as follows.

1. Set a date.
2. Inform family, friends, and coworkers of the decision and request understanding and support.
3. Remove cigarettes from the environment and avoid spending a lot of time in places where smoking is prevalent.
4. Review previous attempts to quit, if applicable, and analyze the factors that caused relapse.
5. Anticipate challenges, particularly during the critical first few weeks.

Training in general problem-solving skills, social support from the clinician, and nicotine replacement therapy are the three main elements of smoking-cessation treatment. Nicotine replacement therapy is recommended as first-line pharmacotherapy

Table 10.7	Symptoms of Nicotine Withdrawal

anxiety
craving for tobacco
decreased blood pressure and heart rate
depression
difficulty in concentrating
drowsiness
frustration, irritability, impatience, restlessness
gastrointestinal disturbances
headache
hostility
increased appetite and weight gain
increased skin temperature
insomnia

for smokers without contraindications to therapy (myocardial infarction in the previous four weeks, serious arrhythmias, severe or worsening angina pectoris).

One major reason smokers do not want to quit is fear of weight gain. Most smokers gain less than ten pounds. Weight gain is caused by both increased caloric intake and metabolic adjustments; it can occur even if caloric intake remains constant or is restricted.

Smoking Cessation Drug Therapy

The most-commonly used agents for smoking cessation are listed in Table 10.8. Patients must understand that nicotine replacement therapy is not a substitute for behavior modification and that success is greatest when the two modes of therapy are used concomitantly. Patients can help by rewarding abstinence and avoiding situations that serve as smoking triggers.

Patients must be strongly advised to stop smoking when initiating nicotine-replacement therapy. Those who continue to smoke may show signs of nicotine excess. The symptoms of nicotine excess and withdrawal often overlap, and are listed in Table 10.9. Dizziness and perspiration are more often associated with excessive nicotine levels; anxiety, depression, and irritability are common symptoms of withdrawal.

Common adverse effects from nicotine chewing gum (usually mild and transient) include mouth soreness, hiccups, dyspepsia, and jaw ache. The patch should be applied daily to a nonhairy, clean, dry site on the upper body or outer arm. Skin reactions from the patches may be prevented by rotating the application site. Adverse effects from the nasal spray include nasal irritation, runny nose, throat irritation, watering eyes, sneezing, and cough. Regular use of the spray during the first week of treatment may help patients adapt to its irritating effects. If patients complain of irritation at first, they should not be told to stop using the drug.

All the listed drugs except the nasal spray and the antidepressant have been approved for OTC drug use. Nicotine nasal spray mimics the effects of cigarette smoking more closely than do transdermal systems or chewing gum because nicotine absorption is more rapid after nasal administration. The gum is recommended for users of smokeless tobacco. Compared with placebo, transdermal nicotine doubles abstinence rates at six and twelve months after initiation of therapy.

Table 10.8   **Most-Commonly Used Agents for Smoking Cessation**

Generic Name	Brand Name	Dosage Form
bupropion (antidepressant)	Zyban (Wellbutrin SR)	tablet
nicotine	Habitrol, Nicoderm, Nicotrol, ProStep	transdermal patch
	Nicorette	gum
	Nicotrol NS	spray

Table 10.9   **Symptoms of Nicotine Excess**

abdominal pain	headache	perspiration
confusion	hearing loss	visual disturbances
diarrhea	hypersalivation	vomiting
dizziness	nausea	weakness

Chapter Summary

Asthma

◇ Chronic obstructive pulmonary disease (COPD) encompasses asthma, emphysema, and chronic bronchitis. Asthma is the only reversible condition.

◇ The asthmatic lung is more sensitive and responds to lower doses of challenge from allergens than do normal lungs.

◇ Asthma is a disease in which inflammation causes the airways to tighten.

◇ Asthma is a pulmonary condition with the following characteristics: reversible small airway obstruction; progressive airway inflammation; increased airway responsiveness to stimuli.

◇ The most useful measure to assess severity and follow the course of asthma is the peak expiratory flow rate (PEFR).

◇ The mainstay of management of asthma is drug therapy.

◇ Asthma is treated in a stepwise fashion:

Step 1. Short-acting oral or inhaled β_2 agonist (less than once a week), no daily medications

Step 2. Short-acting oral or inhaled β_2 agonist (not to exceed three to four times in one day), daily medications (e.g., inhaled corticosteroid)

Step 3. Short-acting oral or inhaled β_2 agonist, daily medications (e.g., inhaled corticosteroid and long-acting bronchodilator)

Step 4. Short-acting oral or inhaled β_2 agonist, daily medications, inhaled corticosteroid, long-acting bronchodilator, long-acting β_2 agonist, and oral corticosteroids, long term

◇ A rescue course of corticosteroids may be needed at any time and any step.

◇ Exercise-induced asthma is best treated with the inhalation of terbutaline or albuterol before exercising. This will provide protection for two hours after inhalation.

◇ Asthmatics should avoid beta blockers, antihistamines in acute attacks, atropine, and ephedrine. Other drugs to be avoided are aspirin, indomethacin, other NSAIDs, penicillins, cephalosporins, and sulfas.

◇ A spacer is recommended to decrease the amount of spray that is deposited on the back of the throat and swallowed.

◇ Nebulizers are effective delivery systems, especially for young children.

◇ Home nebulizers can lead to bronchitis. They can become contaminated easily if not cleaned properly on a daily basis.

◇ Epinephrine is the drug of choice for an acute attack of asthma. Some asthmatics carry an EpiPen for this purpose.

◇ Proventil HFA does not contain chlorofluorocarbons.

◇ Volmax is an extended-release albuterol tablet.

◇ Short-acting inhaled bronchodilators are albuterol, Tornalate, isoetharine, isoproterenol, metaproterenol, and pirbuterol.

◇ Xopenex, the R isomer of albuterol, is more effective and has fewer side effects.

◇ Serevent should be used exactly as directed and never for acute situations.

◇ Long-acting inhaled bronchodilators are salmeterol and terbutaline.

◇ Theophylline should be used only in lung diseases unresponsive to other drugs because of the high interaction profile.

◇ Leukotrienes are 1,000 times more potent than histamine; therefore, when these receptors are antagonized, inflammatory responses do not take place.

Dispensing Medications

1. Mr. Williams brings in the following prescriptions. What areas are a problem here?

R̶ **MT. HOPE MEDICAL PARK**
ST. PAUL, MN (651) 555-3591

DEA# _____

Pt. name __Bob Williams__ Date __6-01-05__

Address _____

Theophylline 50 mg bid #60
Proventil inhaler 1-2 puffs
        every 4-6 hours #2

____ Dispense as written
✓ Fills __5__ times (no refill unless indicated)
__Alex Negal__ M.D.

R̶ **MT. HOPE MEDICAL PARK**
ST. PAUL, MN (651) 555-3591

DEA# _____

Pt. name __Bob Williams__ Date __6-01-05__

Address _____

Eryc 250 mg qid with
        food until finished #20
Inderal 10 mg qid   #28

____ Dispense as written
____ Fills ____ times (no refill unless indicated)
__Alex Negal__ M.D.

2. Create a smoking cessation plan.
3. One inmate from the prison has just been released. While there, he contracted a strain of TB resistant to both isoniazid and rifampin. Describe the treatment you would expect the doctor to prescribe.
4. Mrs. Jones cannot seem to control her asthma. She brings in this new prescription. Where do problems exist in this regimen?

R͓x

MT. HOPE MEDICAL PARK
ST. PAUL, MN (651) 555-3591

DEA#_____

Pt. name _Mary Lou Jones_ Date _6-01-05_

Address _____

Serevent use as directed prn   #3
Azmacort use as directed prn   #3
Ventolin use as directed
                    3-4 Times daily

____ Dispense as written

✓ Fills _5_ times (no refill unless indicated)

_____Kathy Grad_____ M.D.

Internet Research

Use the Internet to complete the following assignments.

1. Find two Internet sites that discuss asthma during pregnancy. List three issues that a woman with asthma must consider if she is, or is considering becoming, pregnant. Does a woman in this situation need to see her physician? List your Internet sources.
2. Find statistics related to tuberculosis in the United States. How many new cases (incidence) are reported each year? Is this number increasing or decreasing? What is the prevalence (existing cases) of tuberculosis in the United States? Which segment of the population has the highest risk of contracting tuberculosis and why? List your Internet sources.

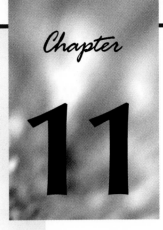

Gastrointestinal Drugs

Learning Objectives

- ◇ Describe gastrointestinal physiology and how it impacts GI disease.
- ◇ Be aware of drug treatments for these diseases.
- ◇ Identify the chemo-receptor trigger zone (CTZ) and its role in nausea.
- ◇ Know which antiemetics act on the CTZ and their mechanisms of action.
- ◇ Describe the role of fiber in the digestive process.
- ◇ Understand gastroesophageal reflux disease and its ramifications.
- ◇ Discuss how antidiarrheals work and the agents in this class.
- ◇ Discuss laxatives, their use and misuse.
- ◇ Explain the use of antiflatulents.
- ◇ Know how to calculate ideal body weight and body mass index, and define obesity.
- ◇ Identify the parasites that invade the human body and treatment for the diseases they cause.

This chapter will discuss the diseases and disorders of the gastrointestinal tract. Problems range from malabsorption syndromes to gastroesophageal reflux; outside triggers can cause ulcers and parasitic disease; fiber deficiency can lead to constipation. Heredity may play a role in obesity. The chemo-receptor trigger zone in the brain can have an effect on emesis. Involved in all this are numerous classes of drugs which can be both cause and treatment.

STRUCTURE AND FUNCTION OF THE GASTROINTESTINAL SYSTEM

The gastrointestinal (GI) tract is a continuous tube that varies in diameter. It begins in the mouth and extends throughout the pharynx, esophagus, stomach, small intestine, and large intestine to end at the anus (see Figure 11.1). The major function of the GI tract is to convert complex food substances into simpler compounds that can be absorbed into the bloodstream and used by the cells of the body. It also excretes solid waste from the body.

GI transit time is the time it takes for material to pass from one end of the GI tract to the other. It is subdivided into gastric emptying time and small intestine and colon transit time. Speeding movement through the intestines, reducing transit time, decreases nutrient and water absorption. Slowing intestinal transit time increases absorption due to increased time at the absorptive surfaces.

Figure 11.1

The Gastrointestinal System

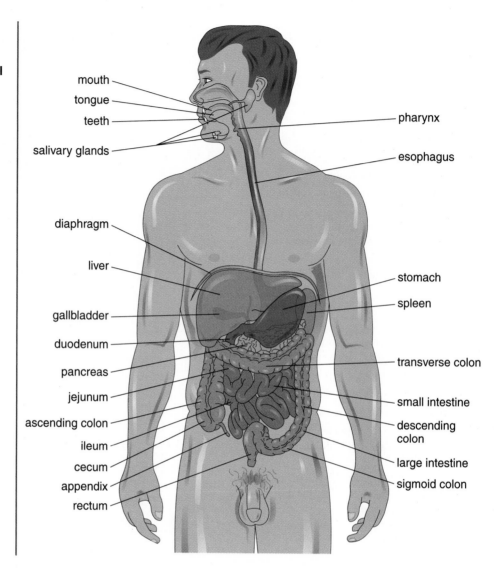

The stomach is composed of layers of smooth muscle lined with glands that secrete gastric juice and hydrochloric acid—enzymes and acid which help break down food. In the large intestine, the material that has not been absorbed will be exposed to bacteria. These bacteria continue some limited digestion. Mucous membranes protect the entire digestive system against abrasion and strong digestive enzymes.

GASTROINTESTINAL DISEASES

Gastritis is an irritation and superficial erosion of the stomach lining. Alcohol is a common causitive factor. The parietal cells of the stomach produce hydrochloric acid (HCl), which converts pepsinogen to pepsin. Acid production is stimulated by acetylcholine (ACh), histamine, and gastrin.

Inflammatory bowel disease has two forms. Ulcerative colitis is an irritation and inflammation of the large bowel, causing it to look scraped and is characterized by bloody mucus leading to watery diarrhea containing blood, mucus, and pus; it is confined to the rectum and colon. Crohn's disease is like ulcerative colitis, but it can affect any portion of the tubular gastrointestinal tract and, therefore, cannot be cured with surgical resection. Malabsorption syndrome is impaired intestinal absorption of nutrients.

Cystic fibrosis is both a GI disease and a pulmonary disease. Involvement of the GI tract is due to increased viscosity of mucous secretions and to relative deficiency of pancreatic enzymes. The backbone of GI therapy in cystic fibrosis is pancreatic enzyme replacement and vitamin supplementation.

Peptic Disease

The term peptic disease refers to disorders of the upper GI tract caused by the action of acid and pepsin. The spectrum of peptic disease is broad and includes mucosal injury, erythema erosions, and frank ulceration. Correlation of symptoms to disease is poor.

An ulcer is a local defect or excavation of the surface of an organ or tissue. There are three common types of GI ulcers: gastric, duodenal, and stress ulcers.

GASTRIC ULCERS Gastric ulcers are local excavations in the gastric mucosa. These lesions have malignant potential, occur more often in men than women, and become more frequent with aging. They are prevalent in smokers and in Western hemisphere populations. They do not necessarily occur in persons who are high acid secretors, but there is usually a family history. A contributing factor for many patients is the bacterium *Helicobacter pylori (H. Pylori)*.

DUODENAL ULCERS Duodenal ulcers are peptic lesions situated in the duodenum. They occur more in hypersecretors and are more difficult to treat than gastric ulcers because of the difficulty of getting medication into the duodenum. Possible causes are increased vagal tone and increased gastrin secretion.

STRESS ULCERS Stress ulcers are peptic ulcers, usually gastric, that occur in the clinical setting. These patients are under severe physiological stress from serious illness, and they are usually in the intensive care units (ICUs). Stress ulcers are caused by the breakdown of natural mucosal resistance. Stressful factors can be due to sepsis, burns, major surgery, chronic disease, or chronic infection. The patient usually has no clinical symptoms but can experience acute hemorrhage. Inserting a nasogastric tube yields blood in the stomach contents' aspirate. Perforations of the stomach wall occur in 8% to 18% of patients, with severe pain radiating toward the back. Therapy includes antacids every three to four hours and histamine$_2$ (H$_2$) blockers intravenously every three to six hours. This is why almost everyone in the ICUs receives an H$_2$ blocker.

GASTROESOPHAGEAL REFLUX DISEASE (GERD) Gastroesophageal reflux disease (GERD), also called heartburn, is a common problem. Symptoms include radiating burning or pain in the chest and an acid taste. Symptomatic relief of mild-to-moderate GERD can be obtained by using a combination of life-style modifications and phase I and II medications. The primary mechanism responsible for meal-related symptoms of esophagitis is the backflow (reflux) of acidic stomach contents across an incompetent valve. The lower esophageal sphincter is normally in a state of relative contraction. During swallowing, this sphincter relaxes enough to allow the forward passage of food and drink into the stomach, after which it contracts again, preventing the reflux of stomach contents. Heartburn occurs when the lower esophageal sphincter becomes incompetent. Several factors contribute to the malfunction of that sphincter, including overeating, eating late at night, consuming certain foods, smoking cigarettes, and drinking alcohol.

Foods known to trigger reflux symptoms include those that contain a high fat content, caffeine (in particular, chocolate, coffee, tea, and colas), citric and other acids, alcohol, and spices. Gas-producing foods also may contribute to heartburn. The likelihood of reflux occurring increases during pregnancy due to upward pressure exerted by the uterus on abdominal organs, including the stomach, in which gastric contents are pushed toward the lower esophageal sphincter and up the esophagus.

GERD is a common, distressing problem compounded by poor eating habits such as overeating, eating on the run, eating late at night, drinking, smoking, and consuming the wrong foods. Patient education remains the cornerstone of preventive therapy. Ideally, persons prone to reflux adopt preventive behavior. However, compliance is difficult to achieve.

The main premise underlying treatment is that many of these patients have a lifelong problem. In order to reduce their discomfort, patients should be instructed not to lie down for at least three hours after a meal. Preventive dietary changes include weight loss if the patient is overweight and restricted intake of foods that tend to produce symptoms. Medications that promote reflux should be avoided (e.g., theophylline and nifedipine). Patients should be advised to stop smoking.

GERD includes all three types of ulcers. Patients with this disease typically describe that they have a mild heartburn associated with anxiety. However, anxiety has little or nothing to do with the formation of the ulcers. GERD patients have recurrent abdominal pain, which may move about in the epigastric area. They may have nonspecific epigastric discomfort (gnawing or burning) that is worse before meals and may awaken the patient from sleep.

There are several complicating and precipitating factors in GERD. Alcohol is the most common cause of gastritis, mucosal irritation, and esophageal varices. Caffeine stimulates acid secretion and is found in coffee, tea, colas, and cocoa. Smoking reduces bicarbonate production in pancreatic juice which neutralizes some acid.

DRUG-INDUCED ULCERS There are several drugs that cause ulcers. They are listed in Table 11.1. Aspirin is the most common cause of drug-induced ulcers.

Pharmacologic Treatment of Gastrointestinal Diseases

The mainstays of therapy for ulcers include antacids, proton pump inhibitors, and H_2 antagonists. Surgery is the last resort when other therapies are unsuccessful.

Table 11.1	Drugs that Cause Ulcers
Drug	**Adverse Effect**
aspirin	irritating to the GI tract

anti-inflammatory drugs
  ibuprofen, fenoprofen,
  naproxen, tolmetin solution
	reduce production of mucus

corticosteroids (often used in inflammatory bowel disease)	reduce the mucosal barrier
potassium chloride (KCl)	irritating to the GI tract
methotrexate	irritating to the GI tract, ulceration, hemorrhage
iron	causes esophageal ulceration (must be taken with food, milk, or lots of water)

Medications used to treat GERD are categorized as phase I and phase II medications. Phase I medications are antacids that neutralize the acidic stomach contents so that if reflux does occur, the contents will be less irritating to the esophageal lining. Fortunately, many patients with acid indigestion or heartburn respond to phase I interventions. Phase I includes life-style modifications and/or use of an antacid.

Phase II medications try to improve gastric motility and decrease acid production in the stomach. These drugs will be used to stimulate cholinergic receptors and to reduce stomach acid production (the H_2 blockers or proton pump inhibitors) in order to block secretion of hydrogen ions into gastric contents.

When treating ulcers, it has been found that it is helpful to eradicate *H. pylori*. Many regimens are being used to eradicate *H. pylori*. The most common combinations of drugs are listed in Table 11.2. If bismuth (Pepto-Bismol) and tetracycline are combined, the doses of the two drugs should be separated by two hours, and the tetracycline should be taken between meals on an empty stomach to prevent an incompatibility problem. The pharmaceutical companies are also developing combinations of these drugs to improve compliance because dosing in their present form is very tedious. Table 11.3 presents the most-commonly used agents for gastrointestinal disease.

ANTACIDS The problem with antacid therapy is the frequency of dosing. For an active bleed, antacids must be given 30 to 60 mL every hour between meals for six to eight weeks. If there is no active bleed, they must be dosed 30 to 60 mL one hour before

Table 11.2	Drug Combinations for Treatment of Gastrointestinal Diseases

amoxicillin, Biaxin, Prevacid
amoxicillin, metronidazole
amoxicillin, metronidazole, ranitidine
amoxicillin, Prilosec
amoxicillin, Prilosec, Biaxin
amoxicillin, Prilosec, metronidazole
Biaxin, Prilosec
Biaxin, Tritec (ranitidine-bismuth complex)
bismuth, Biaxin, amoxicillin
bismuth, Biaxin, Prilosec
bismuth, Biaxin, tetracycline
bismuth, metronidazole, amoxicillin
bismuth, metronidazole, tetracycline
bismuth, metronidazole, tetracycline, and Prilosec
bismuth, tetracycline, Biaxin, ranitidine
bismuth, tetracycline, metronidazole
Helidac Therapy (a kit with a 14-day supply of tetracycline, metronidazole, and bismuth)
metronidazole, Prilosec, Biaxin

Table 11.3	Most-Commonly Used Agents for Gastrointestinal Disease

Generic Name	Brand Name	Dosage Form
Antacids		
aluminum hydroxide	Amphojel	tablet, liquid
aluminum hydroxide- magnesium hydroxide	Maalox Mylanta	tablet, liquid liquid
magnesium hydroxide	Milk of Magnesia (MOM)	tablet, liquid
magnesium trisilicate	Gelusil	tablet

continues

Generic Name	Brand Name	Dosage Form
Histamine₂ Receptor Antagonists		
cimetidine	Tagamet	tablet, liquid, IM, IV
famotidine	Pepcid	tablet, suspension, IM, IV
nizatidine	Axid	tablet, capsule
ranitidine	Zantac	tablet, liquid, IM, IV
Combinations		
ranitidine-bismuth-citrate	Tritec	tablet
tetracycline-metronidazole-bismuth	Helidac	tablet, 14-day kit
Proton Pump Inhibitors		
esomeprazole	Nexium	capsule
lansoprazole	Prevacid	capsule
omeprazole	Prilosec	capsule
pantoprazole	Protonix	tablet
rabeprazole	Aciphex	tablet
Coating Agents		
alginic acid	Gaviscon	tablet, chewable, liquid
sucralfate	Carafate	tablet, liquid
Prostaglandin E Analog		
misoprostol	Cytotec	tablet
Cholinergic Agent		
bethanechol	Urecholine	tablet, injection
Mast Cell Stabilizer		
cromolyn sodium	Intal	nebulizing solution, inhaler
	Nasalcrom	nasal solution
	Gastrocrom	liquid
Pancreatic Enzyme		
pancrelipase	Viokase	tablet, powder
	Cotazym	capsule
	Creon	tablet
Immunosuppression		
azathioprine	Imuran	tablet, IV
Monoclonal Antibody		
infliximab	Remicade	IV
Anti-inflammatories		
balsalazide	Colazal	capsule
mesalamine	Rowasa	suppository, enema
	Asacol, Pentasa	tablet
olsalazine	Dipentum	capsule
sulfasalazine	Azulfidine	tablet, liquid
Gallstone Dissolution		
ursodiol	Actigall	capsule
Antiemetic		
metoclopromide	Reglan	tablet, liquid, IM, IV

meals and at bedtime. Patient compliance is a big problem. **Milk of Magnesia (MOM) (magnesium hydroxide)** has good neutralizing capacity, but diarrhea can be a side effect. **Amphojel (aluminum hydroxide)** can have the side effect of constipation; it also contains aluminum, which can be a problem for some disease states.

HISTAMINE₂ RECEPTOR ANTAGONISTS Histamine₂ (H_2) receptor antagonists block gastric acid and pepsin secretion in response to histamine, gastrin, foods, distention, caffeine, or cholinergic stimulation. The mechanism of action is competitive inhibition of histamine at H_2 receptors on the gastric parietal cells, which inhibits gastric acid secretion. All are available in OTC strengths, but some dosages are prescription form only. The bedtime dose is the most important one for H_2 antagonists.

Tagamet (cimetidine) is indicated for treating ulcers and benign gastric ulcers, gastric hypersecretory states, GERD, postoperative ulcers, upper GI bleeds, and for preventing stress ulcers. It reduces acidity by 70%. Reduced doses are necessary in renal disease. It takes four to six weeks of therapy for ulcers to heal. Cimetidine has many interactions, due to the fact that it is metabolized through the cytochrome P-450 system. Pharmacy technicians should read the warnings carefully.

Axid (nizatidine) is for treating duodenal ulcers and GERD. It may take several days before the patient gets any relief. If an antacid is added to the regimen, the doses of the two agents should be taken at least thirty minutes apart. Nizatidine 100 mg is equivalent to cimetidine 300 mg. The patient should avoid aspirin, alcohol, caffeine, cough and cold preparations, and black pepper and other spices while talking this drug. Drowsiness is a side effect.

Zantac (ranitidine) is used for active duodenal ulcers and benign gastric ulcers, long-term prophylaxis of duodenal ulcers, gastric hypersecretory states, GERD, postoperative ulcers, upper GI bleeding, and preventing stress ulcers. It has fewer interactions than some of the other H_2 blockers. Concomitant administration of an antacid should be separated by thirty to sixty minutes. Constipation seems to be the primary side effect.

Pepcid (famotidine) is indicated for treating duodenal ulcers, gastric ulcers, stress ulcers, GERD, and hypersecretory conditions. It relieves heartburn, acid indigestion, and sour stomach. The dose should be modified in renal impairment, and it should be used cautiously in patients taking a calcium channel blocker.

COMBINATIONS Tritec (rantidine-bismuth-citrate) is a combination of trivalent bismuth citrate and an H_2 blocker. This formulation is an adjunctive therapy to be used in combination with an antibiotic.

PROTON PUMP INHIBITORS Prilosec (omeprazole) blocks gastric acid secretion by inhibiting the parietal cell adenosine triphosphate (ATP) pump. It is indicated for short-term treatment of severe erosive esophagitis, GERD, and hypersecretory conditions. It should be taken before meals. It is also indicated for *H. pylori* in combination with bismuth, tetracycline, Biaxin, and an H_2 antagonist. Diarrhea is a primary side effect, and patients can dehydrate quickly.

Prevacid (lansoprazole) is a proton pump inhibitor and therefore has the same mechanism of action and indications as omeprazole. It is short-term treatment of ulcers (four weeks) and eight weeks for esophagitis. It is also used in long-term treatment of hypersecretory conditions and Zollinger-Ellison syndrome (hypersecretion from a tumor). H_2 blockers and proton pump inhibitors can also be used in this syndrome.

Nexium (esomeprazole) is another proton pump inhibitor very similar to omeprazole. It is the S isomer and is metabolized more slowly. This leads to higher and more prolonged drug concentrations and longer acid suppression. It relieves heartburn faster and is slightly more effective for healing erosive esophagitis. It is used for GERD and in combination with amoxicillin and clarithromycin to treat *H. pylori*. It should be taken on an empty stomach. Since it is in a capsule form, the capsules can be opened and mixed with a small amount of applesauce if patients have difficulty swallowing pills.

Warning

Ranitidine may look like amantadine and/or rimantadine. Zantac and Xanax are similar.

Protonix (pantoprazole), also a proton pump inhibitor, is less expensive than most drugs of this class. It is the drug of choice among many hospitals.

COATING AGENTS **Carafate (sucralfate)** is a complex of aluminum hydroxide and sulfated sucrose with an affinity for proteins. It forms a protective coat over the ulcer, resisting acid-pepsin degradation. It adheres to proteins at the ulcer site, forming a shield against gastric acid, pepsin, and bile salts. It also inhibits pepsin, exhibits a cytoprotective effect, and forms a viscous, adhesive barrier on the surface of the intact intestinal mucosa and stomach. It is used for duodenal ulcers and is dosed every six hours (the duration of the coating action's effectiveness). Patients are often awakened from sleep by the ulcer, so around-the-clock dosing is recommended for the first few days. Once the ulcer is relieved, dosing can be twice daily for better compliance. Sucralfate should be taken on an empty stomach.

Gaviscon (alginic acid), the drug of choice for GERD, contains both an antacid and alginic acid. Together they create "a raft of foam" over the stomach contents. Gaviscon creates a viscous antacid layer on top of the stomach contents so that if reflux does occur, the foam layer precedes the stomach contents, protecting the sensitive esophageal lining. In addition, the viscous foam may act as a barrier, preventing acidic stomach contents from refluxing into the esophagus.

PROSTAGLANDIN E ANALOG **Cytotec (misoprostol)** is a synthetic prostaglandin E for NSAID-induced gastric ulcers. It replaces the protective prostaglandins consumed by such therapies. The primary side effects of this drug are diarrhea and abdominal pain. In other countries it is used for ulcers other than those caused by the nonsteroidal anti-inflammatory drugs (NSAIDs). Pregnant women should not take this drug nor should they handle it with their bare hands.

CHOLINERGIC AGENT **Urecholine (bethanechol)** stimulates cholinergic receptors in the GI tract as well as the urinary tract, resulting in increased peristalsis. It is used primarily for its effect on the urinary tract but is sometimes used to treat GERD. When dispensing the injectable form of this drug be sure to label it subcutaneous. A serious reaction can occur if it is administered intramuscularly or intravenously.

MAST CELL STABILIZER **Gastrocrom (cromolyn sodium)** inhibits release of allergic and inflammatory mediators in the GI tract and is indicated for abdominal pain. The capsule powder should be mixed in water, not fruit juice or milk, and be taken thirty minutes before meals and at bedtime. It reduces diarrhea, flushing, headache, vomiting, rash, abdominal pain, and itch. It is used in inflammatory bowel diseases.

PANCREATIC ENZYME **Viokase, Creon**, and **Cotazym (pancrelipase)** are indicated for replacement therapy in symptomatic treatment of malabsorption syndrome caused by pancreatic insufficiency. Nausea, cramps, constipation, and diarrhea can all be side effects. These drugs can also cause hyperuricemia. Often used in cystic fibrosis patients, they should be taken before or with meals. They can trigger gout attacks because they result in high blood levels of purine, which is converted to uric acid.

IMMUNOSUPPRESSION **Imuran (azathioprine)** is an immunosuppressive agent that interferes with nucleic acid synthesis in both normal and precancer cells. The overall action is the suppression of the immune system. Approved usage is severe arthritis and organ transplant rejection. It is also used as an anti-inflammatory in Crohn's disease, ulcerative colitis, and chronic active hepatitis. It can have serious but reversible forms of bone marrow depression. An allergic response is chills, fever, and arthralgias up to one month after therapy. Rash, alopecia (hair loss), hepatotoxicity, and increased risk of infection are side effects.

MONOCLONAL ANTIBODY **Remicade (infliximab)** binds to tumor necrosis factor (TNF) alpha and neutralizes its activity by preventing it from binding to the cell membrane and in the blood. It decreases infiltration of inflammatory cells and TNF alpha production in inflamed areas of the intestines. It is indicated in the treatment of active Crohn's disease and is generally reserved for moderate to severe cases. Like Imuran, Remicade is an immunosuppressant and will also affect normal immune response. This drug is given either as a single infusion or, for more complicated outbreaks, as a three-dose infusion series. It is also indicated for rheumatoid arthritis because of its action on TNF alpha. The vials should be refrigerated but not frozen. It is reconstituted with sterile water that is directed to the glass wall of the vial. The powder should be gently swirled by rotating the vial. It should not be shaken. It should then be admixed with normal saline. It must be prepared only in glass bottles or polypropylene or polyolefin infusion bags and administered through polyethylene-lined administration sets. It is incompatible with PVC.

ANTI-INFLAMMATORY DRUGS **Rowasa, Asacol,** and **Pentasa (mesalamine)** are used in Crohn's disease and ulcerative colitis. Rowasa is given as a rectal enema. It can cause abdominal pain, headache, flatulence, nausea, and flulike symptoms. It works topically by blocking prostaglandin production and inhibiting inflammation. The tablet and capsule forms of this drug have the same mechanism within the body.

Azulfidine (sulfasalazine) is metabolized by colon bacteria into an active product that penetrates the colon mucosa. It is used in ulcerative colitis and Crohn's disease. It acts in the colon to decrease the inflammatory response and systemically interfere with secretion by inhibiting prostaglandin synthesis. Sulfasalazine is believed to be a prodrug, inactive until bacterial action converts it into an active drug. One metabolite is responsible for the anti-inflammatory effect; the other metabolite may be responsible for the antibacterial action and most of the adverse effects. These effects are dose related. The patient should maintain proper fluid intake and take the drug after meals. The drug can change urine to an orange-yellow color and may permanently stain soft contact lenses yellow. The patient should avoid the sun. It should not be taken for more than two years.

Sulfasalazine is contraindicated in patients allergic to sulfa or salicylates. It should not be given within one hour of iron, as it will bind the iron. Side effects of sulfasalazine are nausea, vomiting, fever, headache, rash, and arthralgias. It can also cause bronchospasm, hepatotoxicity, pancreatitis, neuropathies, and severe anemias.

Dipentum (olsalazine) maintains remission of ulcerative colitis and Crohn's in patients who are resistant to sulfasalazine. This drug should be taken with food in evenly divided doses.

Colazal (balsalazide) is broken down by bacteria in the colon to release mesalamine. It works as well as mesalamine and is better tolerated than sulfasalazine because there is no sulfa entity. It is used to treat ulcerative colitis. Asacol and Pentasa are still preferred to treat colitis higher in the GI tract.

GALLSTONE DISSOLUTION **Actigall (ursodiol)** is a naturally occurring bile acid used as an oral agent to dissolve cholesterol gallstones. It decreases the cholesterol content of bile and bile stones by reducing the secretion of cholesterol from the liver and the fractional reabsorption of cholesterol by the intestines. Frequent blood work is necessary to follow the drug's effects. Persistent nausea, vomiting, and abdominal pain should be reported. Gallstone dissolution can take several months but may never occur. Recurrence of stones within five years has been observed in 50% of patients.

ANTIEMETIC **Reglan (metoclopramide)** promotes GI tract motility by blocking dopamine receptors in the CTZ and thereby enhancing the response to acetylcholine in the upper GI tract. Like urecholine, it increases the pressure at the lower esophageal sphincter, preventing reflux. Metoclopromide is more likely to be useful if the daily dose is divided. It has fewer side effects than the promotility agents, but it does cause sedation.

ANTIDIARRHEALS

Diarrhea can be dangerous because it can quickly lead to dehydration. It decreases GI transit time and will impair absorption of drugs, vitamins, nutrients, and toxins. Antidiarrheals, listed in Table 11.4, should not be used to manage short-term, self-limiting diarrhea. They can also be hazardous in infectious diarrhea by prolonging fever and delaying clearance of organisms. Antidiarrheals should be used in managing chronic disease states, such as inflammatory bowel disease, postvagotomy diarrhea, and ileostomy.

Lomotil (diphenoxylate-atropine) is a C-V narcotic available by prescription only. The opiate in the drug inhibits effective peristalsis. It is 0.25 mg of diphenoxylate with 0.25 mg of atropine. The side effects are anticholinergic effects (dry mouth, blurred vision, flushing, urinary retention), constipation, paralytic ileus, respiratory depression, and sedation. Care should be taken in infectious diarrhea with fever, acute diarrhea, toxic megacolon resulting in perforation, and advanced liver disease.

Motofen (difenoxin) is a metabolite of diphenoxylate and is classified as C-IV. The side effect profile and usage are the same as for diphenoxylate.

Imodium (loperamide) is a synthetic agent similar to diphenoxylate. It acts on the intestinal nerves with antiperistaltic activity. It has provided prolonged use without loss of efficacy or signs of toxicity (eighteen months or longer). Side effects are drowsiness, constipation, and dry mouth. It is available OTC and is replacing diphenoxylate-atropine because it seems to be as efficacious without the addictive side effect profile.

Paregoric (camphorated tincture of opium) is a C-III agent. It increases smooth-muscle tone in the GI tract, decreases motility and peristalsis, and diminishes digestive secretions. The patient should avoid alcohol when taking any opium derivative. Paregoric may cause drowsiness, may impair judgment or coordination, and may cause physical and psychological dependence with prolonged use.

Table 11.4 **Most-Commonly Used Antidiarrheals**

Generic Name	Brand Name	Dosage Form
attapulgite	Kaopectate	liquid
bismuth subsalicylate	Pepto-Bismol	tablet, caplet, liquid
camphorated tincture of opium	Paregoric	liquid
difenoxin	Motofen	tablet
diphenoxylate-atropine	Lomotil	tablet, liquid
loperamide	Imodium	caplet, capsule

Kaopectate (attapulgite) contains 20% kaolin, hydrated aluminum silicate, and 17% pectin. This OTC agent controls diarrhea because of its adsorbent action. If diarrhea is not controlled within twenty-four hours, the physician should be contacted. Kaopectate is an adsorbent which acts by coating the walls of the GI tract, adsorbing the bacteria or toxins causing the diarrhea, and passing them out with the stools. It is usually taken after each loose bowel movement until the diarrhea is controlled. A caution is that Kaopectate may interfere with the absorption of medication given concurrently.

Pepto-Bismol (bismuth subsalicylate) also controls diarrhea through adsorbent action.

FIBER, GI DISEASES, AND CONSTIPATION

Fiber is defined as the undigested residue of fruits, vegetables, and other foods of plant origin after digestion by the human GI enzymes. The most important classification of fiber is by water solubility. Fruits, vegetables, and grains contain both soluble and insoluble fibers. Total fiber is the sum of soluble and insoluble fiber.

In addition to its solubility, fiber is characterized by its fermentability, water-holding capacity, and stool-bulking capacity. Fiber's fermentability is the ability of bacteria to ferment some types of fiber. Soluble fibers are fermented to a greater extent than insoluble ones. The end products are short-chain fatty acids, gases, water, and energy. Fiber's water-holding capacity is the ability of fiber to hold water and make bulking of fecal material possible. Insoluble fibers hold less water than soluble ones. Fiber's stool-bulking capacity is the ability of the fiber to increase the volume of intestinal content because it can absorb and hold water. Bacterial growth in the colon provides additional bulking.

Extended transit time in the colon permits more water to be absorbed, thus producing small, hard stools. Shortening the transit time produces loose, watery stools because too little water is absorbed.

Insoluble fibers speed GI transit time. Some soluble fibers, such as psyllium, work to speed transit. Soluble fibers form gels when mixed with water. In the GI tract they act more like solids than liquids, and thus delay emptying. This is why psyllium can be used as an antidiarrheal as well as fiber. Inactivity or confinement to bed can actually cause constipation when combined with these products. Fiber also provides lubrication.

Chronic constipation has often been associated with low-fiber diets. This is a common problem among the elderly in the United States and other Western countries but does not appear to be a problem in less developed countries. The most widely accepted therapeutic use of high-fiber foods is in managing constipation. Dietary fiber provides bulking, increases colon content, decreases colon pressure, and increases propulsive motility. Bulking agents are considered the safest and most natural of all laxative products.

Soluble fibers exert metabolic effects. Natural soluble fibers delay emptying and absorbing of glucose from the small intestine. High-fiber diets or fiber supplements can help prevent diabetes and coronary artery disease. Fiber may also increase tissue sensitivity to insulin by increasing the number of insulin receptors on target cells. Psyllium, fruit and vegetable fiber, and other soluble fibers bind to bile acids, interrupting enterohepatic circulation of some fatty materials. Soluble fibers bind to the bile acids excreted in the stool. These acids must be replaced to ensure fat metabolism. Bile acids are made from cholesterol and other circulating lipids. Making more bile acids decreases the body's lipoprotein pool, with the end result being to maintain or increase blood levels of high-density lipoproteins (HDLs) and to reduce blood levels of low-density lipoproteins (LDLs).

Fiber Supplementation

Fiber supplementation has been widely used to suppress appetite and achieve weight loss. Fiber helps to produce feelings of fullness, or satiety. The most effective diets are low-calorie, high-residue (high-fiber) ones. Bulk-producing products should be taken with a full glass of water about a half hour before eating. As dietary fiber increases, risk of colorectal cancer is reduced. Colon cancer is more likely to develop when there are high fat levels and low fiber content (the latter raises the risk even more).

Dietary fiber increases the weight and bulk of the stool and alters its consistency through its water-holding capacity and the results of intestinal bacterial fermentation. Most dietary fiber reaches the colon unaltered, where it increases colon content, reduces colon pressure (intraluminal), and increases propulsive motility.

The adverse effects of fiber are distention, excessive gas, and flatulence, but these symptoms usually subside after the first few weeks. These symptoms may also be associated with esophageal, gastric, or small-bowel or rectal obstruction, especially in patients with intestinal stricture or stenosis. They may also interfere with absorbing some drugs and nutrients.

The beneficial fiber intake threshold is about 40 g/day. Most Americans consume only 15 to 20 g/day. Doubling the daily fiber intake could produce a significant health benefit.

Gastrointestinal Diseases

Constipation as a result of low amounts of fiber in the diet is among the causes of several diseases.

DIVERTICULAR DISEASE Diverticular disease is believed to result from a deficiency of fiber over time. It is an out-pocketing from the bowel wall that becomes inflamed (see Figure 11.2). Vegetarians who average a daily fiber intake of about twice (40 g) that of nonvegetarians (20 g) have about one third as much diverticular disease.

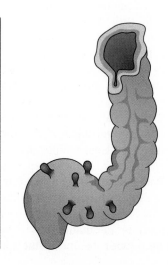

Figure 11.2

Portion of the Colon with Diverticula
In this disease, the muscular layers of the colon wall may become inflamed and herniations form along the mucous membranes, causing pain.

Diverticular disease seems to be related to the predominance of more highly refined carbohydrates and other processed food sources in the modern diet. Colonic segmentation is accompanied by an increase in pressure inside the colon, prolonged GI transit time, and low fecal weight. All of these factors contribute to herniation of weakened areas of the colon walls with accompanying inflammation and pain. Fiber may reduce the pressure generated in the colon.

HIATAL HERNIA Hiatal hernia is related to chronic constipation. Straining to pass small, firm stools can significantly raise intra-abdominal pressures. Over a period of several years, daily straining to pass stools could force the gastroesophageal junction upwards into the thoracic cavity.

IRRITABLE BOWEL SYNDROME (IBS) Irritable bowel syndrome (IBS) is the most common of the GI disorders. As many as 70% of all patients with GI complaints are diagnosed with IBS. IBS is a functional disorder in which the lower GI tract does not have the appropriate tone or spasticity to regulate bowel activity. Some evidence also suggests that patients presenting with IBS have an abnormal sensitivity to neurotransmitter within the GI tract. This disorder affects twice as many women as men. Patients have an increased rate of hospital stays, abdominal surgery, and work absenteeism. A patient may be symptom-free for five years or more. Criteria for diagnosis include

- abdominal distention
- gas
- increased colonic mucus
- irregular bowel habits (diarrhea or constipation more than 25% of the time)
- pain

HEMORRHOIDS Hemorrhoids result from pressure exerted on anal veins while straining to pass a stool, which causes engorgement of the vascular cushions situated within the sphincter muscles. Passing a small, hard stool through the anal canal can abrade the overlying mucosa, causing hemorrhoidal bleeding. Prolapse of the vascular cushions may occur from rupture of their attachments to the surrounding sphincter.

Hemorrhoids are treated with suppositories, ointments, and sometimes surgery. Some medications are **Anusol HC** and **Anucort HC**. Most medications for hemorrhoids include **hydrocortisone**. Modifying diet by increasing fiber can help prevent hemorrhoids.

Pharmacologic Treatment of Constipation

Constipation has many causes, including certain medications and a low-fiber diet. Fiber keeps food moving in the gut, and low fiber intake is related to colon cancer. Everyone over fifty-five years old should have a rectal examination. Another cause of constipation is dehydration, which can be due to fever, hot dry temperature, vomiting, and diarrhea. It is very important to drink six to eight glasses of fluids daily. This alone can often prevent constipation. Bed rest and mucosal damage can also cause constipation. Regular exercise will often help prevent constipation.

Sometimes laxatives are needed to treat constipation and for bowel cleansing prior to colorectal examination. Types of laxatives include stimulants, bulk-forming agents, and emollients/lubricants. Table 11.5 contains the most-commonly used laxatives as well as other agents to treat constipation.

EMOLLIENTS/LUBRICANTS Emollients/lubricants draw water into the colon and thereby stimulate evacuation. For example, glycerin draws fluid into the colon and stimulates

Table 11.5 Most-Commonly Used Agents to Treat Constipation

Generic Name	Brand Name	Dosage Form
Emollients/Lubricants		
dioctyl calcium sulfosuccinate	Surfak	tablet, capsule, liquid
dioctyl potassium sulfosuccinate	Dialose	tablet
dioctyl sodium sulfosuccinate	Colace	tablet, capsule, microenema
glycerin	Fleet	suppository
lactulose	Duphalac, Cephulac	solution
magnesium hydroxide	Milk of Magnesia	liquid
magnesium sulfate	Epsom salts	tablet
sodium phosphate	Fleet Phospho-Soda	solution
Stimulants		
bisacodyl	Dulcolax	tablet, suppository
senna	Senokot	tablet, syrup, granule
Bulk-Forming Agents		
methylcellulose	FiberTrim	tablet
	Citrucel	powder
polycarbophil	Mitrolan	chewable
psyllium hydrophilic mucolloid	Metamucil	powder, wafer
Antiflatulents		
simethicone	Phazyme	
	Gas-X	
	Mylanta	tablet, liquid, gelcap
	Mylicon	drops
Bowel Evacuant		
polyethylene glycol-electrolyte solution	GoLYTELY	powder

evacuation of the lower bowel, so few nutrients are lost. Glycerin suppositories are a fairly quick, effective method to relieve constipation.

Duphalac and **Cephulac (lactulose)** are metabolized by bacteria in the colon, which reduces fecal pH and reduces absorption of ammonia and toxic nitrogenous substances, and have a cathartic effect. Lactulose is used to prevent and treat hepatic-induced encephalopathy. The liver forms nitrogen waste by-products from protein. When the liver is not functioning properly, as in alcoholism, these nitrogen by-products build up, destroying brain cells, which results in encephalopathy. Lactulose reduces ammonia production and absorption from the GI tract. The side effects include nausea and vomiting, cramps, diarrhea, and anorexia.

Magnesium should be used cautiously in renal patients. It is supplied as the citrate, hydroxide, and sulfate (Epsom salts) forms.

Fleet Phospho-Soda (sodium phosphate) is indicated for short-term constipation, evacuation of the colon for treating and testing of hypophosphatemia.

STIMULANTS Stimulants increase gut activity due to mucosal irritation. **Dulcolax (bisacodyl)**, **Doxidan (danthron)**, and **Senokot (senna)** can easily cause diarrhea and allergic reactions that include hives and peripheral swelling. Technicians should be watchful for patients on long-term narcotic pain medication. A tolerance will not be developed for constipation and they should be on a stimulant laxative.

BULK-FORMING AGENTS Bran as a dietary supplement can be acquired through inclusion of whole grains and grain products in the diet. These are naturally occurring bulk materials that appeal to many patients wanting to return to natural foods. Eating bran is an excellent way to increase fiber in the diet and promotes normal gut peristalsis. Bran and other bulking agents are the most natural and safest materials to use.

Metamucil (psyllium hydrophilic mucolloid) increases nonabsorbable bulk to promote soft stools and easy defecation in patients who should avoid straining (e.g., postoperative, post-MI, elderly, pregnant). Patients should drink six to eight glasses of water a day. Patients must be active for this to work; it can cause constipation in a bedridden patient. It is also an excellent cholesterol-lowering agent.

FiberTrim (methylcellulose) and **Mitrolan (polycarbophil)** have the same therapeutic effects as psyllium without the cholesterol lowering.

Patients should maintain adequate fluid intake of six to eight glasses per day. These drugs are recommended for initial therapy. The two most used are psyllium and calcium polycarbophil.

ANTIFLATULENTS **Phazyme**, **Gas-X**, **Mylicon**, and **Mylanta (simethicone)** are inert silicon polymers that are gastric defoaming agents. By reducing surface tension, they cause gas bubbles to be broken or to coalesce into a foam that can be eliminated more easily by belching or passing flatus. They relieve flatulence and functional gastric bloating and postoperative gas pains. Dosage recommendations should not be exceeded, especially in children.

BOWEL EVACUANT **GoLYTELY (polyethylene glycol-electrolyte solution)** stimulates bowel content removal by increasing the osmolarity of bowel fluids. This formulation will be dispensed regularly by the pharmacy technician. It is indicated for bowel cleansing prior to GI examination or in rare cases following toxic ingestion. The recommended dose is 4 L. The patient should fast three to four hours prior to administration and absolutely for two hours; 240 mL (eight ounces) should be consumed every ten minutes until the four liters are gone. The doctor or manufacturer usually supplies a printed informational sheet for the patient with explicit instructions. A powder is dispensed in a liter container. The patient adds a solution of choice.

ANTIEMETICS

Antiemetics are drugs that work primarily in the vomiting center to inhibit impulses going to the stomach which cause vomiting. The chemo-receptor trigger zone (CTZ) is located below the floor of the fourth ventricle (Figure 11.3). Input is received from the cerebral cortex and hypothalamus and also from blood-borne stimuli (bacterial toxins and drugs that have access to the brain via the blood vascular systems). The main neurotransmitters that cause nausea and vomiting are acetylcholine, dopamine, and serotonin. The vomiting center is located in the reticular formation of the medulla. Input is received from the CTZ via the vagus nerve or the tenth cranial nerve.

There are two ways to initiate vomiting. The first is by stimulating the CTZ, which in turn stimulates the GI tract (e.g., narcotics stimulate brain receptors). The second is by stimulating the vagal receptors in the stomach with no CTZ involvement.

Vomiting can cause dehydration, electrolyte imbalance leading to alkalosis (due to loss of Cl^- and H^+), and possible aspiration pneumonia (HCl and gram-positive organisms). It may also cause bradycardia or other arrhythmias due to an electrolyte imbalance.

Emesis often occurs secondary to narcotic intake. Morphine and its derivatives stimulate the CTZ, and vomiting is dose-related. Narcotics increase the vomiting center's sensitivity to vestibular stimuli.

Stimulating the labyrinth system results in impulses being carried via cholinergic and adrenergic tracts to the vestibular nucleus (of the ear), which is near the

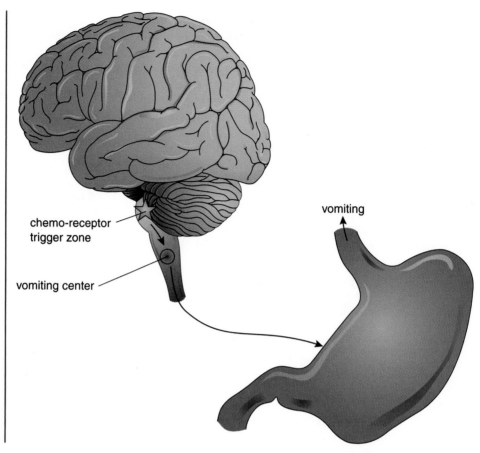

Figure 11.3

Chemo-receptor Trigger Zone and Vomiting Center

chemo-receptor trigger zone

vomiting center

vomiting

vomiting center. This is common in car sickness. Vertigo, the sensation of the room spinning when one gets up or changes positions, is treated with anticholinergic agents.

Table 11.6 presents the most-commonly used antiemetics.

Vomiting can also be induced with ipecac syrup. Ipecac syrup is used in an emergency situation to *cause* vomiting in poisoning cases. It produces vomiting via local irritation of the GI mucosa and stimulation of the CTZ. For anyone over one year old the dose is 15 mL (one tablespoonful) of ipecac followed by one to two glasses of water or milk. Under age one year the dose is 10 mL followed by 100 to 200 mL of water or milk. Patients become sleepy after taking this drug, but they must be kept awake, as they may continue to vomit and could aspirate the vomitus in an unconscious state. Because of this danger, poison centers only recommend this drug when absolutely necessary.

Phenothiazines inhibit the CTZ. They act as a sedative, antiemetic, and anticholinergic (causing dry mouth, blurred vision, and urinary retention). To avoid hypotension, these drugs should not be given by IV push. **Compazine (prochlorperazine)** is the prototype phenothiazine. It is administered orally, by rectal suppository, IM injection, or IV. It must be used with caution in children and is easily overdosed, precipitating seizures.

Reglan (metoclopramide) is used in gastric stasis (lack of stomach motility), GI reflux, and chemotherapeutic-induced emesis. It inhibits or reduces nausea and vomiting by blocking dopamine receptors in the CTZ. It also relieves esophageal

Table 11.6	Most-Commonly Used Antiemetics		
Generic Name		**Brand Name**	**Dosage Form**
cyclizine		Marezine	tablet, IM
dimenhydrinate		Dramamine	tablet, chewable
diphenhydramine		Benadryl	tablet, syrup, capsule, cream, elixir, IM, IV, lotion, solution
granisetron		Kytril	tablet, IV
hydroxyzine		Atarax, Vistaril	tablet, syrup, IM, IV, capsule
meclizine		Antivert, Bonine	capsule, tablet
metoclopramide		Reglan	tablet, syrup, IM, IV
ondansetron		Zofran	tablet, IV
prochlorperazine		Compazine	tablet, capsule, syrup, IM, IV, suppository
promethazine		Phenergan	tablet, syrup, IM, IV, suppository
thiethylperazine		Torecan	tablet, suppository, IM, IV
triflupromazine		Vesprin	tablet, liquid, IM
trimethobenzamide		Tigan	capsule, IM, suppository

reflux by increasing lower-esophageal sphincter tone and reduces gastric stasis by stimulating motility of the upper GI tract, thus reducing gastric emptying time. The side effects are extrapyramidal symptoms (EPS), which are Parkinson-like, especially in children, drowsiness, and depression. Diphenhydramine is used to reduce EPS. The drug should not be used for longer than twelve weeks.

Zofran (ondansetron) blocks serotonin (5-HT) receptors (may do so in CTZ and small-bowel vagal nerve terminals). It is used for chemotherapeutic-induced emesis. Headache is a major side effect. It can also cause either constipation or diarrhea.

Kytril (granisetron) binds to serotonin (5-HT) receptors with little or no affinity for other serotonins (alpha or beta), dopamine D_2, benzodiazepine, or opiate receptors. It blocks the 5-HT receptors both peripherally on vagal nerve terminals and centrally in the CTZ. The side effects can be headache, asthenia (weakness), drowsiness, and diarrhea. It is usually given by the IV route. The drug must be protected from light.

Antihistamines inhibit cholinergic spread of impulses from the vestibular nucleus to the vomiting center. **Antivert** and **Bonine (meclizine)** are used primarily for vertigo. **Tigan (trimethobenzamide)** is structurally related to the antihistamines. It has antinausea activity and is used in Compazine allergies.

OBESITY

Obesity is defined as a state in which an individual's total body weight consists of greater quantities of fat than is considered normal. Obesity in males is 25% of total body weight over ideal body weight; in females the figure is 35%. The normal is defined as the ideal body weight (IBW), and IBW is calculated as follows:

Male IBW kg = 50 + (2.3 × height in inches over 5 feet)
Female IBW kg = 45.5 + (2.3 × height in inches over 5 feet)

Note that IBW is calculated in kilograms, in spite of the fact that the patient's height is measured in feet and inches. Morbid obesity is two to three times the ideal body weight.

Genetic factors play an important role in obesity. A child with one obese parent has a 50% chance of being obese, but that increases to 80% if both parents are obese. Adipocyte cells, known as fat cells, are determined in childhood. The number and size of these fat cells is determined by age two. An obese adult who was not overweight in childhood will more likely be able to sustain a weight loss.

Anxiety, stress, and poor self-image are among the psychological factors experienced by overweight individuals. External factors such as social repugnance and intolerance, discrimination, and emotional reactions to social pressure are correlated with obesity.

Those who strongly believe they can change their eating habits are more likely to be successful in losing weight than those who do not. If patients believe weight loss depends on external circumstances, they are less likely to lose weight. Individuals with weight disorders (obesity, anorexia, bulimia) generally have low self-esteem. External psychological factors include family traits, lifestyle, and customs. Food is usually substituted for manual and oral craving. There may also be craving for certain nutrients (sweets or carbohydrates). Obese persons tend to have poor self-image, greater incidence of cardiovascular disease, and higher incidence of non-insulin-dependent diabetes.

Obesity can be managed by diet, behavioral modification, prescription and nonprescription medications, surgical procedures, and other nondrug therapy.

When a weight-loss diet is initiated, the first loss is retained water, up to six pounds the first week. A decrease in basal metabolic rate and activity levels neutralizes the diet's effectiveness. There is also a roller-coaster syndrome:

1. weight loss
2. plateau
3. cessation of dieting
4. resumption of regular eating habits
5. increase in weight

In order to be effective and permanent, weight loss requires permanent changes in eating habits, behavioral modifications, and regular exercise. Types of diet include

⬦ calorie restriction (To lose one pound, a patient must decrease food intake by 3,500 calories. A decrease of about 500 cal/day can be achieved on a diet of 1,200 to 1,600 cal/day.)
⬦ manipulation of amounts of protein, carbohydrate, and fats but no calorie restriction
⬦ decrease in grams of fat consumed

The most important type of behavior modification for weight-loss is increasing exercise. However, other types of behavior modifications can be helpful such as

⬦ keeping records of what is eaten daily
⬦ restricting cues that signal eating
⬦ slowing the rate of eating
⬦ rewarding appropriate eating behaviors

The decision to treat obesity with drug therapy must be carefully considered. Patients must always be aware of the need for a balanced diet. The body mass index (BMI), which is determined by dividing the patient's weight in kilograms by the patient's height in meters squared (kg/m^2), is used as a guide in deciding whether or not to initiate pharmacologic treatment for this disorder.

Surgical treatment methods are available but have significant side effects and are expensive. These include jaw-wiring (about 50% success), jejunoileal bypass, gastroplasty, and intragastric balloon.

The most-commonly used agents to treat obesity are listed in Table 11.7.

Stimulants

Stimulants are the most-commonly used agents for weight reduction. They work in several ways. **Tenuate (diethylpropion)** and **Fastin (phentermine)** stimulate adrenergic pathways. **Mazanor (mazindol)** stimulates adrenergic and dopaminergic pathways. **Dexedrine (dexatroamphetamine)** and **Desoxyn (methamphetamine)** act on norepinephrine and dopaminergic pathways. **Meridia (sibutramine)** inhibits the reuptake of norepinephrine, serotonin, and dopamine. Preparations usually work for three to four hours; long-acting or sustained-release ones work up to twelve hours. Short-acting agents should be taken thirty to sixty minutes before each meal. Long-acting ones should be taken twelve hours before retiring to prevent insomnia. These drugs are all controlled substances and subject to the laws which govern their dispensing. The adverse effects are

- ◇ CNS stimulation, dizziness, euphoria, dysphoria, fatigue, and insomnia
- ◇ GI symptoms of dry mouth, nausea, abdominal discomfort, and constipation
- ◇ CV hypertension, palpitations, and arrhythmias

Withdrawal from these drugs can cause tremor, confusion, and headache. Most should not be given within fourteen days of a monoamine oxidase inhibitor (MAOI) and are contraindicated in pulmonary hypertension.

Lipase Inhibitor

Xenical (orlistat) has a unique mechanism of action. This drug binds with and inhibits the action of gastric and pancreatic lipases in the lumen of the stomach and small intestine. The fat in the diet cannot be hydrolyzed and absorbed. At the same time, fat soluble vitamins (i.e., A, D, E, and beta carotene) required to maintain good health are also not absorbed. Most patients will need to add a multi-vitamin supplement to their diet. A BMI of at least 30 kg/m^2, or in the presence of other risk factors (e.g., hypertension, diabetes, dyslipidemia) at least 27 kg/m^2, is required to initiate treatment with this drug.

Table 11.7	Most-Commonly Used Agents to Treat Obesity	
Generic Name	**Brand Name**	**Dosage Form**
Stimulants		
dextroamphetamine	Dexedrine	tablet, capsule
diethylpropion	Tenuate	tablet
mazindol	Mazanor	tablet
methamphetamine	Desoxyn	tablet
phentermine	Fastin	capsule
sibutramine	Meridia	capsule
Lipase Inhibitor		
orlistat	Xenical	capsule

Since orlistat and sibutramine have different mechanisms of action, these agents are often used in combination. Patients on orlistat should be on a balanced diet and should spread their fat intake in relatively equal portions over three meals in order to decrease adverse GI events such as oily spotting, flatus with discharge, fecal urgency, fatty or oily stools, increased defecation, and fecal incontinence. Patients should be on a balanced diet that contains 30% of calories from fat. This drug has been shown to decrease low-density lipoprotein (LDL) cholesterol slightly and to increase high-density lipoprotein (HDL) cholesterol.

Fiber Agents

Bulk-producing products provide a sense of fullness and contain active ingredients, which are fibers from natural grain components. The results are a lessened desire to eat and a decrease in calorie intake. These ingredients are not absorbed systemically and are, therefore, considered safe. However, they must be consumed with large quantities of water. They may actually increase peristalsis by moving food faster, but can also have the opposite effect. The accumulation of bulk may result in esophageal, gastric, or small-intestine or rectal obstruction. They should not be used by patients who have preexisting intestinal problems or by those on restricted carbohydrate diets.

PHARMACOLOGIC TREATMENT OF PARASITES

Animal parasites have acquired the ability to live in the body of another animal. Most parasites spend part of their life cycle in one host, such as humans, and another part of the cycle in another animal. Each parasite has its own particular animal host, and these hosts are not interchangeable.

The life cycle of most parasites is complex. The intermediate host is the host the parasite passes through in its larval stage or stages. The definitive host is the one in which the parasite reaches maturity and produces gametes. Parasite spread is encouraged by unsanitary conditions, overcrowding, and warm climate.

Parasitic infections are a worldwide health problem, particularly in less developed countries; they affect a large percentage of all people. Factors supporting infection include population crowding, poor sanitation, inadequate health education, poor parasite vector control, and reservoirs of infection. This is among the most pressing, serious, yet most neglected, public health problems in developing countries.

Management of parasitic disease consists of four approaches.

1. improve hygiene
2. control vector and intermediate hosts
3. vaccines
4. drug therapy

To avoid parasites when traveling, do not drink untreated water, including ice prepared from this water, unpasteurized milk, raw or undercooked meat or freshwater fish (which often contain flukes or tapeworms), or salads washed in local untreated water. Bottled beverages, such as beer and wine, are usually safe. Peelable raw fruit and vegetables are relatively safe when the person eating the food has peeled the fruit or vegetable. Insect bites should be avoided, so wherever possible, wear an insect repellent. Wading or swimming in freshwater streams, lakes, and rivers may lead to schistosome infections.

Drug therapy for travelers includes **Achromycin (tetracycline)** which is often used for prophylaxis of traveler's diarrhea. **Cipro (ciprofloxacin)** as well as **Bactrim** are being used with some success. The concept of prophylaxing traveler's diarrhea is controversial. Table 11.8 presents the most-commonly used antiparasitic drugs.

Platyhelminthes (Flatworms)

FLUKES AND SCHISTOSOMIASIS Flukes (Trematoda) are flat, leaflike, single-sex creatures, 0.16 to 5.7 cm in length, that live in the intestine, liver, lung, or blood. They are named for the organs that they thrive in. Intestinal flukes are found mainly in the Far East. These parasites live in the upper intestine. Lung flukes live in the lung and enter the blood after crossing the intestinal wall. They cause chronic inflammation and fibrosis. Infection comes from eating raw crayfish. Blood flukes enter portal blood vessels (the venous GI drainage) and then flow to the liver. They lay their eggs in vessels around the urinary bladder, destroying surrounding tissue. The mature ova pass into the urine. Ova hatch in freshwater, enter a snail, grow, and then reenter the water, where they pass through the skin of bathers.

Schistosomiasis is the most common disease caused by flukes. The fluke (Schistosoma) lives in veins of the pelvis and bladder. Ova are laid in the bladder wall, causing intense inflammation, passing of blood, and a predisposition to bladder cancer. The fluke infects the liver by traveling up the mesenteric veins from the intestines. It may cause obstruction of the portal vessel branches and fibrosis. Eventually portal hypertension develops, and the patient's general health deteriorates.

TAPEWORMS Tapeworm (Cestoda) is a segmented single-sex parasite. It possesses a small head (scolex), a neck, and varying numbers of proglottides (body segments, each containing numerous ova). It requires two hosts; humans are the definitive hosts.

The beef tapeworm grows up to 30 feet with 2,000 segments. Embryos penetrate beef muscle. Infection comes from eating undercooked infected beef. Symptoms may include abdominal pain and skin eruptions.

The pork tapeworm grows up to 20 feet with 1,000 segments. It lives in pork muscle. Infection occurs from eating undercooked infected pork. Symptoms occur in muscles, heart, brain, skin, and other organs.

Praziquantel (biltricide) is the treatment for intestinal tapeworms. It increases cell permeability of calcium into the worm, causing contractions and paralysis of worm musculature and leading to detachment of suckers from the blood vessel walls and to dislodgment. The tablets should be taken with food. The drug may impair judgment and coordination, so caution should be taken when performing tasks that require mental alertness.

Table 11.8	Most-Commonly Used Antiparasitic Drugs	
Generic Name	**Brand Name**	**Dosage Form**
mebendazole	Vermox	chewable
niclosamide	Niclocide	chewable
praziquantel	Biltricide	tablet
thiabendazole	Mintezol	chewable, suspension

Niclocide (niclosamide) is used to treat beef and fish tapeworm infections. This drug inhibits the synthesis of ATP in these parasites, thereby disabling their metabolism. It affects cestodes of the intestine only. The side effects are nausea, vomiting, and diarrhea. It can also cause dizziness and headache.

Nematodes (Roundworms)

Roundworms (nematodes) can infect any compartment of the body and travel through a host during different segments of their life cycle. They migrate through the intestinal tract, cross the gut wall, and enter the bloodstream. The worm may come to rest in the liver or move on to the lung. From the respiratory tract, the ova or worm may be swallowed. It may also enter and obstruct lymphatics or enter the eye or brain. In the case of roundworms, usually no intermediate host is required to complete the life cycle.

PINWORM Pinworm (Enterobiasis) is the most common type of roundworm and is identified by itching of the anus. It is seen most commonly in children. After the child has gone to sleep, a piece of transparent adhesive tape when touched to the anus will pick up the tiny worms and confirm the diagnosis. The treatment is **Vermox (mebendazole)**. Mebendazole binds to tubular proteins in the parasite and inhibits glucose uptake.

WHIPWORM Whipworm (Trichuriasis) is the most common type of roundworm in the tropics and southeastern United States. There will be symptoms only with heavy infection, especially in children. Nausea, abdominal pain, and diarrhea are associated with this infection. It is treated with **Vermox (mebendazole)**.

HOOKWORM Hookworm (Ascaris) is 15 to 35 cm long (about the size of an earthworm). Ova hatch in soil, reenter by the GI tract, penetrate the gut wall, enter the blood, and then travel to the lungs. They move up the trachea, then travel down the esophagus, causing GI and respiratory problems. Ascarides are treated with **Vermox (mebendazole)**.

TRICHINELLA Trichinella is a parasite primarily of rats. The worm reaches 1.4 to 1.6 mm in length. The female burrows into the intestinal wall and releases larva into the blood. The larva reach muscle, curl up, and form small cysts. Bears and pigs become infected by eating infected rats. Humans become infected by eating undercooked pork. Symptoms include GI effects, fever, generalized edema, and muscle pain. Should the respiratory system and heart muscle become involved, death may occur. The treatment is **Mintezol (thiabendazole)**.

STRONGYLOIDES Strongyloides are tiny roundworms, 2 mm in length, that live in the mucosa of the upper jejunum, generally without symptoms. Larva develop in soil and enter through the skin. From there they pass through the lung, trachea, esophagus, and gut. If the patient is immunocompromised, a massive infection can result, with colitis, pneumonia, and meningitis, complicated by gram-negative bacteremia. At this point the infection becomes lethal. Treatment is **Mintezol (thiabendazole)**. Thiabendazole inhibits ATP synthesis within the parasite. This action blocks cellular metabolism (energy production) and thus leads to the death of the organism.

Chapter Summary

Structure and Function of the Gastrointestinal System

- The gastrointestinal (GI) tract is a tube that begins in the mouth and extends through the pharynx, esophagus, stomach, small intestine, and large intestine and ends at the anus.
- The digestive process takes place in the GI tract.
- Mucous membranes protect the entire digestive system against abrasion and strong digestive chemicals.

Gastrointestinal Diseases

- Gastritis is an irritation and superficial erosion of the intestinal lining. Ulcerative colitis is an irritation of the large bowel.
- The three types of ulcers are: gastric, duodenal, and stress.
- GERD is commonly known as heartburn. Phase I medications are antacids that exert their action by neutralizing the acidic stomach contents so if reflux does occur, the contents will be less irritating to the esophageal lining. Phase II medications serve two functions. First, they improve gastric motility (bethanechol and metoclopramide) and also increase the pressure at the lower esophageal sphincter, preventing reflux. Second, they decrease acid production in the stomach (H_2 blockers, proton pump inhibitors).
- Alcohol, nicotine, and caffeine exacerbate GERD.
- There are drug regimens for the treatment of *Helicobacter pylori (H. pylori)*, understood to be a factor to be eradicated in treating ulcers.
- The antacids in these regimens should be separated from the other drugs when dosing.
- Helidac therapy is a kit with a fourteen-day supply of tetracycline, metronidazole, and bismuth to treat ulcers.
- The bedtime dose of the H_2 blockers is the most important one.
- Gaviscon contains both an antacid and alginic acid, which together create "a raft of foam" over the stomach contents.
- Remicade is an agent used for moderate to severe cases of Crohn's disease. It will affect the normal immune response.
- Rowasa is an enema used in Crohn's disease and ulcerative colitis.
- Azulfidine (sulfasalazine) should not be taken for longer than two years. It decreases inflammatory response in the colon. It can change the color of the urine and stain soft contact lenses.
- Dipentum (olsalazine) is used for patients resistant to sulfasalazine.
- Colazal (balsalazide) is better tolerated than sulfasalazine because there is no sulfa entity.
- Actigall (ursodiol) is used to dissolve gallstones, but it can take several months.

Antidiarrheals

- Lomotil is a combination drug and is a controlled substance that is used for diarrhea.
- Imodium (loperamide) has been found to be as effective as Lomotil and is available OTC.

Fiber, GI Diseases, and Constipation

◇ Chronic constipation is often associated with low-fiber diets.
◇ Dietary fiber increases colon content, decreases colon pressure, and increases propulsive motility.
◇ Simethicone is a gastric defoaming antiflatulent agent. It reduces surface tension, causing bubbles to be broken or coalesced into a foam that can be eliminated more easily by belching or passing flatus.

Antiemetics

◇ The chemotrigger zone (CTZ) is involved in vomiting.
◇ The newer antiemetics bind to serotonin (5-HT) receptors to prevent nausea.

Obesity

◇ Ideal body weight (IBW)
   Males IBW kg = 50 + (2.3 × height in inches over 5 feet)
   Females IBW kg = 45.5 + (2.3 × height in inches over 5 feet)
◇ Morbid obesity is the condition of weighing two or more times the ideal body weight; so called because it results in many serious and life-threatening disorders.
◇ BMI (Body Mass Index) is determined by dividing the patient's weight in kilograms by the patient's height in meters squared (kg/m^2).
◇ The BMI is used as a guide to determine whether or not pharmacological treatment should be used for obesity. A BMI greater than 30, or in the presence of other risk factors 27, would warrant pharmacological intervention, with Xenical (orlistat).
◇ Stimulants are the most-commonly used agents for weight reduction.

Pharmacologic Treatment of Parasites

◇ Tetracycline and quinolones are used for prophylaxis of traveler's diarrhea.

Drug Summary

The following drugs were discussed in this chapter. Each generic drug name is followed in parentheses by one or more brand names. An asterisk (*) indicates drugs frequently written using *either* brand *or* generic name. These need to be memorized.

Gastrointestinal Disease

Antacids
aluminum hydroxide (Amphojel)
aluminum hydroxide-magnesium
    hydroxide (Maalox, Mylanta)
magnesium hydroxide (Milk of
    Magnesia)
magnesium trisilicate (Gelusil)

Histamine$_2$ Receptor Antagonists
cimetidine (Tagamet)*
famotidine (Pepcid)*
nizatidine (Axid)*
ranitidine (Zantac)*

Combinations
ranitidine-bismuth-citrate (Tritec)
tetracycline-metronidazole-bismuth
    (Helidac)

Proton Pump Inhibitors
esomeprazole (Nexium)
lansoprazole (Prevacid)
omeprazole (Prilosec)*
pantoprazole (Protonix)
rabeprazole (Aciphex)

Coating Agents
alginic acid (Gaviscon)
sucralfate (Carafate)*

Prostaglandin E
misoprostol (Cytotec)*

Cholinergic Agent
bethanechol (Urecholine)

Mast Cell Stabilizer
cromolyn sodium (Intal, Nasalcrom,
    Gastrocrom)

Pancreatic Enzyme
pancrelipase (Viokase, Cotazym, Creon)

Immunosuppression
azathioprine (Imuran)*

Monoclonal Antibody
infliximab (Remicade)

Anti-inflammatories
balsalazide (Colazal)
mesalamine (Rowasa, Asacol, Pentasa)
olsalazine (Dipentum)
sulfasalazine (Azulfidine)*

Gallstone Dissolution
ursodiol (Actigall)*

Antiemetic
metoclopromide (Reglan)

Antidiarrheals
attapulgite (Kaopectate)
bismuth subsalicylate (Pepto-Bismol)
camphorated tincture of opium
    (Paregoric)
difenoxin (Motofen)
diphenoxylate-atropine (Lomotil)*
loperamide (Imodium)*

Hemorrhoidal Drugs
hydrocortisone (Anusol HC, Anucort HC)

Constipation
Emollients/Lubricants
dioctyl calcium sulfosuccinate (Surfak)
dioctyl potassium sulfosuccinate
    (Dialose)
dioctyl sodium sulfosuccinate (Colace)
glycerin (Fleet)
lactulose (Duphalac, Cephulac)
magnesium hydroxide (Milk of
    Magnesia)
magnesium sulfate (Epsom salts)
sodium phosphate (Fleet Phospho-Soda)

Stimulants
bisacodyl (Dulcolax)
senna (Senokot)

Bulk-Forming Agents
methylcellulose (FiberTrim, Citrucel)
polycarbophil (Mitrolan)
psyllium hydrophilic mucolloid
    (Metamucil)

Antiflatulents
simethicone (Phazyme, Gas-X, Mylicon,
    Mylanta)

Bowel Evacuant
polyethylene glycol-electrolyte solution
    (GoLYTELY)

OTC Antiemetics
cyclizine (Marezine)
dimenhydrinate (Dramamine)
diphenhydramine (Benadryl)*
meclizine (Antivert, Bonine)*

Prescription Antiemetics
granisetron (Kytril)
hydroxyzine (Atarax, Vistaril)*
metoclopramide (Reglan)*
ondansetron (Zofran)*
prochlorperazine (Compazine)*
promethazine (Phenergan)*
thiethylperazine (Torecan)
triflupromazine (Vesprin)
trimethobenzamide (Tigan)*

Stimulation of Emesis
ipecac syrup

Diet Drugs
dextroamphetamine (Dexedrine)
diethylpropion (Tenuate)
mazindol (Mazanor)
methamphetamine (Desoxyn)
orlistat (Xenical)
phentermine (Fastin)
sibutramine (Meridia)

Antibiotics
ciprofloxacin (Cipro)
tetracycline (Achromycin)

Antiparasitic Drugs
mebendazole (Vermox)
niclosamide (Niclocide)
praziquantel (Biltricide)
thiabendazole (Mintezol)

Chapter Review

Pharmaceuticals and Body Functions

Select the best answer from the choices given.

1. The worst offender of gastritis is
   a. food.
   b. alcohol.
   c. medicine.
   d. All of the above

2. The most common drug-induced cause of ulcers is
   a. alcohol.
   b. aspirin.
   c. NSAIDs.
   d. methotrexate.

3. Which H_2 blocker should be used cautiously in patients taking a calcium channel blocker?
   a. Cimetidine
   b. Pepcid
   c. Axid
   d. Zantac

4. Which drug is a bowel motility stimulant?
   a. Cytotec
   b. Carafate
   c. Ducolax
   d. Prevacid

5. Which drug is a coating agent?
   a. Cytotec
   b. Carafate
   c. Axid
   d. Prevacid

6. Which drug is a prostaglandin analog?
   a. Cytotec
   b. Carafate
   c. Ducolax
   d. Prevacid

7. Which drug is used in cystic fibrosis?
   a. Actigall
   b. Ducolax
   c. Carafate
   d. Cromolyn sodium

8. Which drug is used in Crohn's disease?
   a. Cyclizine
   b. Aspirin
   c. Actigall
   d. Sulfasalazine

9. Which drug is used to treat gallstones?
   a. Imuran
   b. Actigall
   c. Rowasa
   d. Azulfidine

10. Which drug could change the color of urine and stain soft contact lenses?
   a. Imuran
   b. Actigall
   c. Rowasa
   d. Azulfidine

The following statements are true or false. If the answer is false, rewrite the statement so it is true.

_____ 1. Imuran is an enema.

_____ 2. Actigall is an immunosuppressive agent.

_____ 3. Fiber has no adverse effects.

_____ 4. If a child has two obese parents, the percentage chance of that individual being overweight is 20%.

_____ 5. Diethylpropion is a diet medication that stimulates adrenergic pathways.

_____ 6. Loperamide is a narcotic antidiarrheal.

_____ 7. When treating worms, the OTC drugs are often as effective and probably safer than the prescription medications.

_____ 8. Morbid obesity is body weight 30% over the ideal.

_____ 9. Even with drug therapy, diet modification plays an essential role in weight reduction.

_____ 10. Acid production is stimulated by acetylcholine, histamine, and gastrin.

Diseases and Drug Therapies

1. Describe the roller-coaster syndrome.
2. Explain the mechanism of action of Gaviscon.
3. List at least two things for which fiber supplementation has been used.
4. List the symptoms of GERD.
5. Discuss the diet pills listed in the chapter and their mechanism of action.

Dispensing Medications

1. Write protocol for Helidac therapy and detailed instructions for the patient.
2. A patient is in phase I of GERD. He comes into the pharmacy and perfectly describes the symptoms. You would direct the patient to the aisle with which drug? Which is the most important dose?
3. Your patient is going to Mexico and is very concerned about traveler's diarrhea. What would the pharmacist tell that patient?
4. Figure ideal body weight for a male 6 feet 3 inches tall.
5. Figure ideal body weight for a female 5 feet 6 inches tall.
6. Figure the BMI for the above female patient with a weight of 200 pounds. (1 kg = 2.2 lbs; 1 inch = 2.5 cm; 100 cm = 1 m)

Internet Research

Use the Internet to complete the following assignments.

1. Locate information related to ongoing clinical trials aimed at the development of new treatments for Crohn's disease. Create a table listing at least three experimental therapies. Indicate the phase (one through three) of testing presently underway and where (institution and country) the trials are taking place. List your Internet sources.
2. Identify two Internet sites that discuss the role of *Helicobacter pylori* in gastrointestinal disease. What specific disorders does this bacteria affect? List your Internet source(s).

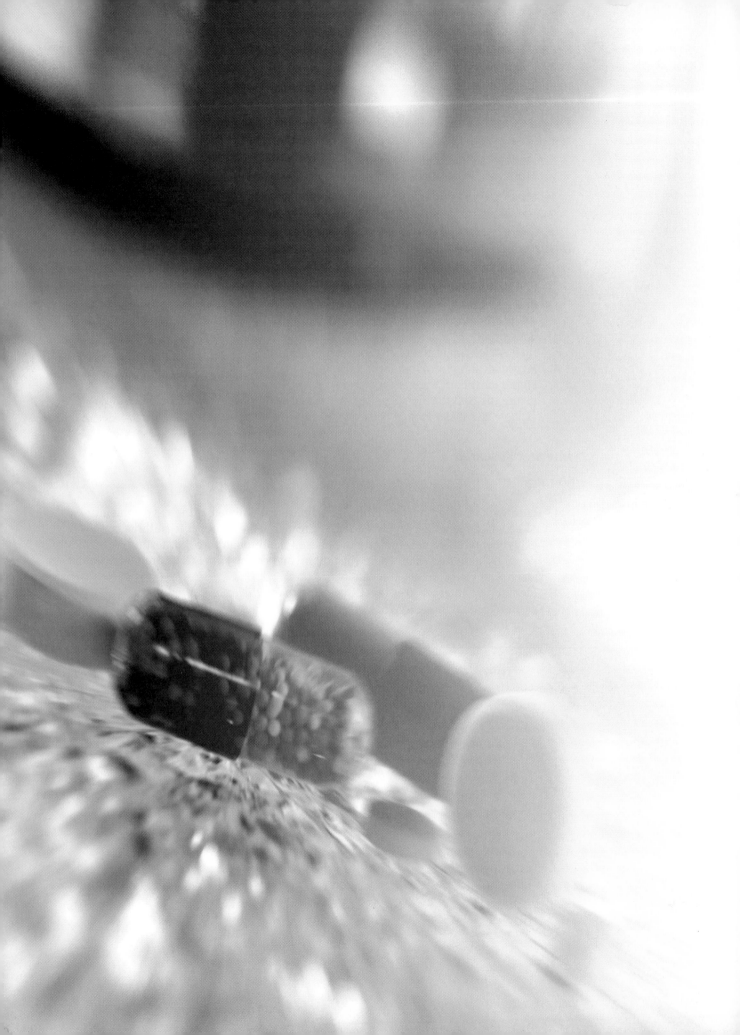

Urinary System Drugs

Chapter

12

Learning Objectives

◇ Understand the renal system, its importance, and how it works.

◇ Differentiate the parts of the renal system.

◇ Recognize renal failure and the agents to treat this progressive disease.

◇ Know the causes and treatment of urinary tract infections.

◇ Understand the classes of diuretics and how they work.

The kidneys, ureters, bladder, and urethra are all part of the urinary tract. Disease in any of these areas of the tract can upset the delicate balance of the body and result in many problems, some of them serious. Kidney disease in particular has disastrous implications, since the kidneys regulate the balance of bodily functions. Although the kidney is most often thought of as an excretory organ, most of the metabolic work of the kidney is directed toward the reclamation of filtered solutes. In addition, the kidney plays an important role in the metabolism of various peptide hormones and is active biosynthetically in the production of renin, ammonia, erythropoietin, and 1-alpha, 25-dihydroxy-vitamin D_3.

RENAL FUNCTION AND DISEASE

The function of the kidneys is to regulate the extra-cellular fluid (plasma and tissue fluid) environment in the body. This function is accomplished through the formation of urine, which is modified filtrate of plasma. Figure 12.1 illustrates the urinary system and renal anatomy. In the process of urine formation, the kidneys regulate (1) the volume of blood plasma and thus contribute significantly to regulation of blood pressure, (2) the concentration of waste products in the blood, (3) the concentration of electrolytes (Na^+, K^+, HCO_3^-, Ca^{++}, and PO_4^{-3}) in the plasma, and (4) the pH of plasma.

Acute renal failure is a rapid reduction in kidney function resulting in accumulation of nitrogen and other waste. Uremia is the clinical syndrome resulting from renal dysfunction. In this syndrome, excessive products of protein metabolism (e.g., urea) are retained in the blood, and the toxic condition produced is marked by nausea, vomiting, vertigo, convulsions, and coma. The normal human kidney contains two million functionally integrated glomerulotubular units called nephrons. These nephrons work in a highly consistent manner to maintain constancy in the body's internal environment. Although the kidney is usually thought of as an excretory organ, most of its metabolic work is directed toward reclamation of filtered

Urinary System Drugs ◇ *Chapter 12* **247**

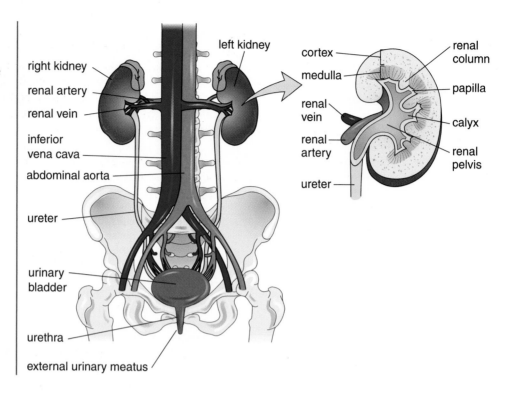

Figure 12.1

The Urinary System and the Renal Anatomy

right kidney
renal artery
renal vein
inferior vena cava
abdominal aorta
ureter
urinary bladder
urethra
external urinary meatus

left kidney

cortex
medulla
renal vein
renal artery
ureter

renal column
papilla
calyx
renal pelvis

solutes. In addition, the kidneys play an important role in the metabolism of various peptide hormones and are active in the biosynthetic production of renin, ammonia, erythropoietin, and 1-alpha, 25-dihydroxy-vitamin D_3.

Stages of Renal Disease

The clinical course of progressive renal disease is classified into four stages.

1. **Loss of Renal Reserve** Patients are generally asymptomatic.
2. **Renal Insufficiency** Patients are still asymptomatic for the most part, but may have nocturia secondary to a loss of urinary concentrating ability, hypertension secondary to volume expansion from impaired sodium excretion, or both. Blood urea nitrogen (BUN) level is mildly elevated, serum creatinine level is increased, and mild anemia is present.
3. **Chronic Renal Failure** Patients are easily fatigued, are intolerant of cold, and have abnormal taste sensation and anorexia. The anemia worsens, and laboratory abnormalities develop, including hyperphosphatemia, hypocalcemia, hyperkalemia, and metabolic acidosis. Uremia develops at this stage. Creatinine clearance drops below 10 mL/min, and the patient has malaise, generalized pruritus, nausea, vomiting, and leg cramps. At this stage before the full syndrome develops, dialysis is indicated to remove the by-products of protein metabolism thought to be responsible for this symptom complex.
4. **End-Stage Renal Disease (ESRD)** The patient requires chronic dialysis.

Causes of Renal Failure

Renal failure is commonly due to prerenal, intrarenal, or postrenal events.

PRERENAL EVENTS Volume problems other than those caused by the kidney can be due to diuretics, vomiting, nasogastric suction, diarrhea, hemorrhage, burns, adrenal insufficiency, or diabetic ketoacidosis. A decreased effective volume may be caused by congestive heart failure (CHF), myocardial infarction (MI), cirrhosis, sepsis, vasodilators, or pulmonary edema. The result is reduced renal blood flow. The kidney usually receives twenty percent of the cardiac output. Reduction in renal blood flow can cause ischemia, cell dysfunction, or even death.

INTRARENAL EVENTS Changes inside the kidney, such as rapidly progressive glomerulonephritis, renal vein thrombosis, vascular obstruction, vasculitis, and hypertension, can all contribute to declining renal function. Causes of ischemia are surgery, hypotension, shock, radiocontrast dyes, emboli, and thrombi. Nephrotoxins can be antibiotics, nonsteroidal anti-inflammatory drugs (NSAIDs), radiocontrast dyes, mismatched transfusions, myoglobin, and mineral precipitates. Glomerular inflammation can cause glomerular membrane rupture, allowing filtrates and blood to flow back into the capsular (Bowman) space and stimulating fibrin formation (fibrin clot). Macrophages are attracted in, and permanent damage results.

Damage to the glomerulus generally results from the following causes.

- **Damage to the Vascular Tree** This can result in occlusive disease.
- **Change in Glomerular Permeability** Damage allows protein and cellular debris to enter the urine and is believed to obstruct blood flow.
- **Immunologic Reactions** The glomerular membrane acts as an antigen; circulating antigen-antibody complex becomes trapped in the glomerular membrane and initiates an immune reaction.

POSTRENAL EVENTS Disease can occur in the structures below the kidney. The urethra and ureter can be damaged by crystals, clots, stones, tumor fibrosis, infection, endometriosis, and papillary necrosis. Bladder disease can be serious, as in prostatic hypertrophy and cancer. Blockage to urine flow may be partial or complete and could involve the renal pelvis, ureters, bladder, or urethra. Initially the obstruction causes vasoconstriction of affected arteries due to feedback information from increased hydrostatic pressure in the tubules. If not corrected, it can lead to defects in the tubes.

Renal Drug Therapy

A diagnosis of renal disease is made by two indicators: signs and evaluations. Signs include orthostatic blood pressure, skin turgor, temperature, color, edema, weight loss, urine volume changes (may not relate directly to disease severity), and bad urine odor. Evaluations of renal disease include filtration rate, urine volume, electrolyte levels and osmolality, urine protein level, measuring of other urine contents, serum creatinine level, and BUN.

Renal therapy is aimed at reestablishing an appropriate intravascular volume and pressure, restricting fluids in volume-overload cases, and treating the underlying problem (fluids, sodium [Na], potassium [K], calcium [Ca], phosphorus [P], magnesium [Mg], and acid-base balance [pH]).

Anemia due to renal failure is caused by decreased erythropoietin. Most renal patients show evidence of erythropoietin deficiency. Inhibitors of erythropoiesis exist in the blood and other body fluids. Patients undergoing hemodialysis or peritoneal dialysis may have a rise in hematocrit (increased red cells) indicating that inhibiting substances are being removed by dialysis. Patients undergoing dialysis also must be watched closely for aluminum intoxication, which interferes with incorporating iron into erythrocytes. Sucralfate and aluminum-containing antacids can be causes. Antacids can also cause iron deficiency by reducing the absorption of iron. Blood loss and reduced dietary intake also lead to iron deficiency. Vitamins are lost, especially the water-soluble ones; pyridoxine (B_6) and folic acid (B_9) are both removed by dialysis.

Table 12.1 presents the most-commonly used agents for renal disease. Appropriate pharmacologic intervention can markedly enhance the quality of life for patients with renal disease. Although drugs can often be the cause, they can also be helpful in treatment. Once a patient is on dialysis, most drugs have to be dosed differently. The technician must be aware of this. If a patient has renal disease, the dosing should always be checked. Drugs that may be used are diuretics, antihypertensives, corticosteroids, and even some cytotoxic agents. Some are discussed in other chapters. The drugs in Table 12.1 are fairly specific to renal disease.

Epogen and **Procrit (epoetin alfa [erythropoietin])** are used to treat anemia associated with end-stage renal disease. These drugs induce release of reticulocytes from bone marrow into the bloodstream, where they mature to erythrocytes. The result is a rise in hematocrit and hemoglobin levels. Frequent blood tests are needed to determine the correct dose. The patient should notify the physician if frequent headaches occur. The drug is produced by animal cell culture into which the human erythropoietin gene has been placed. Adverse effects are hypertension, seizures, increased clotting potential, and allergic reactions.

Folvite (folic acid [vitamin B_9]) should be administered to renal patients daily, as it is required for erythropoiesis.

Nestrex (pyridoxine [vitamin B_6]) should also be administered daily. It is removed by dialysis and must be replaced.

Multiple vitamin complex (MVI) is necessary because of the imbalance of electrolytes (and other substances) which coincides with renal disease, depleting vitamin stores.

InFed (iron dextran injection) releases iron from the plasma and eventually replenishes the iron stores in bone marrow, where it is incorporated into hemoglobin. This complex can be given by deep IM injection into the upper-outer quadrant of the buttocks (never in arm or other area) using the Z-track technique or IV. It must be used with caution, and a test dose should be given before administering the full dose.

Renagel (sevelamer) binds phosphate in the intestinal lumen limiting absorption. The drug has the ability to decrease serum phosphate concentrations without altering calcium, aluminum, or bicarbonate concentrations. The capsules expand in water and are therefore contraindicated in patients with swallowing or GI motility disorders as well as those who have experienced bowel obstruction and/or have undergone GI tract surgery. Renagel can interfere with the absorption of other drugs. Therefore, patients should take other medications at least one hour before or three

Table 12.1	Most-Commonly Used Agents for Renal Disease		
Generic Name		**Brand Name**	**Dosage Form**
epoetin alfa (erythropoietin)		Epogen, Procrit	IV, SC
folic acid (vitamin B_9)		Folvite	tablet, IM, IV, SC
iron dextran injection		INFeD	IM, IV
multiple vitamin complex		MVI	liquid, tablet, IM, IV
pyridoxine (vitamin B_6)		Nestrex	tablet, IM, IV, SC
sevelamer		Renagel	capsule

hours after the administration of this drug. Serum calcium, bicarbonate, and chloride concentrations should be monitored.

Calciferol (ergocalciferol [vitamin D]) supplementation is determined by serum calcium concentrations. It is not routinely given to patients until they begin dialysis.

DRUGS FOR THE URINARY TRACT

Table 12.2 lists the most-commonly used agents for urinary problems.

Urecholine (bethanechol) stimulates cholinergic receptors in the smooth muscle of the urinary bladder and gastrointestinal (GI) tract, resulting in increased peristalsis, increased GI and pancreatic secretions, bladder muscle contraction, and increased ureteral peristaltic waves. This drug should be taken one hour before meals or two hours after meals. It may cause abdominal discomfort, salivation, sweating, or flushing. The patient should notify the physician if these symptoms become pronounced.

Urispas (flavoxate) exerts a direct spasmolytic effect on smooth muscle, primarily in the urinary tract. Acting on the detrussor muscle, this agent increases bladder capacity in patients with bladder spasticity by cholinergic blockage. It also has local anesthetic and analgesic effects. It can cause drowsiness, blurred vision, and GI upset.

Urex and **Hiprex (methenamine)** work primarily as a bactericidal. They should be taken with food to minimize GI upset, with ascorbic acid to acidify urine, and with sufficient fluids to ensure adequate urine flow. Excessive intake of alkalinizing foods (e.g., citrus) or medication (e.g., bicarbonate) should be avoided. Skin rash, painful urination, or excessive abdominal pain should be reported to the physician. Administration with sulfonamides is contraindicated. Hiprex has a dye in the formulation that can cause allergic reactions. Cranberry juice is a good fluid to drink when taking this drug. Alkaline foods and antacids should be avoided.

Pro-Banthine (propantheline) is used to treat bladder spasms. It competitively blocks the action of acetylcholine (ACh) at postganglionic parasympathetic receptor sites. It should be taken thirty minutes before meals and at bedtime. It may cause blurred vision and decreased salivation. Skin rash, flushing, eye pain, difficulty in urination, or sensitivity to light should be reported to the physician.

Pyridium, Azo-Standard, and **Urogesic (phenazopyridine)**, in lower strengths, are OTC agents that have a local anesthetic effect on urinary tract mucosa. Higher strengths require a prescription. They color urine orange and stain anything they contact. They should not be used for more than two days and should be taken with an antibiotic. They are used for symptomatic relief of urinary burning, itching, frequency, and urgency in association with urinary tract infection, or following urologic procedures.

Table 12.2	Most-Commonly Used Agents for Urinary Problems	
Generic Name	**Brand Name**	**Dosage Form**
bethanechol	Urecholine	tablet, SC, IM, IV
flavoxate	Urispas	tablet
methenamine	Urex, Hiprex	tablet
methylene blue	Trac 2-X	tablet
oxybutynin	Ditropan	syrup, tablet
pentosan polysulfate sodium	Elmiron	capsule
phenazopyridine	Pyridium, Azo-Standard, Urogesic	tablet
propantheline	Pro-Banthine	tablet
tolterodine	Detrol	tablet

Elmiron (pentosan polysulfate sodium) is the first oral therapy for interstitial cystitis. It is used for relief of bladder pain, presumably by exerting a protective effect on the bladder wall to reduce irritation and inflammation. Patients need to take it for up to six weeks before they get relief; this is often discouraging and causes poor compliance. It also has a weak anticoagulant effect.

Ditropan (oxybutynin) is a urinary antispasmodic agent used to decrease frequent urination. The antispasmodic works to inhibit the action of acethylcholine. It decreases spasms in smooth muscle without affecting skeletal muscles. This drug also increases bladder capacity and decreases urgency and frequency. Dry mouth is a side effect.

Detrol (tolterodine) is a competitive muscarinic receptor antagonist similar to oxybutynin. It differs in its selectivity for urinary bladder receptors over salivary receptors. As a result, Detrol (tolterodine) has greatly reduced dry mouth effects relative to oxybutynin. This drug also decreases detrussor muscle pressure. Behavioral techniques for this condition should also be considered.

Urinary Tract Infections Drug Therapy

Community-acquired urinary tract infections (UTIs) account for over five million physician visits each year. The presence of bacteria in the urine with localized symptoms is considered symptomatic of UTI. The highest incidence occurs in sexually active women. Incidence is related to the ability of intestinal bacteria to readily colonize the vagina, ascend the short urethra, and gain access to the bladder. UTIs become a problem for males after age fifty because of prostatic obstruction, instrumentation, or surgery. UTIs are classified according to anatomic location in the urinary tract. The classifications are

◇ cystitis
◇ urethritis (lower tract infection)
◇ prostatitis
◇ pyelonephritis (upper tract infection)

UTIs can be described as

◇ uncomplicated: no evidence of underlying structural or neurologic problems of the urinary tract;
◇ complicated: a predisposing lesion of the urinary tract, such as a stone, stricture, neurogenic bladder, prostate hypertrophy, or obstruction.

Even when the urinary tract is healthy, *Escherichia coli* or other bacteria may enter. In UTIs there are many more organisms than normally found. Blood may appear in the urine, and urination may be difficult or painful. Fever is common.

UTIs may be treated with a single dose of medicine or with a three- to fourteen-day course. If several occur in sequence, an antibiotic may be prescribed for six to twelve months to prevent recurrence. Sexual activity can lead to UTI, especially in women. Thus, a female patient with recurrent UTIs may be instructed to urinate and take one dose of an antibiotic right after sexual intercourse.

If an antibiotic is needed, a short course (one to three days) is sometimes all that is needed to clear the infection. UTIs are usually treated with one of the following antibiotics.

◇ **Omnipen (ampicillin)** should be taken on an empty stomach; the primary side effect is skin rash. It is dosed four times a day.

- **Amoxil (amoxicillin)** is taken without regard for food; the primary side effect is skin rash. It is dosed three times a day.
- **Augmentin (amoxicillin-clavulanic acid)** should be taken with food to avoid stomach upset; diarrhea is the primary side effect.
- **Bactrim or Septra (sulfamethoxazole-trimethoprim)** should be taken with plenty of water; a sunscreen should be used.
- **Quinolones** should not be taken with antacids, theophylline, warfarin, magnesium, or calcium; a sunscreen is needed.
- **Cephalosporins** except **Ceftin (cefuroxime)** should be taken without food.
- **Macrodantin (nitrofurantoin)** should be taken with food or milk; it may turn urine brown or dark yellow and alcohol should be avoided. This drug has side effects resembling Antabuse (disulfiram) side effects.

Benign Prostatic Hypertrophy Drug Therapy

Benign prostatic hypertrophy (BPH) is one of the most common medical conditions occurring in older men. This abnormal enlargement of the prostate gland appears to occur with aging in combination with certain pathophysiologic influences. An enlarged prostate becomes a problem when it obstructs urine outflow from the bladder. The prostate is involved primarily in reproduction but may sometimes protect against UTI through the secretion of prostatic antibacterial factor (PAF). Figure 12.2 shows the organs of the male reproductive system.

Increasing evidence shows that nonsurgical interventions, especially drug therapy, may be effective as a primary treatment for selected patients. Alpha blockers and 5-alpha-reductase inhibitors represent promising and innovative approaches to pharmacologic management. The future challenge is to evaluate critically all therapeutic alternatives to identify the optimal treatment for each patient.

Alpha blockers were originally developed for treating hypertension, which, like BPH, is a common disorder in aging men. They cause relaxation of smooth muscles, especially in prostatic tissue, reducing urinary symptoms in BPH. Many older men

Figure 12.2

The Male Reproductive System

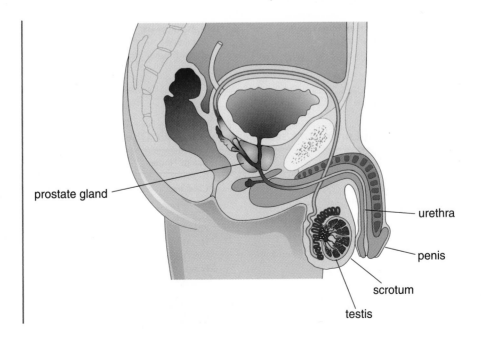

have both conditions. In such cases, it is reasonable to consider using an alpha blocker to treat both the hypertension and the BPH.

Certain drugs affect bladder function and should not be used for patients with BPH. Alternative drugs are preferred. Table 12.3 lists these drugs. Table 12.4 lists the most-commonly used agents for BPH.

Minipress (prazosin) is a selective alpha$_1$ adrenergic antagonist approved for treating hypertension. Several studies have shown benefit in patients with BPH, and the number of patients using this drug is up. Orthostatic hypertension is common, but this effect can sometimes be minimized by initiating the therapy at bedtime.

Hytrin (terazosin) is a long-acting selective alpha$_1$ blocker approved for use as an antihypertensive agent. It produces significant improvement in obstructive symptoms and urinary flow rates. Its primary advantage over prazosin is a longer half-life that allows for once-daily dosing and presumably better rates of compliance. The side effects of tiredness, dizziness, and orthostatic hypotension can be minimized by giving the drug at bedtime. Headache has also been reported. Prophylactic administration of acetaminophen, 650 to 675 mg, a half hour before the terazosin dose may lessen the severity of headache, which usually subsides after several weeks of treatment.

Cardura (doxazosin) exhibits actions similar to terazosin but is not as alpha$_1$ selective. It competitively inhibits postsynaptic alpha-adrenergic receptors which results in vasodilation of veins and arterioles and a decrease in total peripheral resistance and blood pressure. It is approximately fifty percent as potent on a weight-by-weight basis as Hytrin. The side effects are primarily dizziness and painful erections. Both can be avoided by taking before sleep.

Flomax (tamsulosin) is an alpha$_1$ blocker but is more selective than Hytrin. It has little effect on blood pressure but works well for BPH.

Table 12.3	Alternative Drugs for BPH Patients	
	Classification	**Preferred Alternatives**
	anticholinergics	H$_2$ blockers, sucralfate, antacids
	oral bronchodilators	inhalation products
	antidepressants (TCAs)	selective serotonin reuptake inhibitors (SSRIs)
	calcium channel blockers	alpha blockers
	disopyramide	quinidine
	antihistamines	discontinue

Table 12.4	Most-Commonly Used Agents for Prostatic Disease	
	Generic Name	**Brand Name**	**Dosage Form**
	doxazosin	Cardura	tablet
	finasteride	Proscar	tablet
	flutamide	Eulexin	capsule
	goserelin acetate implant	Zoladex	SC
	leuprolide	Lupron Depot	IM, SC
	megestrol	Megace	tablet, oral suspension
	nilutamide	Nilandron	tablet
	prazosin	Minipress	capsule
	tamsulosin	Flomax	tablet
	terazosin	Hytrin	capsule, tablet

Lupron Depot (leuprolide) and **Zoladex (goserelin acetate implant)** are luteinizing hormone blockers that inhibit production of androgen. Monthly injections are necessary. Improvement in symptoms is slow, and with cessation of therapy, the prostate returns to pretreatment size within six months.

Eulexin (flutamide) is an antiandrogen that inhibits androgen uptake or inhibits binding of androgen in target tissues. Used in combination with leuprolide. Both drugs need to be started simultaneously. Over half of study patients reported breast pain or gynecomastia. Half also experienced GI side effects. Flutamide is presently approved for treating symptomatic prostate cancer when used in conjunction with an luteinizing hormone, releasing hormone analogue such as leuprolide or goserelin.

Nilandron (nilutamide) is indicated for use in advanced prostate cancer. It is an antiandrogen similar to Eulexin. It helps reduce metastatic bone pain and improve survival. It is dosed once daily versus three times daily for Eulexin. It causes visual disturbances—mainly a delay in adjusting from light to dark. Patients may need to avoid night driving. It can also cause a disulfiram-like reaction.

Megace (megestrol) is a progestational antiandrogen. It centrally inhibits luteinizing hormone. This inhibition in turn reduces testosterone production, resulting in reduced serum levels and consequently in the adverse effects of decreased libido and impotence.

Proscar and **Propecia (finasteride)** blocks the enzyme that converts testosterone to DHT. The inhibition of only DHT and not testosterone minimizes the side effects of general androgen blockade and results in an increase in intracellular testosterone levels, thereby minimizing sexual dysfunction, the primary drawback of hormonal therapy. Advantageous effects are

- ◇ reduction in prostate size, similar to that with other forms of androgen withdrawal
- ◇ improved urine flow and symptom relief, similar to those with other forms of androgen withdrawal
- ◇ minimal drug-related adverse effects
- ◇ decrease in male pattern baldness

Finasteride is provided in film-coated tablets. Crushed finasteride tablets or finasteride powder should not be handled by a woman who is or may become pregnant because of risk to a male fetus.

DIURETICS

The primary function of the kidney is to maintain the balance of water, electrolytes, and acids and bases in the body (Figure 12.3). Urine formation is essential for normal body function, since it enables the blood to reabsorb necessary nutrients, water, and electrolytes. Large molecules, such as plasma proteins, cannot pass the membranes, whereas small molecules, such as water, ions, and glucose, do pass. The primary action of diuretics on the kidney is to rid the body of excess fluid and electrolytes. A diuretic is often the first drug chosen to treat high blood pressure. Combination with a diuretic enhances the effectiveness of certain drugs. The various causes of edema also may be treated with a diuretic.

The renal tubules produce urine through filtration, reabsorption, and secretion.

- ◇ Filtration takes place in the glomeruli, where substances are removed from the blood.

Figure 12.3

Anatomy of the Nephron

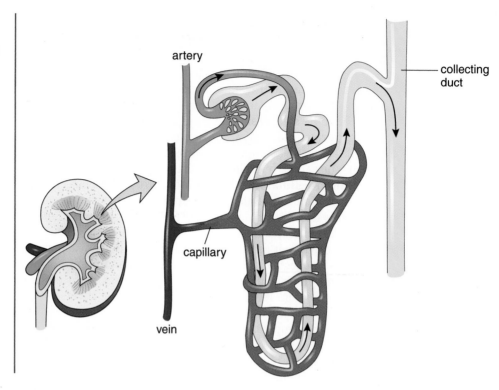

artery

collecting duct

capillary

vein

◇ Reabsorption selectively pulls filtrated substances back into the blood. Sodium (99%) is the principal cation of extracellular fluid (exchange for H^+, K^+, and anion transport Cl^-). Distal tubules secrete K^+ into urine in exchange for sodium. Aldosterone in the distal tubules reacts with receptors, causing potassium secretion. In the loop, sodium is absorbed with chloride.

◇ Secretion of hydrogen ions, potassium ions, weak acids, and weak bases takes place. Hydrogen ion secretion regulates acid-base balance and acidification of urine (blood pH is normally between 7.32 and 7.42).

Table 12.5 presents the most-commonly used diuretics.

Thiazide diuretics promote sodium and water excretion in the urine, lower the sodium level in vessel walls, and reduce vasoconstriction. These drugs are about equivalent in potency, but may differ in onset, peak, and duration of action. The side effects of thiazide diuretics include hypokalemia, hypomagnesia, hyperuricemia, hyperglycemia, and hypercalcemia. Patients should be told to ingest potassium (banana, orange juice, citrus fruits) daily. A few patients become more sensitive to sunlight when taking a thiazide.

Loop diuretics inhibit reabsorption of sodium and chloride in the ascending loop of Henle and distal renal tubules, thus causing increased urinary excretion of water, sodium, chloride, magnesium, calcium, and potassium. Their high degree of efficacy is due to this unique site of action.

Potassium-sparing diuretics result in exchange of the sodium excreted in the urine for the potassium returned to the blood. They should not be administered to patients on ACE inhibitors, since these drugs also have a potassium sparing effect. The side effects are hyperkalemia and gynecomastia in men. Hyperkalemia can lead to serious arrhythmias.

Table 12.5   Most-Commonly Used Diuretics

Generic Name	Brand Name	Dosage Form
Thiazides		
benzthiazide	Hydrex	tablet
hydrochlorothiazide (HCTZ)	Esidrix, HydroDIURIL	tablet
methyclothiazide	Enduron	tablet
trichlormethiazide	Naqua	tablet
Combination		
bisoprolol-hydrochlorothiazide	Ziac	tablet
triamterene-hydrochlorothiazide	Dyazide, Maxzide	capsule, tablet
Related Drug		
chlorthalidone	Hygroton	tablet
Loop		
bumetanide	Bumex	tablet, injection
ethacrynic acid	Edecrin	injection
furosemide	Lasix	tablet, oral solution, IM, IV
torsemide	Demadex	tablet, IV
Potassium-Sparing		
amiloride	Midamor	tablet
spironolactone	Aldactone	tablet
triamterene	Dyrenium	capsule
Carbonic Anhydrase Inhibitors		
acetazolamide	Diamox	capsule, IM, IV
methazolamide	Neptazane	tablet
Osmotic		
mannitol	Osmitrol, Resectisol	IM, IV
Miscellaneous		
indapamide	Lozol	tablet
metolazone	Zaroxolyn	tablet

Carbonic anhydrase inhibitors act in the proximal tubule. Inhibition of the enzyme causes an increase in the urine volume and a change to an alkaline pH, with a subsequent decrease in the excretion of titratable acid and ammonia.

Osmotic diuretics increase the osmotic pressure of glomerular filtrate, which inhibits tubular reabsorption of water and electrolytes and increases urinary output.

Dyazide and **Maxzide (triamterene-hydrochlorothiazide)** are widely used combination drugs. They are among the safest drugs on the market. Even though these drugs are thiazide combinations, they do not waste potassium because of the triamterene. Watch for patients who are taking K^+ supplements or are on an ACE inhibitor. Either can lead to hyperkalemia. The tablet form (Maxzide) gives better absorption. Maxzide can change the urine color to blue-green.

Ziac (bisoprolol-hydrochlorothiazide) is a beta blocker combined with a diuretic. It can cause dizziness, headache, diarrhea, and fatigue.

Hygroton (chlorthalidone) is a related drug that inhibits sodium and chloride reabsorption in the cortical-diluting segment of the ascending loop of Henle. The primary side effect is hypokalemia. It should be taken with food or milk early in the day; with multiple doses, the last should be taken no later than 6 p.m. to avoid nocturia.

Lasix (furosemide), a loop diuretic, is dosed twice daily with doses given six hours apart. The name was designed to indicate the six-hour interval (La*six*). Furosemide should be dosed 20–40 mg at six- to eight-hour intervals twice daily. It gets a better area under the curve (pharmacologic calculation and formula to determine the best way to dose a drug). Also, if the first dose is a morning dose and the next is given six hours later, then the patient is not up going to the bathroom all night, which makes good sense.

Lozol (indapamide) enhances sodium, chloride, and water excretion by interfering with transport of sodium ions across the renal tubular epithelium. The effect is localized at the proximal segment of the distal tubule of the nephron.

Zaroxolyn (metolazone) inhibits sodium reabsorption in the distal tubules, causing increased excretion of sodium, water, and potassium and hydrogen ions. It should be taken with food early in the day to avoid nocturia; take the last dose no later than 6 p.m. It may increase sensitivity to sunlight.

Chapter Summary

Renal Function and Disease

- Acute renal failure is a rapid reduction in kidney function resulting in accumulation of nitrogen and other waste. Uremia is the clinical syndrome resulting from renal dysfunction.
- Renal disease is divided into four stages: (1) loss of renal reserve, (2) renal insufficiency, (3) chronic renal failure, and (4) end-stage renal disease.
- The causes of renal failure are prerenal, intrarenal, or postrenal.
- Most renal patients show evidence of erythropoietin deficiency.
- Sucralfate and aluminum-containing antacids can cause aluminum toxicity in a patient on dialysis.
- Folic acid (vitamin B_9) is required for erythropoiesis.

Drugs for the Urinary Tract

- Pyridium (phenazopyridine) and Urex, Hiprex (methenamine) have a local anesthetic effect on urinary tract mucosa. Phenazopyridine turns the urine orange.
- Elmiron (pentosan polysulfate sodium) is the first oral therapy for interstitial cystitis. It is used for relief of bladder pain, presumably by exerting a protective effect on the bladder wall to reduce irritation and inflammation.
- Ditropan (oxybutin) and Detrol (tolterodine) are urinary antispasmodics used to decrease urinary frequency. Detrol (tolterodine) has greater selectivity for urinary bladder receptors than salivary receptors.
- UTIs are treated with antibiotics, some of which require only a short course to clear the infection.
- Flomax (tamsulosin) is an alpha$_1$ blocker but is more selective than Hytrin.
- Nilandron (nilutamide) is used for advanced prostate cancer.
- Proscar can cause gynecomastia, but so can a lot of other drugs, such as cimetidine, spironolactone, ketoconazole, and others.

Diuretics

- The primary action of diuretics is to rid the body of excess fluid and electrolytes.
- Diuretics have different mechanisms of action. They are classified by where they work in the kidney: thiazide diuretics, loop diuretics, potassium-sparing diuretics, carbonic anhydrase inhibitors, osmotic diuretics, and miscellaneous.
- Dyazide and Maxzide do not waste potassium, and the patient should not be taking potassium with these drugs.

Drug Summary

The following drugs were discussed in this chapter. Each generic drug name is followed in parentheses by one or more brand names. An asterisk (*) indicates drugs frequently written using *either* brand *or* generic name. These need to be memorized.

Renal Disease
epoetin alfa (Epogen, Procrit)*
ergocalciferol (vitamin D) (Calciferol)
folic acid (vitamin B_9) (Folvite)*
iron dextran injection (INFeD)*
multiple vitamins (MVI)*
pyridoxine (vitamin B_6) (Nestrex)*
sevelamer (Renagel)

Urinary Tract Drugs
bethanechol (Urecholine)*
flavoxate (Urispas)
methenamine (Urex, Hiprex)
methylene blue (Trac 2-X)
oxybutynin (Ditropan)
pentosan polysulfate sodium (Elmiron)
phenazopyridine (Pyridium, Azo-
    Standard, Urogesic)
propantheline (Pro-Banthine)*
tolterodine (Detrol)

Antibiotics
amoxicillin (Amoxil)
amoxicillin-clavulanic acid (Augmentin)
ampicillin (Omnipen)
nitrofurantoin (Macrodantin)
sulfamethoxazole-trimethoprim
    (Bactrim, Septra)

Prostatic Disease
doxazosin (Cardura)
finasteride (Proscar)*
flutamide (Eulexin)
goserelin acetate implant (Zoladex)
leuprolide (Lupron Depot)
megestrol (Megace)
nilutamide (Nilandron)
prazosin (Minipress)
tamsulosin (Flomax)
terazosin (Hytrin)

Diuretics
acetazolamide (Diamox)
amiloride (Midamor)
benzthiazide (Hydrex)
bisoprolol-hydrochlorothiazide (Ziac)
bumetanide (Bumex)
chlorthalidone (Hygroton)
ethacrynic acid (Edecrin)
furosemide (Lasix)
hydrochlorothiazide (HCTZ) (Esidrix,
    HydroDIURIL)*
indapamide (Lozol)
mannitol (Osmitrol, Resectisol)
methazolamide (Neptazane)
methyclothiazide (Enduron)
metolazone (Zaroxolyn)
spironolactone (Aldactone)
torsemide (Demadex)
triamterene (Dyrenium)
triamterene-hydrochlorothiazide
    (Dyazide, Maxzide)
trichlormethiazide (Naqua)

Chapter Review

Pharmaceuticals and Body Functions

Select the best answer from the choices given.

1. Anemia due to renal failure is caused by decreased
   a. somatostatin.
   b. erythropoietin.
   c. pyridoxine.
   d. folic acid.

2. Pyridium turns the urine
   a. orange.
   b. blue.
   c. green.
   d. yellow.

3. Elmiron is used as
   a. an aluminum coating antacid.
   b. a urinary agent to relieve bladder pain.
   c. an alpha$_1$ blocker to decrease blood pressure.
   d. a diuretic to rid the body of excess fluid.

4. The primary action of diuretics is on the
   a. feet and hands.
   b. kidney.
   c. heart.
   d. All of the above

5. Which class of diuretics promotes sodium and water excretion in the urine, lowers sodium in vessel walls, and reduces vasoconstriction?
   a. Carbonic anhydrase inhibitors
   b. Loop diuretics
   c. Thiazide diuretics
   d. Potassium-sparing diuretics

6. Which class of diuretics inhibits reabsorption of sodium and chloride in the ascending loop of Henle and distal renal tubule?
   a. Carbonic anhydrase inhibitors
   b. Loop diuretics
   c. Thiazide diuretics
   d. Potassium-sparing diuretics

7. Which diuretic acts as an antagonist of aldosterone?
   a. acetazolamide
   b. furosemide
   c. hydrochlorothiazide
   d. spironolactone

8. Which diuretic's brand name indicates the time between doses?
   a. Furosemide
   b. Indapamide
   c. Benzthiazide
   d. Trichlormethiazide

9. Which drug should *not* be used in a BPH patient?
   a. Terazosin
   b. Benadryl
   c. Phenazopyridine
   d. Finasteride

10. Which diuretic might change the color of the urine?
    a. Furosemide
    b. Lozol
    c. Maxzide
    d. Zaroxolyn

The following statements are true or false. If the answer is false, rewrite the statement so it is true.

_____ 1. Pyridium turns the urine blue.

_____ 2. Minipress (prazosin) has a longer half-life than Hytrin (terazosin).

_____ 3. It is a good idea to give a patient on dialysis an aluminum-containing antacid to prevent stress ulcers.

_____ 4. Renal disease has three stages.

_____ 5. Erythropoietin treats cystic fibrosis.

_____ 6. Patients in end-stage renal disease generally do not need iron replacement.

_____ 7. Methenamine works primarily as a bactericidal.

_____ 8. Urispas exerts a direct spasmolytic effect on smooth muscle, primarily in the urinary tract.

_____ 9. Urecholine is the first oral therapy for interstitial cystitis.

_____ 10. All the cephalosporins should be taken with food.

Diseases and Drug Therapies

1. Define filtration, secretion, excretion, and reabsorption.
2. Why would a patient in end-stage renal disease need iron and folic acid?
3. List the four stages of renal disease.
4. Explain the difference between Urispas and Pro-Banthine.
5. Fill in the following chart.

Thiazides _____

Loop _____

K$^+$-sparing _____

Osmotic _____

Carbonic Anhydrase Inhibitors _____

Misc. _____

Dispensing Medications

1. Mrs. Mary Endres receives furosemide 40 mg q6h bid from Dr. J. Bland. You have furosemide 20 mg tablets available. Dispense one month's supply with four refills.

   —Prepare the label with the patient's name, drug, amount dispensed, sig., name of physician, etc.

   —The Lasix you have in stock has the following label.

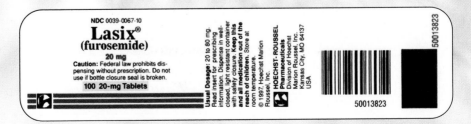

NDC 0039-0067-10

Lasix®
(furosemide)
20 mg

Caution: Federal law prohibits dispensing without prescription. Do not use if bottle closure seal is broken.

100 20-mg Tablets

Usual Dosage: 20 to 80 mg. Read insert for prescribing information. Dispense in well-closed, light resistant container with safety closure. Keep this and all medication out of the reach of children. Store at room temperature.
© 1997, Hoechst Marion Roussel, Inc.

HOECHST- ROUSSEL
Pharmaceuticals
Division of Hoechst
Marion Roussel, Inc.
Kansas City, MO 64137
USA

50013823

2. Dr. J. Bland has prescribed Macrodantin 100 mg qid to Ms. Belinda Bold. You need to dispense a ten-day supply with four refills. How many will you dispense, and which stickers will you put on the bottle? Prepare the label.

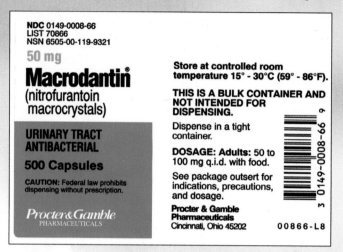

3. You receive the following prescriptions for a dialysis patient. What has the physician left off? How many of each of the following medications will you dispense for eight weeks? Patient weighs 200 lb; what will the dose of Epogen be?

Folic acid comes in tablets of 1 mg.

B_6 comes in 180 mg doses.

Physician forgot _____

# of folic acid _____

of B_6 _____

Amount of Epogen per dose _____

> **R̶**   **MT. HOPE MEDICAL PARK**
>   **ST. PAUL, MN (651) 555-3591**
>
> _____
>
>   DEA# _____
>
> Pt. name __Bill Brown__   Date __6-9-04__
>
> Address _____
>
>   Epogen 3x week for 8 weeks
>   100 units/kg
>   Folic acid 3 mg/day po for 8 weeks
>
> _____ Dispense as written
>
> _____ Fills __5__ times (no refill unless indicated)
>
> _____ *Mary Smith-Chen* _____ M.D.

```
            MT. HOPE MEDICAL PARK
            ST. PAUL, MN (651) 555-3591

                        DEA# _____
Pt. name  Bill Brown _____ Date 6-9-04

Address _____

        Vitamin B6 180 mg po qd
        multi-purpose vitamin qd
              for 8 weeks



_____ Dispense as written
  ✓  Fills 5 times (no refill unless indicated)
        Mary Smith-Chen _____ M.D.
```

Internet Research

Use the Internet to complete the following assignments.

1. Benign prostatic hypertrophy (BHP) is a medical condition which is common in older men. Importantly, this condition must be differentiated from prostate cancer. Use the Internet to find information on prostate cancer screening programs. What is the screening test called and how does it work? Who should be screened? Does BHP affect screening? List your Internet sources.

2. Diuretics are often used to treat high blood pressure. Find one or more Internet sites that describe how diuretics help to treat this condition. Write a paragraph summarizing that information. List your Internet sources.

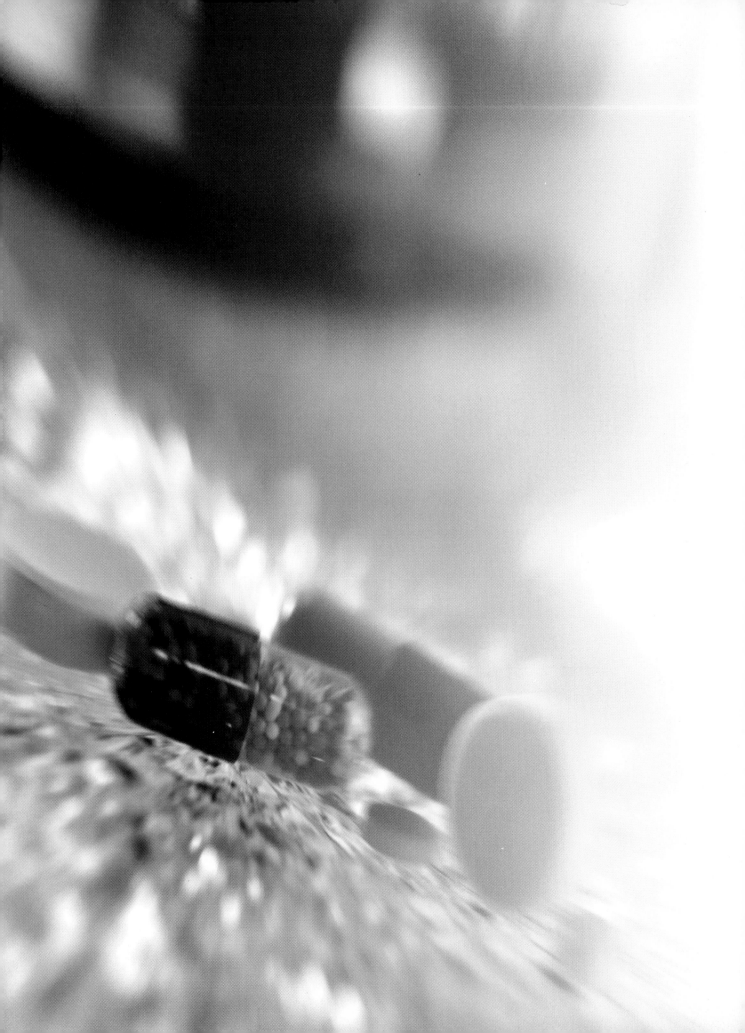

Cardiovascular Drugs

Chapter

13

Learning Objectives

- Understand the cardiovascular system.
- Differentiate arrhythmias, congestive heart failure, myocardial infarction, angina, and hypertension.
- Know the drugs and treatment for each separate aspect of heart disease.
- Recognize anticoagulant and antiplatelet drugs and know their functions.
- Discuss stroke and the drugs used to treat it.
- Identify hyperlipidemia and its role in heart disease and stroke.

Cardiovascular diseases account for significant morbidity and mortality. Many causative factors can be modified by lifestyle changes, and some are amenable to prophylaxis. Drug therapy uses antiarrhythmics, antianginals, antihypertensives, anticoagulants, antiplatelets, and hyperlipidemics.

HEART DISEASE

The heart is a complicated organ. Many things can go wrong. Among the problems are

- arrhythmias
- congestive heart failure
- myocardial infarction (heart attack)
- angina
- hypertension
- coagulation defects
- hypercholesterolemia

Drugs have been developed to help manage these diseases. Many drugs and drug classes are used for more than one problem, so there is overlapping.

The heart has three functional parts, the cardiac muscle, conducting system, and blood supply. Figure 13.1 shows the heart's functional anatomy.

The factors that contribute to heart disease are variable. Some are genetically or naturally ordained, while others are within the individual's control. Most cardiovascular (CV) problems develop because of poor health habits; however, genetics can predispose one to these problems. Proper diet, exercise, and rest can do a lot to keep the heart functioning for a long time.

Predetermined factors include heredity, gender, and increasing age.

- **Heredity** Children of parents with CV disease have a higher risk of developing it. African Americans have high blood pressure two to three times more often than whites.

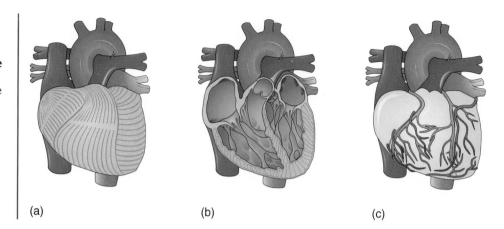

Figure 13.1

Functional Anatomy of the Heart
(a) Cardiac Muscle
(b) Conducting System (c) Blood Supply

(a)　　　　　　　　　(b)　　　　　　　　　(c)

- **Gender** Men have a greater risk of heart attack than women until age fifty-five. At age fifty-five, a woman's risk increases tenfold and may surpass a man's if she smokes or has conditions that cause CV disease.
- **Increasing Age** Almost fifty-five percent of all heart attack victims are age sixty-five or older. Of those who die, more than eighty percent are over age sixty-five.

The following factors can be impacted through lifestyle modification.

- **Cigarette Smoking** Smokers have more than twice the risk of heart attack as nonsmokers. A smoker who has a heart attack is also more likely to die from it.
- **High Blood Pressure** High blood pressure stresses the heart over time and increases the risk of stroke and heart attack. However, drugs, proper diet, weight loss, regular exercise, and reduction of salt intake can lower blood pressure.
- **High Blood Cholesterol Levels** Heart disease is related to rising levels of blood cholesterol. Too much cholesterol in the blood contributes to a buildup of plaque on the inner walls of the arteries feeding the heart, reducing blood flow to the heart. A diet low in cholesterol helps to lower blood cholesterol levels. Drugs can also lower blood cholesterol.
- **Obesity** Obesity, defined as 30% or more above ideal body weight, puts added strain on the heart. It can also increase blood pressure and blood cholesterol levels and lead to diabetes.
- **Diabetes** Type I diabetes occurs in childhood or early adulthood. These patients are insulin dependent. Type II diabetes most often appears during middle age in over-weight persons. More than 90% of diabetics are of this type. Type II diabetics may not have to take insulin. The disease sharply increases the risk of heart attack. Yet proper diet and weight loss, as well as exercise and drugs, can help keep diabetes in check.

It is critical that patients be taught the importance of lifestyle modifications in the treatment of the cardiovascular diseases. The value of dietary modifications, weight control, adherence to drug regimen, and physical exercise cannot be ignored. Therapy requires permanent changes in lifestyle.

ANTIARRHYTHMICS

The various classes of antiarrhythmic drugs have characteristic electrophysiologic effects on the myocardium. Some CV drugs influence the heart by directly or indirectly altering ion movement. Depressant drugs "close" the gate, allowing fewer ions to penetrate the sarcolemma. Stimulating drugs "open" the gate, allowing more ions to penetrate (Figure 13.2).

Normal Cardiac Rhythm

Normal cardiac rhythm is generated by the sinoatrial (SA) node at a rate of about seventy to eighty beats per minute. This rate exceeds the rate of other potential pacemaking automatic cells, such as the atrioventricular (AV) node, the AV bundle (also called the bundle of His), and the Purkinje fibers (Figure 13.3). When the SA

Figure 13.2

The "Gatekeeper" Role of Cardiovascular Drugs

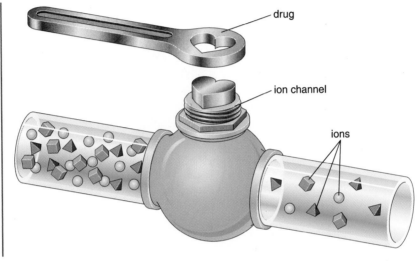

Figure 13.3

Conduction System of the Heart

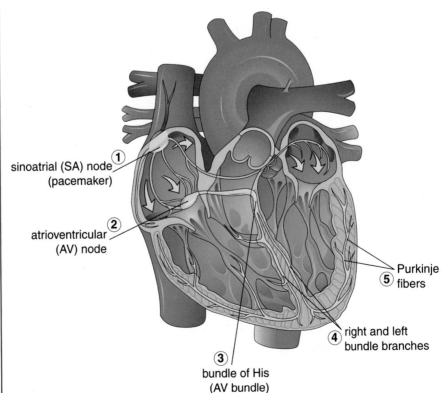

node is suppressed or damaged, conduction is interrupted or other areas become hyperexcitable, another discharging area may then become the dominant pacemaker. This action is termed ectopic pacemaker (i.e., a pacemaker other than the SA node). These conditions may be caused by ischemia, infarction, or alteration of body chemicals resulting in nonautomatic cells becoming automatic cells. Figure 13.4 shows how the heart's conducting system is documented by an electrocardiogram.

Abnormalities in Heart Rate and/or Rhythm

Heart rate and/or rhythm abnormalities occur when the contractions of the ventricles and atria are not synchronized. These abnormalities are rated according to their

Figure 13.4

Electrocardiographic Recording of Normal Electrical Activity in the Heart

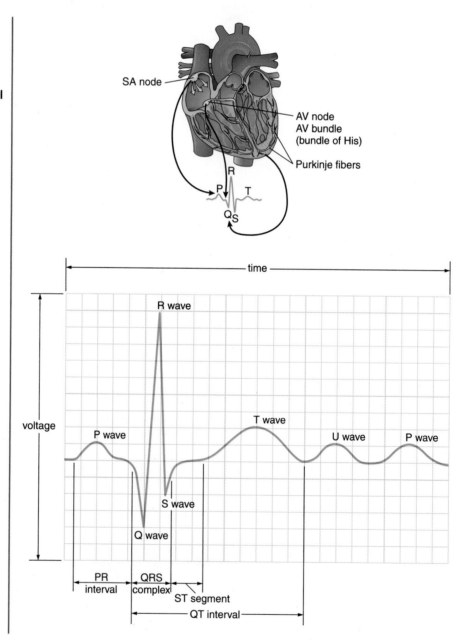

potential for serious outcome. Benign abnormalities have a low likelihood of sudden death. Potentially malignant abnormalities have a moderate risk of sudden death and indicate existing heart disease. Malignant abnormalities indicate an immediate risk and serious heart disease.

Premature contractions result in tachycardia, flutter, or fibrillation. Figure 13.5 shows a premature ventricular contraction. Table 13.1 shows abnormal heart rhythms and rates and their electrocardiogram tracings. The symptoms of abnormal heart rhythms or rates include palpitations, syncope, lightheadedness, visual disturbances, pallor, cyanosis, weakness, sweating, chest pain, and hypotension.

Pharmaceutical Treatment of Abnormal Heart Rates and Rhythms

Pharmaceutical treatment is directed at preventing life-threatening arrhythmias by restoring sinus (normal) rhythm. Table 13.2 lists the most-commonly used antiarrhythmic agents.

Figure 13.5

Premature Ventricular Contraction

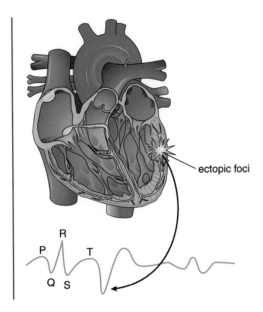

ectopic foci

R

P   T

Q S

Table 13.1   Arrhythmias

Arrhythmia	Beats per Minute	Electrocardiogram
tachycardia	150–250	
bradycardia	< 60	
atrial flutter	200–350	
atrial fibrillation	> 350	
premature atrial contraction	variable	
PVC	variable	
ventricular fibrillation	variable	

Table 13.2 Most-Commonly Used Antiarrhythmic Agents

Generic Name	Brand Name	Dosage Form
Membrane Stabilizing Agents (Class I)		
disopyramide	Norpace	capsule
flecainide	Tambocor	tablet
lidocaine	Xylocaine	IV
mexiletene	Mexitil	capsule
moricizine	Ethmozine	tablet
phenytoin	Dilantin	tablet, capsule, suspension, IV
procainamide	Pronestyl, Procanbid	tablet, capsule, IM, IV
propafenone	Rythmol	tablet
quinidine	Quinaglute, Cardioquin	tablet, IM, IV
tocainide	Tonocard	tablet
Beta Blockers (Class II)		
acebutolol	Sectral	capsule
esmolol	Brevibloc	IV
propranolol	Inderal	capsule, solution, tablet, IV
Inhibitors of Neurotransmitter Release and Reuptake (Class III)		
amiodarone	Cordarone	tablet, IV
bretylium	Bretylol	IM, IV
sotalol	Betapace	tablet
Calcium Channel Blockers (Class IV)		
diltiazem	Cardizem	capsule, tablet, IM, IV
verapamil	Isoptin, Calan, Covera HS, Verelan	tablet, IV, capsule
Other Agents		
amrinone	Inocor	ophthalmic, IV
atropine	Isopto Atropine	IM, IV, solution, tablet
digoxin	Lanoxin	elixir, capsule, tablet, IV
isoproterenol	Isuprel	aerosol, solution, tablet, IV, SC

MEMBRANE STABILIZING AGENTS (CLASS I) Membrane stabilizing agents slow the movement of ions into cardiac cells, thus reducing the action potential. The reduced action potential ability will dampen potential abnormal rhythms and heartbeats.

Quinaglute and **Cardioquin (quinidine)** act to slow SA node rate and AV conduction in atrial and ventricular arrhythmias. Adverse effects include thrombocytopenia and cinchonism (headache, blurred vision, tinnitus, confusion, and nausea).

Pronestyl and **Procanbid (procainamide)** have the same action as quinidine, but they are less effective for atrial arrhythmias. Procainamide and quinidine are so similar that they can be used interchangeably. Adverse effects include anorexia, nausea, vomiting, diarrhea, leukopenia, agranulocytosis, and a lupus-like syndrome.

Norpace (disopyramide) is similar to quinidine. It is used primarily on ventricular arrhythmias but is avoided in patients with heart failure. It is a strong anticholinergic, so dry mouth, urinary retention, constipation, and blurred vision are side effects. Other side effects include hypotension, heart block, fibrillation, and myocardial depression.

Rythmol (propafenone) is acceptable only for life-threatening arrhythmias. May cause new or worsen arrhythmias. It may also worsen CHF and alter pacemakers. Patients should be on a cardiac monitor at the beginning of therapy or any increase in dosage.

Ethmozine (moricizine) is used only in life-threatening ventricular arrhythmias. It slows conduction through nodes and bundle; however, it may cause new arrhythmias, hypotension, tremor, anxiety, urinary retention, hyperventilation, apnea, and asthma.

Xylocaine (lidocaine) reduces the ability of myocardial cells to respond to stimulation. It is the drug of choice for emergency IV therapy. It is effective on ventricles but has little effect on the atria. It must be given IV for premature ventricular contractions (PVCs) associated with myocardial infarction (MI). It can cause dizziness, confusion, and paresthesia (sensation of numbness, prickling, and tingling), delirium, stupor, and seizure.

Mexitil (mexiletene) has action similar to lidocaine. It is used for ventricular tachycardia but is more effective when used with another drug. Adverse effects include gastrointestinal and neurologic symptoms and elevated liver enzyme levels.

Dilantin (phenytoin) decreases the refractory period, action potential duration, and QT interval. It is used on resistant arrhythmias and arrhythmias due to digitalis toxicity. Adverse effects include cardiovascular collapse and central nervous system (CNS) and respiratory depression. (Phenytoin is also an anticonvulsant agent.)

Tonocard (tocainide) suppresses and prevents symptomatic life-threatening ventricular arrhythmias. It blocks both the initiation and conduction of nerve impulses by decreasing the neuronal membrane's permeability to sodium ions, which results in inhibition of depolarization with resultant blockade of conduction. The primary side effects are tremor, nausea, dizziness, and confusion.

Tambocor (flecainide) prolongs refractory periods, action potential duration, and QT interval. It is used for ventricular arrhythmias. The side effects are dizziness, blurred vision, tremor, nausea, and vomiting.

BETA BLOCKERS (CLASS II) These drugs competitively block response to beta stimulation, which results in decreases in heart rate, myocardial contractility, blood pressure, and myocardial oxygen demand. Since there are two types of beta receptors (β_1 and β_2), a drug that blocks both is considered to be nonselective. In choosing a drug for the heart, one with more β_1 than β_2 blockage is preferred, as β_1 receptors are found more abundantly in the heart.

These drugs slow conduction through the AV node and inhibit sympathetic neurotransmission. During exercise or stress, they slow ventricular response to atrial flutter. They are used for ventricular arrhythmias. Side effects are heart depression, bronchoconstriction, impotence, depression, and fatigue. They may also mask signs and symptoms of hypoglycemia and cause bradycardia. Sudden withdrawal may lead to recurrence of angina or even sudden death.

INHIBITORS OF NEUROTRANSMITTER RELEASE AND REUPTAKE (CLASS III) These drugs prevent release of neurotransmitters and reuptake and prolong the action potential.

Cordarone (amiodarone) is used for atrial and ventricular arrhythmias not responding to other medications. It is very effective, but is also almost toxic. It may take several days to several weeks before control is established. It can take up to one to four weeks before the oral dose takes effect. Many patients experience hypotension. The IV drip must be mixed in a glass bottle in D_5W. During a crisis, the "push" will be put in a bag of D_5W, then the drip will be mixed in glass.

Betapace (sotalol) is a beta blocker. It is indicated for treatment of documented ventricular arrhythmias (e.g., sustained ventricular tachycardia) that in the judgment of the physician are life-threatening. An unapproved use of this drug is supraventricular arrhythmias. The side effects are bradycardia, mental depression, and decreased sexual ability.

CALCIUM CHANNEL BLOCKERS (CLASS IV) The calcium channel blockers prevent movement of calcium ions through slow channels. These are the agents of choice for most supraventricular tachyarrhythmias and successfully convert most to normal sinus rhythm. They slow conduction through the AV node, slow SA node action, and relax coronary artery smooth muscle. They are used to control fast ventricular rates in patients with atrial flutter and atrial fibrillation. The side effects are bradycardia, hypotension, heart block, cardiac failure, nausea, constipation, headache, dizziness, and fatigue.

OTHER AGENTS There are other agents used to treat abnormalities in heart rate that have different mechanisms of action. **Lanoxin (digoxin)** is the most important drug in managing atrial flutter and fibrillation. It does not convert atrial fibrillation to sinus rhythm, but slows ventricular rate and treats cardiac failure.

Isuprel (isoproterenol) may constrict some blood vessels, but dilates coronary vessels. It is used parenterally in ventricular arrhythmias due to AV nodal block, hemodynamically compromised bradyarrhythmias, or atropine-resistant bradyarrhythmias. It may be used temporarily in third-degree AV block until pacemaker insertion. It increases heart rate and contractility.

Isopto Atropine (atropine) is an anticholinergic agent that decreases parasympathetic tone by suppressing the vagus nerve, allowing sympathetic action to take over. It is used in slow rates often associated with MI and other forms of bradycardia that is described as heart rates below sixty beats per minute. Low doses may worsen the bradycardia. High doses may cause cardioacceleration; too high a rate increases oxygen demand, resulting in ischemia and leading to arrhythmias. It is used to treat sinus bradycardia and as preoperative medication to inhibit salivation and secretions.

DRUGS FOR CONGESTIVE HEART FAILURE (CHF)

Figure 13.6 shows the normal flow of blood through the heart. When the pumping ability of the heart can no longer meet the metabolic needs of the body's tissues, the heart pumps less blood than it receives. Blood accumulates in the chambers and stretches the walls. Less blood circulates to organs. Kidneys, sensitive to reduced oxygen, retain water and electrolytes to increase blood volume. The result is edema.

In the normal heart, contraction is directly proportional to the length or stretch of the cardiac muscle cells. After accelerated stimulation and/or excessive ventricular filling, two changes will occur in the heart. Cardiomegaly is enlargement of the heart due to overwork from overstimulation. The muscle stretches and loses elasticity. Myocardial hypertrophy is a thickening of the heart muscle in response to overstimulation.

Congestive heart failure (CHF) involves ten percent of the population over seventy-five years of age. Its causes are listed in Table 13.3.

In left-sided failure, fluid accumulates in the lungs, causing pulmonary edema, reduced gas exchange, shortness of breath, cough, memory loss and confusion, anorexia, and profuse sweating. Right-sided failure results in fluids collecting in abdominal organs (ascites) and the lower extremities, causing weight gain, anorexia, and nausea.

The causes of death are progressive failure of the pump and sudden cardiac death. The goals of therapy are to preserve and prolong the quality of life, avoid hospitalization, and slow left-ventricle deterioration.

Treatment of CHF involves use of combinations of diuretics, digoxin, and angiotensin-converting enzyme (ACE) inhibitors. Calcium channel blockers are contraindicated. The most-commonly used agents for CHF are listed in Table 13.4.

Figure 13.6

Blood Flow Through the Heart

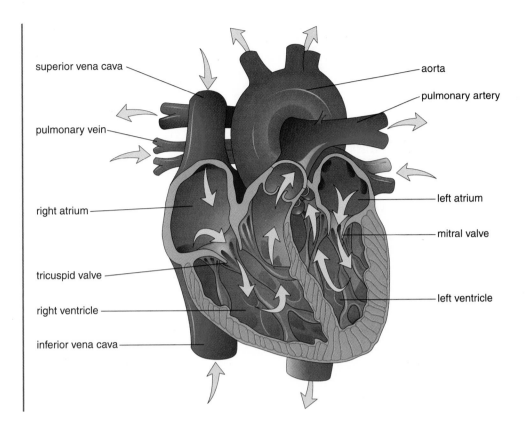

superior vena cava

aorta

pulmonary artery

pulmonary vein

left atrium

right atrium

mitral valve

tricuspid valve

left ventricle

right ventricle

inferior vena cava

Table 13.3	Causes of Congestive Heart Failure	
Primary Causes	**Secondary Causes**
cardiomyopathy	high salt intake
coronary artery disease	noncompliance to treatment
hypertension	side effects to drug therapy
	kidney failure
	stress
	infection and inflammation
	cigarette smoking

Antiarrhythmics

Lanoxin (digoxin) is a much-used drug for treating congestive heart failure and atrial fibrillation and flutter. It has the following mechanisms of action.

⋄ It increases the force of contraction.
⋄ It increases the effective refractory period of the AV node (slows AV node stimulation).
⋄ It affects the SA node, increasing automaticity due to ion imbalance (direct stimulation).

Digoxin is used to restore the force of myocardial contraction without increasing oxygen demands and to slow ventricle response to stimulation by reducing AV node stimulation. Digoxin should be used with caution because of the possibility of

Table 13.4 **Most-Commonly Used Agents for Congestive Heart Failure**

Generic Name	Brand Name	Dosage Form
Antiarrhythmics		
amrinone	Inocor	IV
digoxin	Lanoxin	capsule, tablet, elixir, IV
Vasodilators		
milrinone	Primacor	IV
nitroprusside	Nitropress	IV
ACE Inhibitors		
benazepril	Lotensin	tablet
captopril	Capoten	tablet
enalapril	Vasotec	tablet, IV
fosinopril	Monopril	tablet
lisinopril	Prinivil, Zestril	tablet
moexipril	Univasc	tablet
quinapril	Accupril	tablet
ramipril	Altace	capsule
trandolapril	Mavik	tablet
Angiotensin II Antagonists		
losartan	Cozaar	tablet
valsartan	Diovan	capsule

systemic accumulation. Digitalis toxicity is commonly referred to as "dig toxicity." When this occurs the patient becomes very nauseous, has vertigo, experiences general weakness, and may see yellow-green halos around objects. The three primary signs of digitalis toxicity are nausea, vomiting, and arrhythmias. If this occurs, the drug should be withdrawn immediately.

Inocor (amrinone) is a phosphodiesterase inhibitor. It increases resting cardiac output while decreasing systemic vascular resistance as well as left ventricular end-diastolic, pulmonary capillary wedge, and right atrial pressures. It also is used only IV and in patients resistant to digitalis, diuretics, and vasodilators.

Vasodilators

Primacor (milrinone) is a phosphodiesterase inhibitor resulting in vasodilation. It is used for short-term IV therapy of CHF and for calcium antagonist intoxication. Milrinone is closely related to amrinone, but is fifteen times more potent with fewer side effects.

ACE Inhibitors

ACE inhibitors competitively inhibit conversion of angiotensin I to angiotensin II, a potent vasoconstrictor, through the angiotensin-converting enzyme activity, with resultant lower levels of angiotensin II. Lower angiotensin II levels increases plasma renin activity and reduces aldosterone secretion. CHF is especially responsive to ACE inhibitors. Some examples are **Lotensin (benazepril)**, **Capoten (captopril)**, **Vasotec (enalapril)**, **Monopril (fosinopril)**, **Prinivil** and **Zestril (lisinopril)**, **Univasc (moexipril)**, **Accupril (quinapril)**, **Altace (ramipril)**, and **Mavik (trandolapril)**.

Warning

Prinivil, Plendil, Prevacid, and Prilosec often look and sound alike.

Warning

Zestril and Vistaril are alike.

A persistent cough seems to be the most troublesome side effect. It is a dry, unproductive cough, but is extremely annoying. Many patients refuse to take the drug because of this aggravation. The drug should be taken one hour before meals. It may cause dizziness, especially the first few days. The patient should be told to arise slowly to avoid orthostatic hypotension, and to not add salt substitutes, which contain potassium, to the diet. ACE inhibitors have a potassium-preserving effect. If the patient is taking a potassium-sparing diuretic or potassium supplements or salt substitutes, the patient will become hyperkalemic. ACE inhibitors should be given with caution to patients taking lithium.

Angiotensin II Antagonists

Angiotensin II antagonists seem to work as well as ACE inhibitors to lower blood pressure. ACE inhibitors reduce the production of angiotensin II. Angiotensin antagonists block the action of angiotensin II at its receptors. There is less cough, angioedema, etc., so they are better tolerated. Two drugs on the market are **Cozaar (losartan)** and **Diovan (valsartan)**.

MYOCARDIAL INFARCTION (MI)

Myocardial infarction (MI), most commonly known as a heart attack, is the leading cause of death in industrialized nations. When the heart muscle is deprived of oxygen because of reduced blood supply, muscle cells die (necrosis). This is an infarct. Lesser infarcts undergo healing; muscle is replaced by connective tissue (scar), thus contractility of the heart is reduced around scarring. Treatment is aimed at allowing the heart to rest and undergo normal healing.

Causes of a Heart Attack

MI may occur when there is a prolonged decrease in oxygen delivery to a region of cardiac muscle. There is substantial narrowing of the artery lumen equal to or greater than seventy percent in one or more of the three major arteries. Factors that increase risk of MI include a history of angina, alcohol consumption, dyspnea on exertion, reduced pulmonary vital capacity, cigarette smoking, and atherosclerosis.

The recommendations for risk reduction are to

- eliminate smoking
- control diabetes
- reduce hypertension by diet, medication, or both
- exercise moderately at least three times weekly
- adjust calories to achieve ideal body weight
- decrease alcohol consumption
- use aspirin therapy
- reduce dietary cholesterol/triglycerides

Symptoms of a Heart Attack

Symptoms of a heart attack are described as oppressive or burning tightness or squeezing in the chest, choking and indigestion-like expansion, a sense of "impending doom," and substernal pain with varying radiations to the neck, throat, jaw, shoulders, and one or both arms. The pain lasts thirty minutes to several hours and can be severe. It may occur at rest, does not subside with rest, and may not be relieved completely with nitroglycerin. Half the patients admit to having some symptoms in the day or days before the attack: vague chest discomfort, weakness, fatigue, or sweating.

Myocardial Drug Therapy

Beta blockers are frequently prescribed to reduce the risk of death or recurrence following an MI event. Table 13.5 lists these drugs.

Most of the adverse reactions to these drugs are mild and transient and rarely require withdrawal of therapy. The most common is tiredness. Beta blockers should not be withdrawn abruptly. Dosage should be reduced gradually over one to two weeks.

ANGINA PECTORIS

Angina pectoris is the occurrence of chest pain and is due to an imbalance between oxygen supply and oxygen demand. Oxygen demand is directly related to heart rate, strength of contraction, and resistance to blood flow. In angina, the diminished blood supply to the heart does not cause irreversible changes related to obstruction or narrowing of coronary arteries as occur in atherosclerosis, arterial spasm, pulmonary hypertension, or cardiac hypertrophy.

There are three types of angina.

◇ Stable angina is effort-induced pain from physical activity or emotional stress. This pain is relieved by rest and is usually predictable and reproducible.
◇ Unstable angina is pain that occurs with increasing frequency that diminishes the patient's ability to work and decreases response to treatment. It may signal an oncoming MI.
◇ Variant angina is pain due to coronary artery spasm. The ST segment is elevated and prolonged during pain. This pain may occur at certain times of the day, but is not stress-induced.

The Symptoms and Risk Factors of Angina Pectoris

The characteristic symptom of angina pectoris is severe chest discomfort, which may be described as heaviness, pressure, tightness, choking, a squeezing sensation, or a combination of these. Other symptoms may include sweating, dizziness, and dyspnea. Diagnosis is made from the physical examination, resting and exercise

Table 13.5   **Most-Commonly Used Beta Blockers for Reducing Risk of Death After an MI**

Generic Name	Brand Name	Dosage Form
atenolol	Tenormin	tablet, IV
metoprolol	Lopressor	tablet, IV
	Toprol XL	tablet
nadolol	Corgard	tablet
propranolol	Inderal	capsule, tablet, solution, IV

ECGs, coronary angiogram, and radioisotope study. The ECG may be normal, but usually the T wave is flat or inverted. Anginal pain is usually brief and precipitated by exercise or emotional stress.

The risk factors for angina are

⋄ hypertension
⋄ increased serum lipoprotein levels
⋄ smoking
⋄ increased serum glucose levels (diabetes)
⋄ type A personality
⋄ advanced age
⋄ coronary artery disease
⋄ obesity

Factors that initiate an attack of angina are

⋄ emotions
⋄ pain
⋄ cold weather
⋄ heavy meals, which causes blood flow to the gut to increase, resulting in decreased flow to the brain and heart
⋄ hypoglycemia
⋄ smoking

Nicotine causes arterial constriction and contributes to arteriosclerosis.

Antianginal Drugs

Table 13.6 presents the most-commonly used agents for angina.

NITRATES Nitrates relax vascular smooth muscle (venous more than arterial), which reduces venous return and cardiac filling and decreases tension in the heart walls. Nitrates dilate coronary vessels, allowing blood flow to redistribute to ischemic tissues. Because peripheral vasodilation decreases venous return to the heart (preload), nitroglycerin also helps to treat pulmonary edema in CHF. Arterial vasodilation decreases arterial impedance (afterload), thereby lessening left ventricular work and aiding the failing heart. Nitroglycerin is approved for angina and CHF.

Nitroglycerin may also be used as prophylaxis, by taking the drug a few minutes before the activity or stress that might cause the attack. This is the drug of choice for acute attacks and is taken sublingually. If the pain does not subside in five minutes, the patient should take a second tablet. This may be repeated every five minutes for fifteen minutes with a maximum of three doses in fifteen minutes. If there is still no relief within fifteen minutes, the patient should go immediately to the hospital. The spray is applied under the tongue, one to two sprays every three to five minutes, with a maximum of three doses in a fifteen-minute period. Both the spray and the tablets produce a stinging sensation under the tongue. Only the sublingual and translingual routes should be used for acute attacks.

Nitroglycerin patches should not be allowed to remain on the skin for twenty-four hours. There should be a free time, usually when the patient is sleeping, or tolerance will develop. The label should instruct the patient in this procedure.

Nitroglycerin can cause severe headaches when first given; aspirin or acetaminophen may provide relief. The dose of nitroglycerin may be reduced; if it is given as a patch or ointment, it can be placed lower on the body and gradually moved back to

Table 13.6   Most-Commonly Used Agents for Angina

Generic Name	Brand Name	Dosage Form
Nitrates		
isosorbide dinitrate	Isordil	tablet, capsule
	Dilatrate-SR	capsule
isosorbide mononitrate	Imdur, ISMO	tablet
nitroglycerin	Nitrolingual	spray
	Nitrostat	tablet
	Nitro-Bid	capsule
	Nitro-Bid, Nitrol	ointment
	Nitro-Bid IV	injection, IV
	Nitro-Dur, Nitrodisc, Transderm Nitro, Minitran	transdermal patch
	Nitrostat IV, Tridil	IV
Calcium Channel Blockers		
amlodipine	Norvasc	tablet
bepridil	Vascor	tablet
diltiazem	Cardizem, Dilacor XR	capsule, tablet, IV
felodipine	Plendil	tablet
isradipine	DynaCirc	capsule
nicardipine	Cardene	capsule, injection
nifedipine	Adalat, Procardia	capsule, IV
nisoldipine	Sular	tablet
verapamil	Calan, Isoptin, Verelan, Covera HS	tablet, capsule, IV
Beta Blockers		
acebutolol	Sectral	capsule
atenolol	Tenormin	tablet, IV
metoprolol	Lopressor, Toprol XL	tablet, IV
nadolol	Corgard	tablet
propranolol	Inderal	capsule, solution, tablet, IV

Warning

Nicardipine, nifedipine, and nimodipine could easily be confused.

Warning

Cardene and Cardizem are often confused.

Warning

Cardene can look like codeine.

the chest. Nitroglycerin can also cause orthostatic hypotension when first used, so patients should be advised to move slowly, especially when changing from a sitting or lying position. The drug can also cause flushing. The drug should not be stopped abruptly, but tapered.

Nitroglycerin is sold, and should be stored, in an amber glass container. The patient should replenish the prescription every three months and discard any remaining drug.

Dilatrate-SR (isosorbide dinitrate) is used for the same purposes as nitroglycerin, the prevention of angina and CHF. It is easily confused with Dilacor XR. Dilacor XR is diltiazem, a calcium channel blocker. The technician should be careful, as they are very different drugs.

Warning

Dilatrate-SR and Dilacor XR are often confused.

CALCIUM CHANNEL BLOCKERS Calcium channel blockers inhibit the calcium ion from entering the "slow channels," or select voltage-sensitive areas of vascular smooth muscle and myocardium, during depolarization, producing relaxation of coronary vascular smooth muscle and coronary vasodilation, which in turn increases oxygen delivery. Sodium and calcium ions cross the cell membranes through openings called channels. Sodium ions cross rapidly through fast channels, while calcium ions cross more slowly through separate openings (the slow channels). The action potential regulates calcium entry during its plateau phase; calcium crosses the membrane and releases large amounts of calcium from internal stores; activation energy is needed for muscle contraction. Blockage of the slow channels reduces calcium influx; therefore, cell contractility is reduced. The cell's energy requirements and oxygen demand also are reduced, dilating coronary arteries and arterioles.

Some of these drugs should be taken with food, and caffeine should be limited. The most common side effect is constipation. The patient should notify the physician in the event of swelling hands and feet or shortness of breath. Some patients experience drowsiness when they begin taking a calcium channel blocker.

Covera HS (verapamil) is a timed-release product designed for bedtime dosing. It is approved for either hypertension or angina. The tablets do not release until about four to five hours after they have been swallowed. The drug is pumped out of two laser holes in the tablet. Patients may see an empty shell of ghost tablet in their stool, as with Procardia (nifedipine).

BETA BLOCKERS Beta blockers are used in angina for their effectiveness in slowing the heart rate, decreasing myocardial contractility, and lowering blood pressure, particularly during exercise. All of these actions reduce oxygen demand, and thus beta blockers reduce frequency and severity of attacks. Beta blockers are similar in molecular structure to the catecholamines and compete for the same receptor sites. In response to increased anxiety, physical activity, or emotional stress, the sympathetic nervous system stimulates the release of catecholamines, which increases heart rate and contractile force.

The primary side effect of beta blockers is bradycardia; they also mask symptoms of hypoglycemia and hyperthyroidism. They should be used with caution in patients with bronchospastic disease because they may inhibit the bronchodilating effects of endogenous catecholamines. They should not be discontinued abruptly.

HYPERTENSION

Blood pressure (BP) is defined as the product of cardiac output (CO) and total peripheral resistance (TPR) and is expressed as the systolic reading over the diastolic reading. Even though there is really no "normal" reading, 120/80 is referred to as such. Hypertension is defined arbitrarily as a disease in which the systolic blood pressure is greater than 140 mm Hg (top number) and the diastolic pressure is greater than 90 mm Hg (bottom number). Table 13.7 describes the staging of blood pressure in adults. Cardiac output is the major determinant of systolic pressure, while total peripheral resistance largely determines the level of diastolic pressure.

The primary cause of hypertension is unknown, although family history, cigarette smoking, and a high-fat diet are definite factors. Secondary causes can be kidney disease, decreased pressure or delayed pulse in the lower extremities, truncal obesity, adrenal tumor, and drugs such as oral contraceptives, corticosteroids, nonsteroidal anti-inflammatory drugs (NSAIDs), nasal decongestants, and appetite suppressants.

Vasoconstriction, caused by the sympathetic nervous system, is the main factor that increases peripheral resistance. Cardiac output, the product of heart rate and stroke volume, is determined by three aspects: preload, afterload, and contractility. Additional factors involved in determining blood pressure are blood viscosity, blood volume, and various nerve controls.

Untreated Hypertension

Untreated hypertension can have devastating results. Some of these results follow.

Table 13.7 **Staging of Blood Pressure in Adults**

Category	Systolic (mm Hg)	Diastolic (mm Hg)
Normal	< 130	< 85
High normal	130–139	85–89
Hypertension		
Stage 1 (mild)	140–159	90–99
Stage 2 (moderate)	160–179	100–109
Stage 3 (severe)	180–209	110–119
Stage 4 (very severe)	210	120

◇ Cardiovascular disease is characterized by enlargement of the heart (cardiomegaly), cardiac hypertrophy, and thickening of the cardiac wall, with loss of elasticity. Cardiac output is reduced, along with the heart's ability to push blood through the body to perfuse tissue. The left ventricle does most of the work.

◇ CHF results in inadequate perfusion, cold extremities (toes and fingers), pitting or whole-body edema (especially in the feet and legs), and increased bronchial secretions.

◇ Renal insufficiency can be the result of high blood pressure. The higher the pressure, the more the kidney reduces renal blood flow and renal function. Renin is released to form angiotensin, which causes vasoconstriction and release of aldosterone.

◇ Accelerated cardiac and peripheral vascular disease can also result from high blood pressure. In general, the higher the pressure, the greater the risk. Hypertension alters capillaries, venules, and arterioles. Blood cholesterol collects in arterial walls, reducing the size of the lumen and, therefore, the blood flow, with loss of feeling, increased potential for infection, vascular problems (as in diabetes), and deterioration of nerves from diminished blood supply.

Hypertension Therapy

Hypertension control begins with detection and continued surveillance. Initial readings should be confirmed with subsequent readings for several weeks, unless the pressure is dangerously high at the first reading.

The goal of therapy is to prevent morbidity and mortality associated with high blood pressure and reduce the pressure by the least offensive means possible. A four-step regimen is needed. This regimen is presented in Table 13.8.

Table 13.8 **Regimen for Reducing Blood Pressure**

Step 1	Modify lifestyle factors.		
	high sodium intake	to	moderate sodium intake
	excess consumption of calories	to	weight reduction
	physical inactivity	to	regular aerobic physical activity
	excess alcohol consumption	to	moderate alcohol consumption
	nicotine usage	to	cessation of nicotine usage
	high stress	to	control stress
Step 2	Monotherapy; use a single drug, usually a diuretic, beta blocker, ACE inhibitor, or calcium channel blocker.		
Step 3	Add a diuretic if it was not the drug used to begin therapy in step 2 of the regimen.		
Step 4	Add a third agent that will be synergistic with the other two in reducing blood pressure.		

Antihypertensive Therapeutics

Table 13.9 gives an overview of the main drug classes used in the treatment of hypertension and Table 13.10 lists the most commonly prescribed agents for this disease state.

DIURETICS Diuretics are a first-line drug for treating hypertension. They reduce the cardiac output by increasing the elimination of urine and reducing the volume of fluid in the body, thereby reducing total peripheral resistance. However, the most important effect of diuretics on lowering blood pressure appears to be due to their ability to reduce sodium load.

Table 13.9   Pharmacologic Antihypertensive Therapies

Drug Class	Mechanism of Action
diuretics	First-line therapy (discussed in Chapter 12). Reduces total peripheral resistance.
calcium channel blockers	First-line therapy. Dilates the aterioles thereby reducing peripheral resistance, energy consumption, and oxygen requirements. Reduces heart action.
ACE inhibitors (Angiotensin Converting Enzyme)	Acts by blocking angiotensin-converting enzymes to prevent the conversion of angiotensin I to angiotensin II, which is a potent vasoconstrictor. The decrease in blood pressure is accompanied by a reduction in peripheral resistance and an increase in the elasticity of the large arteries suggesting a direct effect on aterial smooth muscle.
angiotensin II-receptor antagonists	Binds to the antiotensin II receptors thereby blocking the vasoconstriction effects of these receptors. Unlike ACE inhibitors bradykinin-altered responses are not affected (therefore no cough).
beta blockers	Blocks beta receptor response to adrenergic stimulation which decreases heart rate, myocardial contractility, blood pressure, and myocardial oxygen demand. Agents selective to $beta_1$ act specifically on the heart and are said to be cardio-specific. Agents that act at either $beta_1$ or $beta_2$ receptors are said to be nonspecific.
CNS agents	Stimulates the $alpha_2$ adrenergic receptors in the brain and thereby reduces the sympathetic outflow from the vasomotor center in the brain. Thus, heart rate is decreased, cardiac output decreases slightly, and total peripheral vascular resistance is lowered due to reduced stimulation of vascular muscle.
peripheral acting agents	Blocks alpha stimulation to peripheral nerves and innervates vessels. Leads indirectly to vasodilation and hypotension.
vasodilators	Relaxes arterial smooth muscle and lowers peripheral resistance via direct mechanism.
combination drugs	Second line therapy. Additive effects to lower blood pressures. Two low doses of different drugs usually cause fewer side effects than pushing the dose of either drug.

Table 13.10   Most-Commonly Used Antihypertensive Therapeutics

Generic Name	Brand Name	Dosage Form
Calcium Channel Blockers		
amlodipine	Norvasc	tablet
diltiazem	Cardizem, Dilacor XR	capsule, tablet, IV
felodipine	Plendil	tablet
isradipine	DynaCirc	capsule
nicardipine	Cardene	capsule, injection
nifedipine	Adalat, Procardia	capsule, tablet
nisoldipine	Sular	tablet
verpamil	Calan, Covera-HS, Isoptin, Verelan	tablet, capsule, IV
ACE Inhibitors		
benazepril	Lotensin	tablet
captopril	Capoten	tablet
enalapril	Vasotec	tablet, IV
fosinopril	Monopril	tablet
lisinopril	Prinivil, Zestril	tablet
moexipril	Univasc	tablet
perindopril	Aceon	tablet
quinapril	Accupril	tablet
ramipril	Altace	capsule
trandolapril	Mavik	tablet
Angiotensin II-Receptor Antagonists		
candesartan	Atacand	tablet
eprosartan	Tevetan	tablet
irbesartan	Avapro	tablet
losartan	Cozaar	tablet
telmisartan	Micardis	tablet
valsartan	Diovan	capsule
Cardio-Selective Beta Blockers		
acebutolol	Sectral	capsule
atenolol	Tenormin	tablet, IV
betaxolol	Kerlone	tablet, ophthalmic
bisoprolol	Zebeta	tablet
metoprolol	Lopressor	tablet, IV
	Toprol XL	tablet
Beta Blockers		
carvedilol	Coreg	tablet
esmolol	Brevibloc	IV
labetalol	Normodyne, Trandate	tablet, IV
nadolol	Corgard	tablet
pindolol	Visken	tablet
propranolol	Inderal	capsule, solution, tablet, IV
timolol	Blocadren	tablet, opthalmic
CNS Agents		
clonidine	Catapres	tablet, patch, IV
guanfacine	Tenex	tablet, liquid
methyldopa	Aldomet	tablet, oral suspension, IV
Peripheral Acting Agents		
doxazosin	Cardura	tablet
guanethidine	Ismelin	tablet
prazosin	Minipress	capsule
terazosin	Hytrin	capsule

continues

Generic Name	Brand Name	Dosage Form
Vasodilators		
epoprostenol	Flolan	IV
fenoldopam	Corlopam	IV
hydralazine	Apresoline	tablet, IV
minoxidil	Loniten, Rogaine	tablet, topical
Combination Drugs		
benzapril-hydrochlorothiazide	Lotensin HCT	tablet
enalapril-diltiazem	Teczem	tablet
enalapril-hydrochlorothiazide	Vaseretic	tablet
losartan-hydrochlorothiazide	Hyzaar	tablet
trandolapril-verapamil	Tarka	tablet

CALCIUM CHANNEL BLOCKERS   Calcium channel blockers are also first-line therapy. They reduce blood pressure by dilating the arterioles, which leads to reduced peripheral resistance and reduced energy consumption and oxygen requirements. Calcium movement into myocardial cells is slowed, thus reducing contraction ability, coupled with lower energy and oxygen usage.

ACE INHIBITORS (ANGIOTENSIN CONVERTING ENZYME)   ACE inhibitors act by competitive inhibition of angiotensin-converting enzyme to prevent the conversion of angiotensin I to angiotensin II, a potent vasoconstrictor. This results in lower levels of angiotensin II, which increases plasma renin activity and reduces aldosterone secretion. The decrease in blood pressure is accompanied by a reduction in peripheral resistance and an increase in the elasticity of large arteries suggesting a direct effect on arterial smooth muscle. These drugs should not be given in conjunction with antacids, phenothiazines, indomethacin, allopurinol, digoxin, lithium, potassium, or potassium-sparing diuretics. ACE inhibitors have a potassium-sparing element. These drugs are less effective in African American patients. It is recommended that a thiazide diuretic be used in conjunction with most ACE inhibitors. The most common side effect is an irritating cough which will often cause the patient to discontinue the drug.

ANGIOTENSIN II-RECEPTOR ANTAGONISTS   Angiotensin II-receptor antagonists bind to the angiotensin II receptors and prevent the binding of angiotensin II, thereby blocking the vasoconstriction and aldosterone-secreting effects of angiotensin II. It has no effects on angiotensin-converting enzyme, therefore bradykinin-altered responses are not affected. This is why the cough associated with ACE inhibitors is substantially lower in patients receiving this drug class. Side effects include diarrhea, leg pain, dizziness, insomnia, nasal congestion, and sinusitis. These drugs should not be given with phenothiazines, antacids, or indomethacin. Angiotensin II-receptor antagonists can be given alone or in combination therapy with other drugs.

BETA BLOCKERS   Beta blockers competitively block the beta receptors, which results in a blocked response to adrenergic stimulation and decreases heart rate, myocardial contractility, blood pressure, and myocardial oxygen demand. Some beta blockers are more selective to β_1 than β_2 and this is desirable because these are more cardioselective. Membrane-stabilizing and intrinsic sympathomimetic activity are exhibited by certain agents in this class.

     Sectral (acebutolol) and **Visken (pindolol)** are blockers with intrinsic sympathomimetic activity (ISA) and so produce less reduction in heart rate. Side effects are bradycardia, increased airway resistance, fluid retention, masked signs of hypoglycemia, and depression.

Coreg (carvedilol), the first beta blocker for CHF, is a nonselective beta blocker with vasodilating effects. Physicians usually avoid beta blockers in CHF because they slow the heart and make CHF worse. However, studies indicate that left ventricular function can be improved by blocking excessive adrenergic stimulation. The patients are started on a low dose, which is slowly increased. If taken with food, dizziness will be reduced.

Normodyne and **Trandate (labetalol)** are both alpha blockers and nonspecific beta blockers. Pharmacy technicians should watch for a patient with prescriptions for both of these brands. Prescribers often do not realize the two brands are the same drug, so a patient could risk getting a double dose. Side effects are the same as for acebutolol and pindolol.

CNS AGENTS CNS agents stimulate the $alpha_2$ adrenergic receptors in the brain. This leads to reduction in sympathetic outflow from the vasomotor center in the brain and an associated increase in vagal tone. As a consequence of reduced sympathetic activity, together with some enhancement of parasympathetic activity, heart rate is decreased, cardiac output decreases slightly, total peripheral resistance is lowered, plasma renin activity is reduced, and baroreceptor reflexes are blunted.

Catapres (clonidine) is the only antihypertensive supplied as a transdermal delivery system, and this delivery form seems to have fewer side effects than the other forms. It is also used in patients undergoing withdrawal to treat hypertension, especially in alcoholics.

Tenex (guanfacine) is more effective than clonidine, with less sedation. Its side effects are drowsiness, fatigue, dry mouth, depression, and fluid retention.

PERIPHERAL ACTING AGENTS Peripheral acting agents block alpha stimulation to peripheral nerves, which innervate vessels. This action leads indirectly to vasodilation and hypotension, known as the first dose phenomenon.

Minipress (prazosin) blocks impulses at the neurovascular junction and vascular smooth muscle. The side effect is orthostatic hypotension which is severe on the first few doses. The patient should be told to take the drug at bedtime. Other side effects are dizziness, weakness, and headache.

Hytrin (terazosin) blocks impulses at vascular smooth muscle. The side effects are orthostatic hypotension with the first dose.

Cardura (doxazosin) selectively blocks $alpha_1$ receptors which results in vasodilation of veins and arterioles. It has the same effects as Minipress and Hytrin. On a weight-to-weight basis, doxazosin is fifty percent more potent than prazosin.

Ismelin (guanethidine) prevents storage of norepinephrine in peripheral nerves by an alpha blockade, thus reducing sympathetic outflow and producing a decrease in vasomotor tone and heart rate. The primary side effects are postural hypotension and impaired sexual function.

VASODILATORS Vasodilators have a direct relaxant effect on arterial smooth muscle, which provides reduced peripheral resistance.

Apresoline (hydralazine) has to be given three to four times a day, so compliance is a problem. Side effects are reflex sympathetic stimulation associated with vasodilation, which leads to tachycardia, palpitations, flushing, and headache. Patients often complain of a racing heart. Less common is a lupus-like disorder. Somehow the drug stimulates the production of antibodies that cause the lupus symptoms (butterfly rash, joint pain, and stiffness). This antibody may also attack the kidney. If all of these symptoms occur, the drug must be stopped immediately.

Loniten and **Rogaine (minoxidil)** relax arteriolar smooth muscle with little effect on veins. Stimulation of hair growth is secondary to vasodilation. Other side effects are temporary edema, nausea, vomiting, and rash. This drug lowers blood pressure, even when applied topically, and the patient could easily become hypotensive. This is why it has been a prescription-only drug for so long. The topical form of Rogaine is indicated for male pattern baldness.

Flolan (epoprostenol) is a prostacyclin (PGI-2) used only in pulmonary hypertension. It is a strong vasodilator of all vascular beds, including the pulmonary vessels. In addition, it is a potent endogenous inhibitor of platelet aggregation so it can prevent thrombogenesis and platelet clumping in the lungs by inhibiting platelet aggregation.

Corlopam (fenoldopam) is a dopamine D_1 receptor agonist that exhibits a vasodilating action. It is a racemic mixture but the R isomer is responsible for its biological activity. It is indicated for the in-hospital, short-term (up to forty-eight hours) management of severe hypertension when rapid, but quickly reversible, emergency reduction of blood pressure is clinically indicated. It increases renal blood flow and diuresis. The most common adverse events are hypotension, headache, flushing, and nausea. It should not be used concurrently with a beta blocker. An infusion can be abruptly stopped or tapered. Oral anti-hypertensive agents can be administered during an infusion. It has an elimination half-life of about five minutes. It can be mixed with either D_5W or normal saline and is stable under normal light and temperature for twenty-four hours. It does contain metabisulfite which may cause an allergic reaction.

COMBINATION DRUGS Combination drugs have additive effects to relax blood vessels and lower pressure. Two low doses of different drugs usually cause fewer side effects than pushing the dose of either drug. This is still second-line therapy.

ANTICOAGULANTS AND ANTIPLATELETS

Anticoagulants prevent clot formation; antiplatelets reduce the risk of forming clots by inhibiting platelet aggregation. These classes of drugs are used to prevent blood clots (thrombi). Thrombi develop from abnormalities in

- ◇ blood flow (stasis)
- ◇ vessel walls (from damage, surgery)
- ◇ platelet adhesiveness (hypercoagulability)
- ◇ blood coagulation (hypercoagulability)

About ten percent of patients with a pulmonary embolism die; two thirds have an undiagnosed deep-vein thrombosis (DVT). A proximal DVT (at the level of the knee or above) is the most serious.

Risk factors for DVT are

- ◇ age over forty years
- ◇ high-dose estrogen therapy
- ◇ obesity
- ◇ estrogen combined with nicotine
- ◇ varicose veins
- ◇ previous DVT
- ◇ bed rest for over four days
- ◇ trauma
- ◇ pregnancy
- ◇ surgery
- ◇ parturition
- ◇ major illness

The therapy is either low-dose heparin, adjusted-dose heparin, or low-molecular-weight heparin, and Coumadin. The purpose is to prevent fatal blood clotting while ensuring adequate coagulation.

The blood should be monitored to prevent future emboli and minimize risk of hemorrhage. The following are the most-frequently used laboratory tests.

⬦ Prothrombin time (PT) assesses the function of the extrinsic and common pathways of the coagulation system; in particular it measures the activity of the vitamin K-dependent factor. (PT is affected by warfarin.)
⬦ Partial thromboplastin time (PTT) measures the function of the intrinsic and common pathways. (PTT is affected by heparin.)

Anticoagulant Agents

Table 13.11 presents the most-commonly used anticoagulant agents. Anticoagulant therapy should be started with IV heparin, then overlapped a few days with warfarin, then switched to warfarin only. The warfarin dose is based on PTT results. The patient should take the dose without food, report any signs of bleeding, avoid hazardous activities, avoid foods high in vitamin K, use a soft toothbrush, and carry a Medi-Alert device. The urine may turn red-orange; the physician should be notified if the urine turns dark brown or if red or tar-black stools occur. Warfarin has a very large number of interactions with other drugs, so the technician should always check the patient's drug profile before dispensing the drug.

Heparin inhibits thrombin formation, but the objective is to prevent clot formation. Heparin does not dissolve a clot once it has already formed. Heparin is usually found in mast cells. It does nothing to an existing clot, but reduces the ability to clot and prevents formation of another clot. Heparin is the only anticoagulant that can be used in pregnancy because it does not cross the placenta. Heparin should be used with caution, since hemorrhaging may easily occur. Some common side effects are bleeding from gums and unexplained bruising. Heparin can be given only IV or SC, but never IM because IM injection will cause a hematoma. Heparin dosage should be titrated according to PTT results. Heparin flushes are dilute solutions used to keep IV lines open. Low-dose heparin is used for prophylaxis of DVT or pulmonary embolism (PE) in postoperative patients, bedridden patients, obese patients, multiple bone fractures, hip prothesis insertion, MI, and gynecologic or abdominothoracic surgery (for surgery when limbs are not moving to assist blood flow).

Refludan (lepirudin) is an alternative anticoagulant for patients who cannot tolerate heparin. This agent is a direct inhibitor of thrombin. As with all anticoagulants, excessive bleeding is the most important side effect. A concentration of 5 mg/mL is used for IV bolus, whereas solutions of 0.2 mg/mL or 0.4 mg/mL are recommended for continuous infusion.

Table 13.11   Most-Commonly Used Anticoagulant Agents

Generic Name	Brand Name	Dosage Form
heparin		IV, SC
lepirudin	Refludan	IV
warfarin	Coumadin, Dicumarol	tablet
Low Molecular Weight Heparins		
dalteperin	Fragmin	SC
enoxaparin	Lovenox	SC
tinzaparin	Innohep	SC

Coumadin and **Dicumarol (warfarin)** work on the liver to prevent production of vitamin K-dependent clotting factors. It takes three to four days to achieve the effect. It is a vitamin K antagonist and inhibits vitamin K-dependent clotting factors II, VII, IX, and X. The objective is to prevent future clots. Like heparin, it has no effect on existing clots, but it can prevent clot formation, extension of formed clots, and secondary complications of thrombosis. It is rapidly and completely absorbed from the GI tract. Minor hemorrhage is not an indication to stop warfarin therapy. Concomitant use with NSAIDs or aspirin increases the risk of bleeding due to impaired platelet function. The first home monitor for "clotting time" has been approved. It is called CoaguChek.

Protamine sulfate is the antidote for heparin. 1 mg neutralizes 90 to 120 units of heparin or 1 mg per 100 units of heparin.

Mephyton (phytonadione, vitamin K) is an antagonist to warfarin. Charts are available to indicate the amount to administer based on the PTT. In severe hemorrhage, fresh whole blood is given, which contains the clotting factors necessary to stop blood loss.

Low molecular weight heparins present less likelihood of bleeding. They are generally administered twelve hours after surgery. There is no protein-binding problem as with regular heparin. The advantages to these heparins are

- reduced bleeding
- reliable dose response
- longer plasma half-life
- no effects on platelets

Lovenox (enoxaparin) is used to prevent DVT after orthopedic surgery. It is administered SC. It does not bind to heparin-binding proteins, and the half-life is two to four times that of heparin. It is about half the molecular weight of heparin. At the recommended dose, single injections do not significantly influence platelet aggregation or affect global clotting time. Platelet counts and the possibility of occult blood should be monitored, but it is not necessary to monitor PT or PTT. Side effects are hemorrhage and thrombocytopenia.

Fragmin (dalteparin) is used to prevent DVT, which may lead to pulmonary embolism (PE), in patients undergoing abdominal surgery who are at risk for thromboembolism complications. This group includes those over forty years of age, the obese, patients with malignancy, those with a history of DVT or PE, and those undergoing surgical procedures requiring general anesthesia and lasting longer than thirty minutes.

Innohep (tinzaparin) uses a portion of the larger heparin molecule. Innohep should not be interchanged with the other low molecular weight heparins as these agents differ in dose, duration of action, as well as activity on various clotting factors. Innohep is given once daily.

Antiplatelet Agents

Table 13.12 presents the most-commonly used antiplatelet agents.

GLYCOPROTEIN ANTAGONISTS Glycoprotein antagonists bind to receptors on platelets preventing platelet aggregation as well as the binding of fibrinogen and other adhesive molecules. The action of these antagonists is reversible. Glycoprotein antagonists are indicated for acute coronary syndrome and are administered during invasive procedures to prevent artery closure.

Table 13.12 Most-Commonly Used Antiplatelet Agents

Generic Name	Brand Name	Dosage Form
Glycoprotein Antagonists		
abciximab	ReoPro	IV
eptifibatide	Integrilin	IV
tirofiban	Aggrastat	IV
Fibrinolytic Agents		
alteplase	Activase	IV, vial
anistreplase	Eminase	IV
reteplase	Retavase	IV
streptokinase	Streptase	IV
urokinase	Abbokinase	IV

ReoPro (abciximab) is a monoclonal antibody to reduce acute cardiac complications in angioplasty patients at high risk for abrupt artery closure. The most common adverse effects are bleeding and thrombocytopenia. It is coadministered with aspirin postangioplasty and heparin infused and weight-adjusted to maintain a therapeutic bleeding time.

Aggrastat (tirofiban) and **Integrelin (eptifibatide)** mimic native protein sequences in the platelet receptors. These agents are used in conjunction with heparin and aspirin. The primary side effects associated with these antagonists are bleeding and thrombocytopenia (a decrease in blood platelet levels). Both agents must be protected from light.

FIBRINOLYTIC AGENTS Fibrinolytic agents dissolve clots. They are used for massive PE and MI.

Streptase (streptokinase) is used as an IV injection only. It is prepared from type C beta-hemolytic streptococci. It may stimulate antibody production. Clinical uses include PE, MI, and hemorrhagic complications with clot stabilizers. It may cause mild increase in temperature, may alter platelet function, and should not be given if the patient is taking antiplatelet drugs.

Abbokinase (urokinase) is an IV-only thrombolytic agent. It is an enzyme obtained from a cultural fraction of fetal kidney cells which have been selected for their ability to break down fibrin clots. The clinical use is for PE and MI.

Activase (alteplase) is a tissue plasminogen activator (TPA) that dissolves clots as well as streptokinase. It is a recombinant technology product. The side effects include bleeding, arrhythmias associated with reperfusion, allergy, nausea, vomiting, hypotension, and fever. Alteplase is most effective when administered within the first three hours post stroke or MI.

Eminase (anistreplase) is an inactive plasminogen-streptokinase complex activated in the bloodstream. It is used to dissolve coronary artery clots. Side effects include arrhythmias, hypotension, allergy, and viral transmission. It is contraindicated in patients who have undergone surgery or biopsy within the last ten days and in those with a history of stroke or severe hypertension (could cause bleeding through surgical wounds or in stroke could bleed into the head). It can reduce heart damage if given in the first three hours after onset of symptoms of MI.

Retavase (reteplase) binds to fibrin in a thrombus (clot) and thereby converts entrapped plasminogen to plasmin and dissolves the clots. The drug must be refrigerated and must remain sealed to protect it from light. No other medication should be added to the IV solution line. Bleeding is the most pronounced side effect.

STROKE

Under normal circumstances, the brain is one of the most oxygen-enriched organs in the human body. If cerebral circulation is abruptly stopped, the brain exhausts its supply of oxygen in about ten seconds. Loss of consciousness quickly follows. The death of brain tissue is particularly tragic because the brain is incapable of cell regeneration.

Stroke is the result of an event that interrupts the oxygen supply to a localized area of the brain; a stroke by definition implies hypoxic insult. A stroke may be caused by one of two primary events: cerebral infarction (by far the most common) or cerebral hemorrhage.

Stroke can be seen as a finite event, an ongoing event, or a series of protracted occurrences. A stroke may evolve over several months, over days, or over hours. A transient ischemic attack (TIA) refers to an attack of temporary neurologic changes that an individual may experience during a time period. TIAs may be important warning signs and predictors of imminent stroke. Reversible ischemic neurologic deficits (RINDs) are events that reverse spontaneously but less rapidly than a TIA. RINDs last more than twenty-four hours and resolve in less than twenty-one days. In most cases, however, RINDs resolve within a matter of days, rather than weeks.

Causes of a Stroke

The risk factors for stroke are advanced age (risk doubles every ten years after age fifty-five), male gender (24% higher risk than in females), hypertension, smoking, alcohol abuse, diabetes, and high cholesterol levels. Coronary artery disease appears to be the major cause of death among stroke survivors. Among the other important factors to the risk of a stroke are left ventricular hypertrophy and CHF.

A newly formed thrombus may remain lodged at its site of origin in a cerebral blood vessel. As the lumen of the vessel narrows and becomes obstructed, blood flow through the vessel slows, diminishes, and in some cases, even ceases. Cerebral ischemia is the result of reduced blood supply to the brain, and infarction with tissue necrosis may follow.

Emboli that move from one cerebral vessel to another are known as artery-to-artery emboli. Both cardiogenic and artery-to-artery emboli can ultimately lodge in distal vessels, causing TIAs or infarction. Regardless of the source of the ischemia, the diminished blood flow results in less oxygen reaching the cerebral tissues.

Several factors in a person's history are highly significant in the pathogenesis of cardiogenic embolic cardiovascular accidents (CVAs). First is the history of nonrheumatic atrial fibrillations. Very rapid contractions of cardiac muscle lead to incomplete emptying of the atria. The blood that remains pooled in the atria has a propensity to clot. A portion of the clot may leave the heart and move into the vessels of the head and neck. Other factors that may predispose to the occurrence of a CVA include rheumatic heart disease, acute MI, prosthetic heart valves, and left ventricular thrombi.

Several other causes are responsible for 5% of ischemic strokes. Among them are oral contraceptive use by smokers, substance abuse, migraine headaches, and various cellular anomalies.

Types of Stroke

Ischemia and intracranial hemorrhage differ significantly. Ischemia is the result of obstruction to flow; hemorrhage involves primary rupture of a blood vessel.

Hemorrhagic stroke may be marked by the sudden onset of severe headache, stiff neck, stupor, or a combination of these. Its effects are likely to be long lasting and irreversible. Intracerebral hemorrhage is most likely due to hypertension, cerebral amyloid angiopathy, or arteriovenous malformation. Hypertensive hemorrhage and saccular ("berry") aneurysms occur in separate parts of the brain with such predictability that the location itself is helpful in differential diagnosis of the stroke. They are usually found in the thalamus, pons, cerebellum, or putamen. Saccular aneurysms are thin-walled dilations that protrude off one of the arteries or proximate branches. When one of these weakened sacs ruptures, blood flows into the subarachnoid space. They carry a high risk of death.

Stroke Prevention and Management

In managing stroke, emphasis is on prevention. Some patient risk factors can be modified; some cannot (Table 13.13).

The six major options in stroke management are antiplatelet therapy, anticoagulant therapy, fibrinolytic intervention, cerebrovascular surgery, nonpharmacologic therapy, and post-stroke management. Pharmacologic treatment options for TIAs and prevention of initial strokes include antiplatelet and anticoagulant agents. Pharmacologic treatment for prevention of recurrent stroke may include antiplatelet and anticoagulant agents (Table 3.14).

ANTIPLATELET AND ANTICOAGULANT AGENTS Antiplatelet agents prevent platelet activation and formation of the platelet plug in one of two primary ways. They may interfere with the platelet aggregation induced by adenosine diphosphate (ADP), or they

Table 13.13   Stroke Risk Factors

Modifiable	Not Modifiable
cigarette smoking	age
coronary artery disease	gender
diabetes	genetic predisposition
excessive alcohol intake	prior stroke
hyperlipidemia	race
hypertension	
obesity	
physical inactivity	

Table 13.14   Most-Commonly Used Agents for TIAs and Stroke Prevention

Generic Name	Brand Name	Dosage Form
aspirin		tablet
aspirin-dipyridamole	Aggrenox	capsule
clopidogrel	Plavix	capsule
dipyridamole	Persantine	tablet
pentoxifylline	Trental	tablet
sulfinpyrazone	Anturane	tablet, capsule
ticlopidine	Ticlid	tablet

may interfere with the synthesis of thromboxane. Chemical compounds that interfere with thromboxane formation are aspirin, Anturane (sulfinpyrazone), and Persantine (dipyridamole). Ticlid (ticlopidine) and Plavix (clopidogrel) are chemical compounds that inhibit platelet aggregation through interference with ADP-induced platelet activity. Anticoagulant agents interfere with the synthesis or activation of the blood's coagulation factors.

Antiplatelet agents are most often used to prevent initial and recurrent thrombotic stroke. Anticoagulant agents are used for deep-vein thromboses and pulmonary emboli, as well as in preventing and treating cardiogenic stroke.

Determining the cause of a stroke is critical. To treat hemorrhage with anticoagulant agents or fibrinolytic agents would be detrimental. Treatment goals should confirm the diagnosis, evaluate the cause, stabilize the event, and then establish a plan to prevent further loss to the brain.

ANTICOAGULANT AND FIBRINOLYTIC AGENTS Treatment options for acute thrombotic stroke include anticoagulant agents and fibrinolytic agents. Formed clots have the potential to continue to expand and cause greater neurologic damage; anticoagulant agents may prevent existing clots from expanding. In some settings, fibrinolytic agents have been used to dissolve formed thrombi and emboli found in other circulations. Anticoagulant agents have been routinely used to treat acute cardiogenic stroke.

Fibrinolytic agents, also known as thrombolytic agents, differ from anticoagulant agents in one important aspect. Whereas anticoagulant agents can help prevent existing emboli and thrombi from expanding, fibrinolytic agents actually dissolve existing emboli and thrombi.

Primarily, indications for fibrinolytic therapy include

- DVT (deep vein thrombosis)
- acute peripheral occlusion
- acute MI with embolization
- PE (pulmonary embolism)
- coronary embolus

The major fibrinolytic agents include tissue plasminogen activator (TPA), urokinase, and streptokinase.

Dissolution of the emboli and thrombi would appear to be clearly preferable to simple containment. However, adoption of fibrinolytic agents as the pharmaceutical therapy of choice has been slow, even though clinical trials have demonstrated the efficacy of fibrinolytics in dissolution of arterial and venous thrombosis.

SIDE EFFECTS AND DISPENSING ISSUES FOR TIA AND STROKE PREVENTION AGENTS **Ticlid (ticlopidine)** is indicated to reduce the risk of thoracic stroke (fatal or nonfatal) in patients who have experienced stroke precursors and those who have had a completed thrombotic stroke. Because a risk of neutropenia and/or agranulocytosis has been associated with Ticlid, the drug should be reserved for cases in which aspirin cannot be used because the patient cannot tolerate it. Ticlid therapy may begin as soon as the diagnosis of TIA or thrombotic stroke has been made and cerebral hemorrhage has been ruled out. It may be used indefinitely. Adverse effects may include neutropenia and thrombocytopenia, diarrhea, nausea, and rash. The established protocol includes routine monitoring of CBC and white cell differentials during the first three months of therapy. After that, CBCs need to be obtained only when signs or symptoms suggest infection.

Plavix (clopidogrel) is chemically related to Ticlid. By blocking the ADP receptors, this drug prevents fibrinogen binding at that site and thus reduces platelet adhesion and aggregation. Plavix is approved to prevent the recurrence of atherosclerotic events such as MI and stroke. The major side effect of this drug is bleeding. Consequently, it should be discontinued seven days before surgery. Platelet transfusion may be appropriate if rapid reversal of the pharmacological effects of the drug is warranted. Plavix can be taken without regard to food.

Aspirin interferes with the enzyme cyclooxygenase and thereby disrupts production of thromboxane, prostacyclin, and prostaglandin. There are many side effects, especially GI symptoms. A patient with a history of peptic ulceration or other bleeding disorder should not take aspirin. The labeled use of aspirin for stroke is only for reduction of recurrent TIAs or stroke in patients who have had transient ischemia of the brain due to fibrin platelet emboli.

Anturane (sulfinpyrazone) inhibits ADP and 5-HT, resulting in decreased platelet adhesiveness and increased platelet survival time. Renal function and CBCs should be monitored routinely. The drug is taken with food; adequate hydration and high fluid intake are needed to prevent formation of uric acid kidney stones. Alcohol should be avoided. The drug should not be given to patients with peptic ulcer disease or those taking diabetic medication, diuretics, nitrofurantoin, or cholestyramine. Nausea and vomiting are primary side effects.

Persantine (dipyridamole) inhibits platelet aggregation and may cause vasodilation. It maintains patency after surgical grafting procedures, including coronary artery bypass. It is used with warfarin to prevent other thromboembolic disorders. The primary side effect is dizziness. The technician should notify the physician or pharmacist if the patient is taking other medications that affect bleeding, such as NSAIDs or warfarin.

Trental (pentoxifylline) improves capillary blood flow by increasing erythrocyte flexibility and reducing blood viscosity. Tablets are time-released, so it is important that the patient swallow them whole. They should be taken with food. Dizziness, headache, nausea, and vomiting are the primary side effects.

Aggrenox (aspirin-dipyridamole) is approved to help prevent the recurrence of stroke or TIA. Each dose contains 25 mg of aspirin and 200 mg of extended-release dipyridamole and is taken twice daily. The daily dose falls short of the 75 mg of aspirin that is recommended to prevent heart attacks.

HYPERLIPIDEMIA

Cholesterol is essential for good health. It circulates continuously in the blood for use by all body cells. The liver is responsible for making new cholesterol when needed and for processing cholesterol from food. This process is summarized in the following steps.

1. The liver puts together packages containing triglycerides, cholesterol, and carrier proteins called lipoproteins and sends them out into the bloodstream.
2. The fat is drawn off for energy or storage. The low-density lipoproteins (LDLs) that are left continue circulating to bring needed cholesterol to the body's cells.
3. LDLs not used by the cells may be deposited in artery walls, restricting blood flow; if arteries are clogged, a heart attack occurs.

High-density lipoprotein (HDL) may prevent cholesterol buildup in arteries by removing already formed deposits and delivering them to the liver for processing.

Hyperlipidemia is a condition in which there is an elevation in one or more of the lipoprotein levels. Lipoproteins are spherical particles that contain a core of triglycerides and cholesterol, in varying proportions, surrounded by a surface coat of phospholipids so they can remain in solution. Total cholesterol increases throughout life in men and women. It enhances other risk factors for coronary artery disease. Evidence collected over the last three decades has linked elevated low-density lipoprotein (LDL) and reduced high-density lipoprotein (HDL) to the development of coronary artery disease. Premature atherosclerosis is the most common and signifi-cant consequence of hyperlipidemia. These disorders are genetically determined, but may be secondary to diabetes, obesity, alcoholism, hypothyroidism, liver disease, or kidney disease. Figure 13.7 illustrates normal and clogged arteries.

There are four classes of soluble lipoproteins (lipids bound to proteins).

1. Chylomicrons are very large lipoproteins. They are 90% triglycerides and 5% cholesterol. They are absorbed into the lymphatic system from the GI tract and show up in blood eight to twelve hours after a meal.
2. Very-low-density lipoproteins (VLDLs) are 60% triglycerides and 12% choles-terol. Fatty acids are produced in the liver, transported as triglycerides by VLDL, and deposited in adipose tissues. Fatty acids are used by muscle and other cells as fuel. Remnants of VLDL are transformed into cholesterol-rich LDL.
3. Low-density lipoproteins (LDLs) are 6% triglycerides and 65% cholesterol. LDLs are the major carrier of cholesterol. Cholesterol is an odorless, white, waxlike, powdery substance present in all foods of animal origin, but absent in foods of

Figure 13.7

Cross Section of Arteries
(a) Normal Artery
(b) Clogged Artery

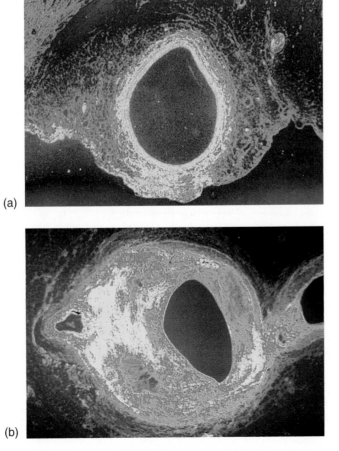

(a)

(b)

plant origin. LDLs bind to receptors and are taken into the cells. Receptors are synthesized as the cell needs cholesterol, which is used by lymphocytes, adrenal cortical cells, muscle, and renal cells to make cell membranes and steroid hormones and used by the liver to make bile acids. Atherosclerosis is a narrowing of the arteries due to deposits of cholesterol and fat in the inner surface lining of the vessel, resulting in stroke, MI, or limbs lost to gangrene.

4. High-density lipoproteins (HDLs) are 5% triglycerides, 25% cholesterol, and 50% protein. They remove cholesterol from cells to be transported back to the liver for reprocessing or removal and inhibit cellular uptake of LDLs. High HDL levels lower the incidence of atherosclerosis with related heart and stroke problems.

Food fats contain a mixture of three fatty acids: saturated, monounsaturated, and polyunsaturated. Saturated fat raises blood cholesterol levels more than anything else in the diet. Most patients can achieve an average cholesterol reduction of ten to fifteen percent through diet. The major dietary recommendation is to reduce the amount of total and saturated fats in the diet. The total intake should not exceed thirty percent of total calories.

Evidence now shows that lowering the blood lipid concentrations in a patient with atherosclerosis halts the process. Physicians recommend treatment for patients with hyperlipidemia because they are at increased risk and because the increased plasma lipid levels can be reduced somewhat by therapy with diet, drugs, or both.

The treatment goals for cholesterol and LDL levels are as follows.

- ◇ blood cholesterol levels per 100 mL of blood
   - 240 mg, at risk
   - less than 200 mg, desirable
   - 135 mg, more desirable
- ◇ blood LDL levels per 100 mL of blood
   - 160 mg, high risk
   - 139–159 mg, borderline risk
   - less than 139 mg, desirable

Hyperlipidemic Agents

Cholesterol-lowering drugs are always used as an adjunct to proper diet control. Table 13.15 presents the most-commonly used hyperlipidemic agents. Drugs from different classifications are often prescribed together because they are synergistic (e.g., the bile acids and niacin, Mevacor and niacin, and Mevacor and Questran). However, interactions between these and other drugs can cause serious muscle problems. Any symptom of myalgia (muscle pain) should be reported to the physician immediately.

Some drugs increase cholesterol; obviously patients with hyperlipidemia should avoid them. As in other situations, the advantages must be weighed against the disadvantages. For example, birth control pills increase cholesterol levels. Estrogens increase HDL, and progestins decrease HDL. Depending on the combination in the birth control product, lipid profiles could increase unfavorably. Estrogen given alone would have a favorable effect on the profile. Thiazide diuretics, loop diuretics, and glucocorticoids all increase the lipid profile unfavorably. Prazosin, clonidine, and calcium channel blockers increase HDL, so they would be good choices for someone with hyperlipidemia. If a patient is taking a cholesterol-lowering drug, the technician should always check the profile for other drugs with adverse interactions.

HMG-CoA Reductase Inhibitors HMG-CoA reductase inhibitors inhibit the enzyme that catalyzes the rate-limiting step in cholesterol biosynthesis. The side effects

Table 13.15   Most-Commonly Used Hyperlipidemic Agents

Generic Name	Brand Name	Dosage Form
HMG-CoA Reductase Inhibitors		
atorvastatin	Lipitor	tablet
fluvastatin	Lescol	capsule
lovastatin	Mevacor	tablet
pravastatin	Pravachol	tablet
simvastatin	Zocor	tablet
Fibric Acid Derivatives		
clofibrate	Atromid-S	capsule
fenofibrate	TriCor	capsule
gemfibrozil	Lopid	tablet, capsule
Bile Acid Sequestrants		
cholestyramine	Questran	suspension, powder
colestipol	Colestid	tablet, granule
Other Cholesterol-Lowering Agents		
niacin	Nicobid, Nicolar	capsule, elixir, tablet, IM, IV, SC
psyllium	Metamucil, Fiberall	powder, wafer

include GI upset and headache, which may dissipate with time. Any unexplained muscle pain or weakness, especially with fever, should be reported to the physician immediately. Liver enzymes should also be monitored regularly.

Zocor (simvastatin) acts on the enzyme that catalyzes the rate-limiting step in cholesterol biosynthesis. It should be taken with meals and patients should report any muslce pain that is accompanied by fever. Zocor should be stored in well-sealed containers.

Lipitor (atorvastatin) is a potent lipid-lowering drug. It lowers LDL significantly. It also lowers triglycerides. Until now, physicians had to resort to niacin or gemfibrozil to reduce triglyceride levels.

When required, a prescriber may switch a patient from one statin to another. The estimated equivalencies between the HMG-CoA reductase inhibitors are Zocor 10 mg, Mevacor 20 mg, Pravachol 20 mg, Lescol 40 mg, and Lipitor 5 mg. Patients should be monitored after a switch and doses adjusted as needed.

The dietary supplement Cholestin claims to lower cholesterol. It contains lovastatin, an HMG-CoA reductase inhibitor. It lowers total cholesterol by twenty-five to forty points. The manufacturer cannot claim that it treats heart disease. It is marketed as a food supplement.

FIBRIC ACID DERIVATIVES The exact mechanism of action for fibric acid derivatives is unknown.

TriCor (fenofibrate) increases the catabolism (breakdown) of VLDLs by enhancing the synthesis of lipoprotein lipase. This drug is indicated as adjunctive therapy to dietary modification. As with the statins, TriCor may be associated with muscle pain. Dosages of oral anticoagulant being taken concurrently should be decreased accordingly. If, after six to eight weeks of therapy, only marginal changes in total serum cholesterol and triglyceride concentrations can be observed, TriCor should be discontinued. The primary side effects of TriCor are mild GI disturbances such as gas, diarrhea, or constipation. It should be taken with food.

Atromid-S (clofibrate) inhibits triglyceride synthesis in the liver and inhibits the breakdown of triglycerides in fat tissue. Adverse effects are headache, nausea, diarrhea, skin rash, and alteration of liver and kidney function.

Lopid (gemfibrozil) lowers triglyceride and VLDL levels while increasing HDL levels by reducing liver triglyceride production. Adverse effects are GI symptoms (abdominal pain, diarrhea, nausea, vomiting), CNS symptoms (vertigo, headache), alteration in taste, and skin rash.

BILE ACID SEQUESTRANTS Bile acid sequestrants form a nonabsorbable complex with bile acids in the intestine. If a second medication is being used, it should be taken one hour before or four to six hours after the bile acid sequestrant. Constipation is the primary side effect.

Questran (cholestyramine) stays in the intestines and combines with bile salts by combining with cholesterol and other fats that are then removed in the feces. Adverse effects are nausea and vomiting due to the large doses required and pooling in the GI tract. Other effects are GI disturbances and binding to medication and fat-soluble vitamins (A, D, E, K). For this reason, vitamin supplementation may be necessary.

Colestid (colestipol) binds with bile acids to form an insoluble complex eliminated in the feces, thereby increasing fecal loss of LDL. This drug should be taken with water or fruit juice or sprinkled on food. After taking the granular form, the patient should rinse the glass with a full amount of liquid and drink the contents to ensure that the full dose is taken. Other drugs should be taken at least one hour before or four hours after. Side effects are primarily gastrointestinal, including constipation.

OTHER CHOLESTEROL-LOWERING AGENTS **Nicobid** and **Nicolar (niacin)** are vitamin B_3 and inhibit synthesis of VLDL by the liver and lower triglyceride and LDL cholesterol levels. This drug induces a strange phenomenon of extreme skin flushing when first taken. This is avoidable with aspirin prophylaxis thirty minutes before taking the drug, by taking with food, and by increasing the dose very slowly. Other side effects are nausea, vomiting, diarrhea, and an increase in uric acid levels, which can produce symptoms of gout.

Metamucil and **Fiberall (psyllium)** lower cholesterol when used daily. They have the same effect as a high-fiber diet.

Chapter Summary

The Causes of Heart Disease

- ◇ The heart is a complicated organ. Many things can go wrong.
- ◇ Proper diet, exercise, and rest can do a lot to keep the heart functioning for a long time.

Antiarrhythmics

- ◇ The various classes of antiarrhythmic drugs have characteristic electrophysiologic effects on the myocardium.
- ◇ Dilantin (phenytoin) is an antiarrhythmic drug that is also used to control seizures.
- ◇ Betapace (sotalol) is a beta blocker.
- ◇ Lanoxin (digoxin) is an important drug in managing atrial flutter, fibrillation, and congestive heart failure.
- ◇ Bradycardia exists when the heart rate is below sixty beats per minute.
- ◇ Isopto Atropine (atropine) is used for heart rates less than sixty beats per minute. It is also used preoperatively to inhibit salivation and secretions.

Drugs for Congestive Heart Failure (CHF)

- ◇ CHF is treated with combinations of diuretics, digoxin, and ACE inhibitors. Beta blockers and calcium channel blockers should not be used.
- ◇ "Dig toxicity" is common in patients taking digitalis, especially the elderly. They may see yellow-green halos around objects. The three primary signs are nausea, vomiting, and arrhythmias.
- ◇ CHF is especially responsive to ACE inhibitors. ACE inhibitors are potassium-preserving, so it is very easy for the patient to become hyperkalemic if other potassium-sparing drugs or potassium supplements are taken.

Myocardial Infarction (MI)

- ◇ MI is the leading cause of death in industrialized nations.
- ◇ MIs occur when there is a prolonged decrease in oxygen delivery to a region of cardiac muscle.
- ◇ Symptoms are described as oppressive or burning tightness or squeezing in the chest, choking and indigestion-like expansion, a sense of "impending doom," and substernal pain, which may radiate to the neck, throat, jaw, shoulders, and one or both arms.
- ◇ Beta blockers are prescribed for reducing the risk of death or recurrence following an MI.

Angina Pectoris

- ◇ Angina pectoris is an imbalance between oxygen supply and oxygen demand. The three types are: stable, unstable, and variant.
- ◇ Nitrates are the drugs most used for angina; they dilate coronary vessels leading to redistribution of blood flow to ischemic tissues. They reduce preload on the heart, which reduces cardiac workload.

- A transdermal nitroglycerin patch should be removed at night to avoid development of tolerance of the drug. The label should instruct the patient in this procedure.
- When patients begin using these drugs, it is common for them to experience a severe headache.
- Nitroglycerin should be sold and stored in an amber glass bottle.
- Nitroglycerin should be replaced at least every three months; the patient should discard any remaining drug.
- Covera HS is a timed-release verapamil designed for bedtime dosing. It is approved for either hypertension or angina. The tablets do not release until about four to five hours after they have been swallowed. The drug is pumped out of two laser holes in the tablet. Patients may see an empty shell of ghost tablet in their stool, as with Procardia.
- Beta blockers may mask symptoms of hypoglycemia; therefore, diabetics should avoid them.

Hypertension

- Hypertension is treated in stepwise fashion.
  Step 1. Change lifestyle.
  Step 2. Add a first-line drug.
  Step 3. Add a diuretic if not given in step 2.
  Step 4. Add a third drug that is synergistic with the others.
- High blood pressure should be treated with salt restriction, weight control, regular exercise, reduction of alcohol consumption, cessation of smoking, stress control, and medicine as prescribed.
- The first-line drug for hypertension can be a diuretic, a beta blocker, an ACE inhibitor, or a calcium channel blocker.
- Calcium channel blockers reduce blood pressure by arteriolar dilation, which leads to reduced peripheral resistance.
- ACE inhibitors reduce blood pressure by competitive inhibition of angiotensin-converting enzyme (ACE); they prevent the conversion of angiotensin I to angiotensin II, a potent vasoconstrictor.
- Beta blockers have many other unapproved uses, such as treating migraine headache and test anxiety.
- Coreg is the first beta blocker for CHF. It is a nonselective beta blocker with vasodilating effects. Physicians usually avoid beta blockers because they slow the heart and make CHF worse. However, studies indicate that they can improve left ventricular function by blocking excessive adrenergic stimulation. They are started with a very low dose, which is slowly increased. They should be taken with food to reduce dizziness.
- Aldomet (methyldopa) is the only drug approved to treat hypertension in pregnancy.
- Catapres (clonidine) is the only high blood pressure medication that has a transdermal delivery system.
- Loniten (minoxidil) reduces blood pressure and grows hair.
- ACE inhibitors and calcium channel blockers have additive effects to relax blood vessels and lower pressure. Also, two low doses of different drugs usually cause fewer side effects than pushing the dose of either drug. This is still second-line therapy.

Anticoagulants and Antiplatelets

- ◇ The therapy for preventing blood clots is low-dose heparin, adjusted-dose heparin, low molecular weight heparin, and Coumadin. The purpose is to prevent abnormal blood clotting without exposing the patient to complications from excessive bleeding.
- ◇ Anticoagulants prevent clot formation; antiplatelets dissolve clots once formed.
- ◇ PTT measures the function of the intrinsic and common pathways and is affected by heparin.
- ◇ Heparin inhibits thrombin formation. It prevents clot formation; it does not dissolve a clot already formed.
- ◇ Refludan (lepirudin) is an alternative anticoagulant for patients who cannot tolerate heparin.
- ◇ Protamine sulfate is the antidote for heparin.
- ◇ Mephyton (phytonadione, vitamin K) is an antidote for warfarin.
- ◇ Two low molecular weight heparins on the market are Lovenox and Fragmin. Lovenox is approved only for hip or knee surgery.
- ◇ These heparins are given twelve hours after surgery and have better bioavailability. The advantages are reduced bleeding, reliable dose response, longer plasma half-life, and no effects on platelets.
- ◇ The first home monitor for Coumadin was CoaguChek.
- ◇ Innohep (tinzaparin) cannot be interchanged with the other low molecular weight heparins.
- ◇ Aggrastat and Integrilin mimic native protein sequences in the platelet receptors. They are used in conjunction with heparin and aspirin.

Stroke

- ◇ A stroke may be caused by one of two primary events: cerebral hemorrhage and cerebral infarction.
- ◇ Risk factors for stroke are advanced age, male gender, hypertension, smoking, alcohol abuse, diabetes, and high cholesterol levels.
- ◇ A TIA is a very strong predictor of an impending stroke.
- ◇ "White" thrombi originate in the arteries; "red" thrombi are formed in slow-moving fluid environments.
- ◇ Emphasis should be on stroke prevention.

Hyperlipidemia

- ◇ Lipids occur in the blood in the form of fatty acids, triglycerides, lipoproteins, and cholesterol.
- ◇ Food fats contain a mixture of three fatty acids: saturated, monosaturated, and polysaturated.
- ◇ LDLs (low-density lipoproteins) can deposit in artery walls, restricting blood flow and clogging arteries so a heart attack occurs.
- ◇ HDLs (high-density lipoproteins) may prevent cholesterol buildup in arteries and may remove deposits already formed.
- ◇ Drugs are used as an adjunct to proper diet to prevent buildup of LDLs.
- ◇ When patients are taking these drugs, any symptoms of myalgia should be reported to the physician immediately. Some combinations of these drugs are synergistic; others can be dangerous.
- ◇ Thiazide diuretics, loop diuretics, and corticosteroids all increase cholesterol.

- Zocor (simvastatin) acts on the enzyme that catalyzes the rate-limiting step in cholesterol biosynthesis.
- Lipitor (atorvastatin) is a potent new lipid-lowering drug. It lowers LDLs significantly. It also lowers triglycerides. Until now, physicians had to resort to niacin or gemfibrozil to reduce triglyceride levels.
- Tricor (fenofibrate) increases the catabolism of LDLs.

Drug Summary

The following drugs were discussed in this chapter. Each generic drug name is followed in parentheses by one or more brand names. An asterisk (*) indicates drugs frequently written using *either* brand *or* generic name. These need to be memorized.

Antiarrhythmic Agents
amiodarone (Cordarone)
amrinone (Inocor)
atropine (Isopto)
bretylium (Bretylol)
digoxin (Lanoxin)*
disopyramide (Norpace)*
flecainide (Tambocor)
isoproterenol (Isuprel)
lidocaine (Xylocaine)*
mexiletene (Mexitil)*
moricizine (Ethmozine)
phenytoin (Dilantin)*
propafenone (Rythmol)
procainamide (Pronestyl, Procanbid)*
quinidine (Quinaglute, Cardioquin)*
tocainide (Tonocard)*

Beta Blockers
acebutolol (Sectral)
atenolol (Tenormin)*
betaxolol (Kerlone)
bisoprolol (Zebeta)
carvedilol (Coreg)
esmolol (Brevibloc)
labetalol (Normodyne, Trandate)
metoprolol (Lopressor, Toprol XL)*
nadolol (Corgard)*
pindolol (Visken)*
propranolol (Inderal, Betachron)*
sotalol (Betapace)

Calcium Channel Blockers
amlodipine (Norvasc)*
bepridil (Vascor)
diltiazem (Cardizem, Dilacor XR)*
felodipine (Plendil)
isradipine (DynaCirc)
nicardipine (Cardene)
nifedipine (Adalat, Procardia)*
nisoldipine (Sular)
verapamil (Calan, Isoptin, Verelan,
    Covera HS)*

ACE Inhibitors
benazepril (Lotensin)
captopril (Capoten)*
enalapril (Vasotec)*
fosinopril (Monopril)
lisinopril (Prinivil, Zestril)*
moexipril (Univasc)
perindopril (Aceon)
quinapril (Accupril)
ramipril (Altace)
trandolapril (Mavik)

Angiotensin II-Receptor Antagonists
candesartan (Atacand)
eprosartan (Tevetan)
irbesartan (Avapro)
losartan (Cozaar)*
telmisartan (Micardis)
valsartan (Diovan)

Centrally Acting
clonidine (Catapres)*
guanfacine (Tenex)
methyldopa (Aldomet)*

Alpha Blockers
doxazosin (Cardura)
guanethidine (Ismelin)
phentolamine (Regitine)
prazosin (Minipress)*
terazosin (Hytrin)*

Peripheral Vasodilators
diazoxide (Hyperstat)
hydralazine (Apresoline)*
minoxidil (Loniten)*

Vasodilators
fenoldopam (Corlopam)
isoproterenol (Isuprel)
isosorbide dinitrate (Isordil, Dilatrate-SR)
isosorbide mononitrate (Imdur, ISMO)
milrinone (Primacor)
nitroprusside (Nitropress)

nitroglycerin (Nitrostat, Nitro-Bid, Nitro-
    Bid IV, Nitro-Dur, Nitrodisc,
    Transderm Nitro, Minitran, Nitrol,
    Nitrostat IV, Tridil)*
nitroprusside (Nipride)

Combinations
enalapril-diltiazem (Teczem)
losartan-hydrochlorothiazide (Hyzaar)
trandolapril-verapamil (Tarka)

Low Molecular Weight Heparins
dalteparin (Fragmin)
enoxaparin (Lovenox)
tinzaparin (Innohep)

Antidote for Warfarin
phytonadione (vitamin K)

**Anticoagulants, Antiplatelets,
Fibrinolytic Agents**
alteplase (Activase)
anistreplase (Eminase)
aspirin
aspirin-dipyridamole (Aggrenox)
clopidogrel (Plavix)
dipyridamole (Persantine)*
heparin
lepirudin (Refludan)
pentoxifylline (Trental)*
reteplase (Retavase)
streptokinase (Streptase)
sulfinpyrazone (Anturane)
ticlopidine (Ticlid)*
urokinase (Abbokinase)
warfarin (Coumadin)*

Antidote for Heparin
protamine sulfate

Glycoprotein Antagonists
abciximab (ReoPro)
eptifibatide (Integrilin)
reteplase (Retavase)
tirofiban (Aggrastat)

Pulmonary Hypertension
epoprostenol (Flolan)

HMG-CoA Reductase Inhibitors
atorvastatin (Lipitor)*
fluvastatin (Lescol)
lovastatin (Mevacor)*
pravastatin (Pravachol)*
simvastatin (Zocor)*

Fibric Acid Derivatives
clofibrate (Atromid-S)
fenofibrate (TriCor)
gemfibrozil (Lopid)*

Bile Acid Sequestrants
cholestyramine (Questran)*
colestipol (Colestid)

**Miscellaneous Cholesterol-Lowering
Drugs**
niacin (Nicobid)*
psyllium (Metamucil, Fiberall,
    Cholestin)

Chapter Review

Pharmaceuticals and Body Functions

Select the best answer from the choices given.

1. Quinidine is more effective than procainamide for
    a. headaches.
    b. cinchonism.
    c. atrial arrhythmias.
    d. nausea and vomiting.

2. Which agent is often the first used for emergency therapy of arrhythmias?
    a. Lidocaine
    b. Mexitil
    c. Dilantin
    d. Tocainide

3. Which drug must be combined with another drug to be effective?
    a. Lidocaine
    b. Mexitil
    c. Dilantin
    d. Tocainide

4. Which drug is used on digitalis-induced arrhythmias?
    a. Lidocaine
    b. Mexitil
    c. Dilantin
    d. Tocainide

5. Which beta blocker is preferred for the heart?
    a. β_1
    b. β_2
    c. Nonselective
    d. All of the above

6. Which drug is used only for life-threatening arrhythmias?
    a. Cordarone
    b. Betapace
    c. Bretylol
    d. All of the above

7. Which drug class is preferred for most supraventricular tachyarrhythmias?
    a. Beta blockers
    b. Calcium channel blockers
    c. Membrane-stabilizing agents
    d. All of the above

8. The leading cause of death in industrialized nations is
   a. cancer.
   b. MI.
   c. stroke.
   d. a and b.

9. Which factor(s) increase risk of heart attack?
   a. Proper diet
   b. Appropriate rest
   c. Cigarette smoking
   d. All of the above

10. A beta blocker is given after an MI to
    a. speed heart action.
    b. reduce risk of death.
    c. prevent stroke.
    d. improve breathing.

The following statements are true or false. If the answer is false, rewrite the statement so it is true.

_____ 1. The drug of choice for acute angina attacks is Lanoxin.

_____ 2. A nitroglycerin patch should be left on twenty-four hours.

_____ 3. Blocadren is the only drug approved to treat high blood pressure in pregnancy.

_____ 4. Heparin inhibits thrombin formation and dissolves a clot after it has formed.

_____ 5. Nutrition guidelines indicate that the total intake of fat should not exceed sixty-five percent of the diet.

_____ 6. Intracranial hemorrhage differs significantly from ischemia. Ischemia is the result of obstruction to flow; hemorrhage involves primary rupture of a blood vessel.

_____ 7. Lidocaine is never used as an antiarrhythmic agent.

_____ 8. The advantages of low molecular weight heparins are reduced bleeding, reliable dose response, and longer plasma half-life.

_____ 9. Emboli can be of several types: fat, air, and accumulation of debris.

_____ 10. Captopril directly inhibits angiotensin II.

Place the correct letter in each blank.

a. ACE inhibitor   b. beta blocker   c. calcium channel blocker

1. Inderal _____
2. Adalat _____
3. Calan _____
4. DynaCirc _____
5. Betapace _____
6. captopril _____
7. Lotensin _____
8. Visken _____
9. Vasotec _____
10. Accupril _____

11. Toprol XL _____
12. Normodyne _____
13. Altace _____
14. acebutolol _____
15. propranolol _____
16. bepridil _____
17. lisinopril _____
18. quinapril _____
19. verapamil _____
20. metoprolol _____

Diseases and Drug Therapies

1. Identify four types of drugs used to treat arrhythmias. List two drugs per group.
2. Discuss the stepwise treatment of hypertension.
3. What is the difference between anticoagulants and antiplatelets? List the ones discussed and designate their class.
4. Classify the lipid-lowering drugs.

HMG-CoA Reductase	Fibric Acid Derivatives	Bile Acid Sequestrants	Miscellaneous

Dispensing Medications

1. Mr. Bob Day receives Lanoxin 0.25 mg po qd for atrial fibrillation.
   Prepare the label to dispense a thirty-day supply (six refills, Dr. J. Crews).

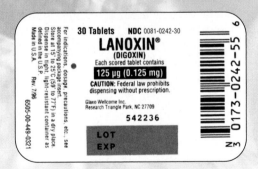

Sample: for educational use only.
Reproduced with permission of Glaxo Wellcome Inc.

2. The intern sent the following orders down:
   Mr. Brown, 50 mg Protamine stat.
   You check Mr. Brown's chart, and he received 3,000 units of heparin. What would be the correct dosage for the Protamine?

3. Mrs. Jones brings in the following prescription. Is this a good combination? Why or why not?

```
        MT. HOPE MEDICAL PARK
Rx      ST. PAUL, MN (651) 555-3591
        _____

                        DEA#_____
Pt. name  Bill Jones        Date  Aug. 5, 05
Address _____

        Mevacor 20 mg with
                evening meal #30

        Questran 4 g bid #60


_____ Dispense as written

_____ Fills_____times (no refill unless indicated)
_____  J.Cruns  _____ M.D.
```

Internet Research

Use the Internet to complete the following assignments.

1. Locate statistics on heart disease. What is the yearly incidence of myocardial infarction in the United States? How many individuals are currently living with congestive heart failure? Coronary artery disease? Make sure to include the date associated with your data source(s). List your Internet sources.
2. Research common cardiovascular procedures. Create a table explaining three common procedures. Your table should include a brief description of the procedure and identify the condition(s) the procedure is intended to treat.

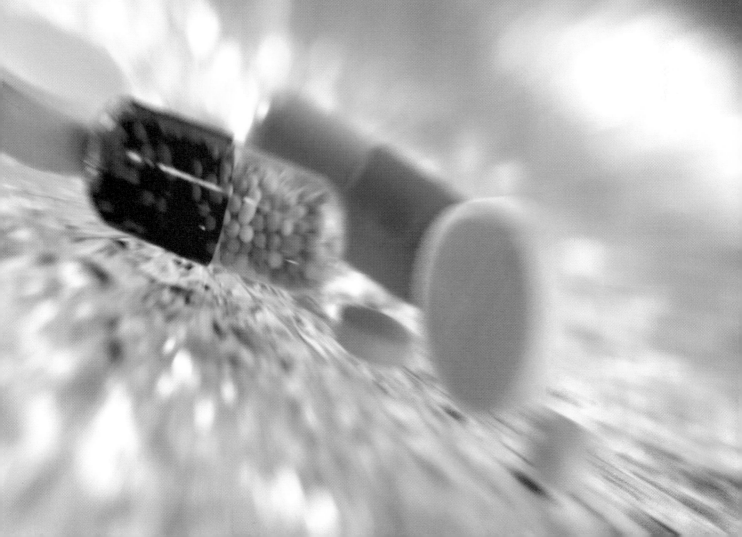

Nonnarcotic Analgesics, Muscle Relaxants, Hormones, and Topicals

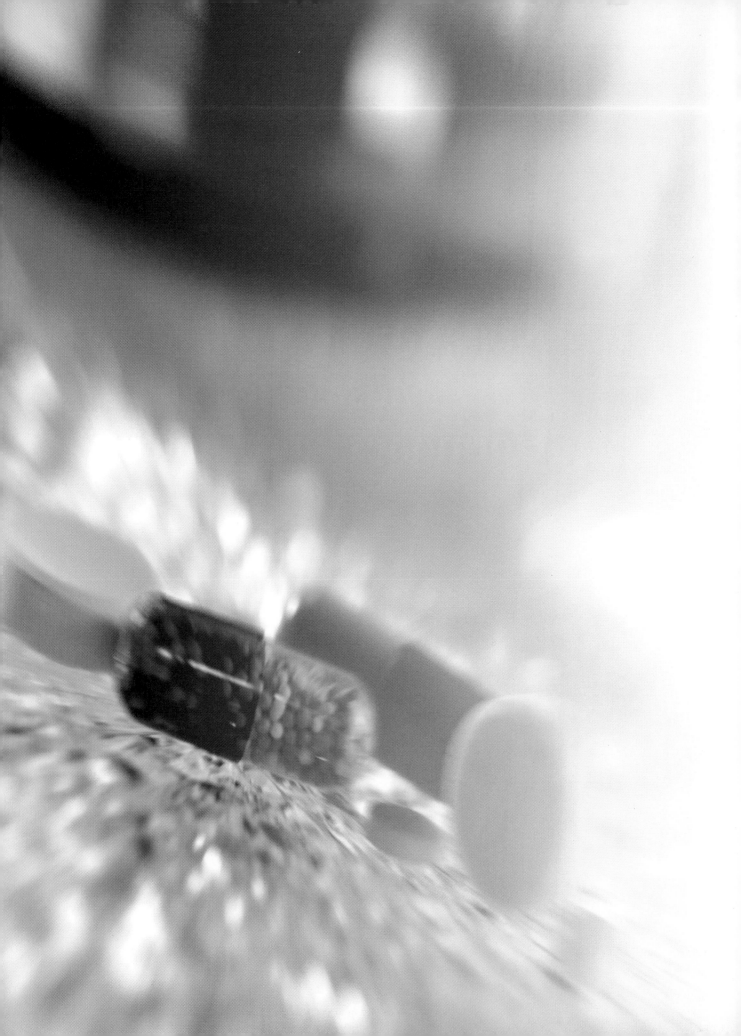

Muscle Relaxants, Nonnarcotic Analgesics, and Drugs for Arthritis

Learning Objectives

⬦ Define muscle relaxants.

⬦ Identify muscle relaxants and their various mechanisms of action.

⬦ Identify the nonnarcotic analgesics, and describe their uses and mechanisms of action.

⬦ Define rheumatoid arthritis and gout.

⬦ Identify agents used to treat arthritis, rheumatoid arthritis, and gout; their usage; and side effects.

Muscle relaxants are used to reduce spasticity in multiple sclerosis, cerebral palsy, skeletal muscle injuries, orthopedic surgery, postoperative recovery, and spinal cord injury. Other serious problems can involve the muscles and joints and are treated with nonsteroidal anti-inflammatory drugs (NSAIDs). Aspirin, acetaminophen, and ibuprofen do not require prescriptions. Other NSAIDs are achieving OTC status and are being added to that list. This means that more drugs will be used to self-medicate. The pharmacy technician must be aware of the side effects and proper use of these drugs.

MUSCLE RELAXANTS

Skeletal muscles are voluntarily controlled by impulses originating in the central nervous system (CNS). Impulses are conducted through the spinal cord in somatic neurons that eventually synapse with the muscle in a neuromuscular junction. The neurotransmitter acetylcholine (ACh) is released to combine with ACh receptors on the muscle cell membrane. When an adequate number of ACh receptors are bound, the cell then experiences sodium ion influx, causing an impulse to travel over the cell and into the T tubules, releasing calcium, which causes a contraction. Relaxation occurs when ACh is broken down by acetylcholinesterase. The anatomy of a muscle was illustrated in Chapter 9.

Types of skeletal muscle contraction are

⬦ voluntary (movement)
⬦ involuntary (tone; posture)

Ways to block normal muscle function are to

⬦ block release of ACh (to date no agent can do this)
⬦ prevent destruction of ACh (continuous depolarization leads to paralysis by fatigue)
⬦ prevent ACh from reaching receptors (competitive nondepolarizing inhibitors)

Agents that continuously bind to ACh receptors (depolarizing agents, paralysis by fatigue) can also block normal muscle function.

Table 14.1 presents the most-commonly used muscle relaxants.

It is always important for the prescriber to get a drug history from the patient before any of these drugs are administered in order to avoid possible drug interactions. The pharmacy technician will often obtain this history as well.

Centrally acting muscle relaxants do not directly relax muscles. Instead, they depress the CNS which reduces the anxiety that increases muscle tone. Sedative properties cause the patient to relax, which in turn reduces reflex impulse conduction. Side effects of the muscle relaxants are sedation, reduced mental alertness, reduced motor abilities, and GI upset. Patients taking these drugs should avoid alcohol.

Dantrium (dantrolene) reduces calcium release from sacs of T tubules, which reduces muscle responsiveness to stimulation with reduced force of contraction. It is used in treating spasticity related to spinal cord injuries, stroke, cerebral palsy, and multiple sclerosis. The side effects are malaise, weakness, fatigue, possible liver toxicity, and photosensitivity. Alcohol and other CNS depressants should be avoided. The drug acts on skeletal muscle beyond the neuromuscular junctions. It is given before surgery to patients susceptible to malignant hyperthermia. The use of dantrolene in the treatment of malignant hyperthermia was covered in greater detail in Chapter 7.

Valium (diazepam) is a benzodiazepine. Some authorities consider it to be the best muscle relaxer. It should not be discontinued abruptly after prolonged use. The addictive qualities of this drug restrict its use.

Robaxin (methocarbamol) is used to treat muscle spasms associated with acute painful musculoskeletal conditions and as supportive therapy in tetanus. It causes skeletal muscle relaxation by reducing the transmission of impulses from the spinal cord to skeletal muscles. It may cause drowsiness or impair judgment or coordination. Patients should avoid alcohol or other CNS depressants and notify the physician of rash, itching, or nasal congestion. The drug may turn urine brown, black, or green.

Norflex (orphenadrine) is indicated to treat muscle spasms and to provide supportive therapy in tetanus. It is an indirect skeletal muscle relaxant thought to work by central atropine-like effects; it has some euphorigenic and analgesic properties. It may cause drowsiness. The tablet should be swallowed whole, not crushed or chewed. The patient should avoid alcohol as it may impair coordination and judgment.

Soma (carisoprodol) is a skeletal muscle relaxant subject to much abuse. Once the drug is ingested, the molecules are cleaved to meprobamate, a scheduled substance. Because of the abuse potential, there is an effort to change the status of this drug to a scheduled substance. It causes drowsiness and dizziness. Use with alcohol and other CNS depressants increases the risk of toxicity; it also interacts with clindamycin, phenothiazines, and monoamine oxidase inhibitors (MAOIs).

Table 14.1	Most-Commonly Used Muscle Relaxants	
Generic Name	**Brand Name**	**Dosage Form**
baclofen	Lioresal	tablet, intrathecal
carisoprodol	Soma	tablet
chlorzoxazone	Paraflex, Parafon Forte DSC	tablet, caplet, capsule
cyclobenzaprine	Flexeril	tablet
dantrolene	Dantrium	capsule, IV
diazepam	Valium	tablet, solution, IM, IV
metaxalone	Skelaxin	tablet
methocarbamol	Robaxin	tablet, IM, IV
orphenadrine	Norflex	tablet, IM, IV

Paraflex (chlorzoxazone) is for symptomatic treatment of muscle spasms and pain associated with acute musculoskeletal conditions. It acts on the spinal cord and subcortical levels by depressing polysynaptic reflexes. It may cause drowsiness and dizziness. Alcohol should be avoided.

Flexeril (cyclobenzaprine) is for treating muscle spasms associated with acute painful musculoskeletal conditions and for supportive therapy in tetanus. It is a centrally acting skeletal muscle relaxant pharmacologically related to tricyclic antidepressants. It reduces tonic somatic motor activity influencing both alpha and gamma motor neurons. Onset of action is usually within one hour, and the drug should not be used for more than two to three weeks. It may impair ability to perform hazardous activities requiring physical coordination.

Skelaxin (metaxalone) is available in 400 mg tablets. The drug has no direct action on muscle, endplate, or fiber. It probably relaxes muscle through general CNS depression and may cause drowsiness. The patient should notify the physician if skin rash or yellowish discoloration of the skin and/or eyes occur.

Lioresal (baclofen) is indicated for treating reversible spasticity or spinal cord lesions. It is used in treating multiple sclerosis. A number of unlabeled uses for this drug include hiccups and bladder spasticity. It inhibits transmission of monosynaptic and polysynaptic reflexes at the spinal cord level, possibly by hyperpolarization of primary afferent fiber terminals, with resultant relief of muscle spasticity. The drug should be taken with food or milk and may impair coordination and judgment. Abrupt withdrawal after prolonged use may cause hallucinations, tachycardia, or spasticity.

DIGESTIVE THERAPY FOR HERNIATED DISC

Chymodiactin (chymopapain) is digestive therapy used to treat a herniated lumbar disc in patients not responsive to other conservative therapy. It is not a muscle relaxer. Hydrolysis of chondromucoprotein decreases intradiscal osmotic pressure and fluid accumulation, thereby reducing symptoms of compression. The drug has no effect on collagen. Concomitant use of radiographic contrast media increases risk of neurotoxicity. Pretreatment with histamine-receptor H_1 and H_2 antagonists is recommended. The drug is given only in a hospital by a trained clinician. It is injected into the subarachnoid space through the dural canal, so it must be mixed exactly as directed. Up to fifty percent of patients who take this drug experience back pain, stiffness, and soreness, and up to thirty percent have post-treatment spasm that may last for several days.

NONNARCOTIC ANALGESICS

Nonnarcotic analgesics are used for mild to moderate pain, inflammation, and fever. A widely accepted mechanism for many of their actions in relieving pain is their ability to inhibit the enzyme cyclooxygenase and thereby decrease the conversion of arachidonic acid to prostaglandins (PGs), thromboxane A_2, and prostacyclin. Somatic pain from skin, muscle, and bone is dull and throbbing, while visceral pain from the organs is sharp and stabbing.

Fever is a response by the body temperature regulating center (hypothalamus) to substances called endogenous pyrogens produced as a result of bacterial or viral infections. The subsequent release of PGs from the brain causes the body "thermostat" to reset at a higher temperature. Figure 14.1 shows the pathway of inflammation and pain that occurs when the tissue is injured.

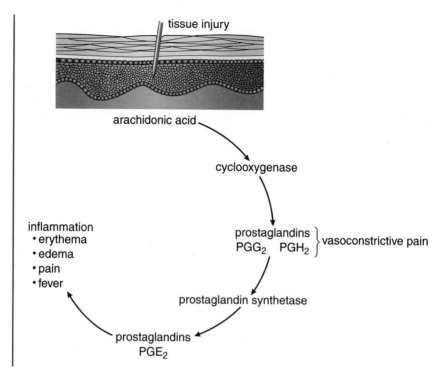

Figure 14.1

Pain Pathway in Tissue Injury

Adverse gastrointestinal (GI) effects may limit the use of nonnarcotic analgesics. These products also elevate serum concentrations of hepatic enzymes, promote water and electrolyte retention, and cause acute renal insufficiency. They can displace oral anticoagulants, sulfonylureas, phenytoin, and sulfonamides from binding to plasma proteins. Since PGs are not stored, their release during inflammation depends on synthesis. The inhibition of cyclooxygenase reduces the influence of PGs at sites of inflammation and tissue damage. Table 14.2 lists the most-commonly used nonnarcotic analgesics.

Salicylates

Salicylates were first discovered and isolated from the bark of the white willow tree. They were first used for rheumatic fever. They have both analgesic (pain-relieving)

Table 14.2   Most-Commonly Used Nonnarcotic Analgesics

Generic Name	Brand Name	Dosage Form
Salicylates		
aspirin (acetylsalicylic acid)	(many)	tablet, liquid, capsule, gum, suppository
buffered aspirin	Bufferin, Ascriptin	tablet
choline magnesium salicylate	Trilisate	tablet, liquid
magnesium salicylate	Magan	tablet
salsalate	Disalcid	tablet, capsule
Antipyretic Analgesic		
acetaminophen	Tylenol	various tablets, liquid, suppository

and antipyretic (fever-reducing) properties. They reduce fever by increasing blood flow to the skin and inhibiting prostaglandin synthesis. The primary analgesic action is peripheral rather than central. In contrast, the primary antipyretic action is central, presumably in the hypothalamus. PGs maintain the integrity of gastric mucosa. They promote mucosal production in the stomach, protecting the gastric lining from autodigestion by acids. Salicylates prevent the production of PGs and, therefore, open the stomach to ulceration.

Salicylates are indicated for

- simple headache
- muscular aches and pains
- arthritis
- menstrual cramps
- pain and fever of influenza or other infections
- inflammation of arthritis and rheumatism

Salicylates should be avoided in patients with asthma, nasal polyps, chronic sinusitis, bleeding ulcers, and hemophilia and after surgery or tooth extraction.

If used during pregnancy, salicylates may result in anemia, prolonged pregnancy and labor, and excessive bleeding before, during, and after delivery. Prostaglandins stimulate uterine contraction. That's why Cytotec (misoprostol), a prostaglandin analog, should never be given to pregnant women. Use in the last trimester results in prematurity, stillbirth, newborn death, low birth weight, and bleeding into the fetal brain. The drugs can also cause closure of the ductus arteriosus, causing premature distribution of blood to the lungs.

Patients taking probenecid or sulfinpyrazone should not take a salicylate. It can prevent the excretion of uric acid and precipitate an attack of gout. Salicylates should not be taken with methotrexate because they can increase methotrexate levels to a toxic life-threatening range. If a patient taking Coumadin (warfarin) is taking aspirin, the pharmacy technician should alert the pharmacist. Some prescribers are using the two drugs in combination, but this does increase bleeding times.

Low dosages (300–900 mg per day) of salicylate can be taken safely. More than 4 g/day can cause problems; 10 g per day can be lethal. It is not uncommon, however, for a patient with rheumatoid arthritis to take 3 g to 6 g per day under a physician's supervision.

Salicylates have side effects that include GI upset, tinnitus, and platelet changes. The nonionized portion of the acetylsalicylic acid is lipid soluble and easily absorbed into the gastric mucosal cells. Within the gastric mucosal cell this same acid becomes ionized and causes cellular damage. This allows hydrogen ions to diffuse in the gastric mucosa, which in turn causes further damage. It actually disrupts the integrity of the gastric mucosal barrier.

Aspirin has some serious side effects often overlooked. Mild salicylate intoxication (salicylism) is characterized by ringing in the ears (tinnitus), dizziness, headache, and mental confusion. Severe intoxication is characterized by hyperpnea, nausea, vomiting, acid-base disturbances, petechial hemorrhages, hyperthermia, delirium, convulsions, and coma. The lethal dose for aspirin is usually over 10 g for an adult. The advent of childproof caps for medicine has reduced the incidence of pediatric intoxication.

Aspirin should not be given to children. Reye's syndrome can develop in children who have been exposed to chicken pox. This syndrome includes a range of mental changes (mild amnesia, lethargy, disorientation, and agitation) that can culminate in coma and progressive unresponsiveness, seizures, relaxed muscles, dilated pupils, and respiratory failure.

Antipyretic Analgesic

Tylenol (acetaminophen) is an effective analgesic and antipyretic without the anti-inflammatory, antirheumatic, or uric acid excretory effects of aspirin. The mechanism and site of action have not been established, but they appear to involve central PG inhibition. Like salicylates, acetaminophen acts centrally to cause antipyresis.

Acetaminophen is given in the same doses as aspirin and is equipotent to aspirin as an antipyretic or for simple analgesia. It can be especially useful in patients

- with peptic ulcer
- taking a uricosuric agent for gout
- taking oral anticoagulants
- with clotting disorders
- at risk for Reye's syndrome
- intolerant to aspirin (still a 6% chance of cross-intolerance)

A study suggests acetaminophen increases the risk of bleeding in warfarin patients. It is still safer than aspirin or NSAIDs with warfarin. We do sometimes see aspirin used in combination with warfarin. Patients who take more than two to four tablets daily or a combination drug should be monitored.

Acetaminophen does not cause GI irritation, bleeding, alteration of platelet adhesiveness, or potentiation of oral anticoagulants. There are few interactions. However, it should not be taken if a patient has severe liver disease or is an alcoholic. At a dosage of about 10 g per day, liver damage can occur.

Mixed Analgesics

The National Kidney Foundation is urging the Food and Drug Administration (FDA) to require a prescription for mixed analgesics. Chronic use can lead to kidney failure because these drugs have additive toxic effects on the kidneys. Also important is the fact that any of the OTC analgesics can cause problems for persons who drink alcohol daily. The FDA wants manufacturers of all OTC analgesics to put an alcohol warning on their labels. For acetaminophen the problem is liver toxicity; for ibuprofen it is increased GI bleeding.

Combination drugs containing a narcotic combined with aspirin or acetaminophen are often prescribed without regard for the acetaminophen dose. The pharmacy technician can play a critical role here. When a prescription for any of these drugs is received, it would be prudent to calculate the dose of the nonnarcotic to see if it exceeds the toxicity dosage.

Nonsteroidal Anti-Inflammatory Drugs (NSAIDs)

Nonsteroidal anti-inflammatory drugs (NSAIDs) are anti-inflammatory, analgesic, and antipyretic. Inflammation occurs from tissue damage, which releases histamine, bradykinins, PGs, and serotonin. The result is vasodilation and increased permeability of capillary walls; leakage of cells, fluids, and plasma proteins into tissue; and subsequent stimulation of pain receptors. The mechanism of action is inhibition of PG synthesis; however, it is unlikely that all NSAIDs act only on PGs and by only one mechanism.

Clinical trials have not shown any of these agents to be superior to the others for managing rheumatoid arthritis. Response to these drugs varies widely. Inadequate response or loss of response to one NSAID does not imply inefficacy of others. Treatment with another NSAID is appropriate in these instances before considering adding other agents. Rotating these agents is common, and patients seem to get better results.

DRUGS FOR ARTHRITIS AND RELATED DISORDERS

Arthritis can present itself in many forms, and the most common complaint from patients with any form of arthritis is the persistent pain. This pain is caused by functional problems of the joints. Figure 14.2 shows the anatomy of a healthy joint.

Osteoarthritis is a degenerative joint disease resulting in loss of cartilage, elasticity, and thickness, and causing bone to wear and become deformed. The most commonly affected joints are the sternoclavicular joint, spine, hips, knees, finger joints, and great toes. Joints carrying large loads (knees) or those under stress (fingers) are most often affected. This disease generally appears after age forty. In the disease process, cartilage appears to be very dynamic, not stable like normal cartilage, which suggests abnormal chondrocyte activity. Disease is characterized by progressive pain, stiffness, limitations of motion, and deformed joints. Stiffness in the morning is the most prevalent complaint; it is also common after inactivity like sitting.

Bursitis is inflammation of a bursa, a saclike pouch filled with synovial fluid and located at a site of friction, such as passage of muscle or tendon over bone. The cause of bursitis is usually unknown, although trauma, overuse, chronic infection, arthritis, or gout may be involved.

Rheumatoid arthritis is an autoimmune disease in which the body's immune system attacks its own connective tissue, causing destruction. The synovium swells and becomes thickened. Finger-like projections grow from the synovium into joint spaces and cartilage, bone, and tendon, causing bone and cartilage reabsorption. Bone-to-bone contact occurs, with eventual joint fusion. The initiating antigen is unknown. Joint antigens are attacked by the inflammatory leukocytes that activate and release mediators, chemotactic substances, enzymes, and other substances capable of sustaining an inflammatory response; thus the disease becomes self-sustaining.

Cytokine-activated macrophages present in joints release two substances which are important in sustaining the inflammatory condition responsible for the progression of rheumatoid arthritis. These substances, interleukin I and tumor necrosis factor, stimulate the destructive growth of the synovial membrane which leads to the deterioration of the bone and cartilage tissue.

Two enzymes have been found to have a critical role in the inflammation process. These are cyclooxygenase-1 (COX-1) and cyclooxygenase-2 (COX-2). Both are present in the synovial fluid of patients with arthritis. It is COX-2 which is associated with pain and inflammation, whereas COX-1 has a more extensive role in the body including protection of the gastrointestinal lining.

Figure 14.2

Anatomy of a Joint

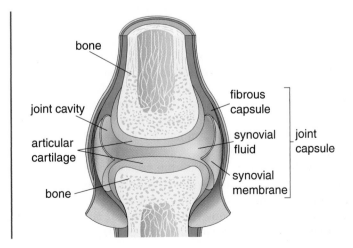

bone
joint cavity
articular cartilage
bone
fibrous capsule
synovial fluid
synovial membrane
joint capsule

Rhematoid arthritis is typically insidious, with fatigue, anorexia, weight loss, and fever (high and unexplained in children). Only about twenty percent of cases have a sudden onset. Because cartilage has no nerves, pain originates from surrounding joint structures, such as bone, tendon, ligament, and muscle. Morning stiffness is usually symmetric and lasts longer than sixty minutes. The same joints on both sides are affected about seventy percent of the time. The small joints of the hand usually are affected first, followed by feet, ankles, knees, wrists, elbows, shoulders, temporomandibular joints, and the vertebral column. Fingers become immobile and clawlike. Other organs may become involved, resulting in anemia, vasculitis, subcutaneous nodules (firm, rounded masses usually found subcutaneously in tissue exposed to pressure), pericarditis, and ocular changes. Symptoms may remit during pregnancy because of hormone activity. Patients are prone to cold and feel changes in barometric pressure.

Laboratory studies for rheumatoid arthritis are the erythrocyte sedimentation rate (ESR), which indicates the presence of inflammation, and the rheumatoid factor (RF), to which eighty percent of arthritis patients have a positive reaction. Criteria for a diagnosis of rheumatoid arthritis are

◇ morning stiffness
◇ presence of RF
◇ joint tenderness or pain on motion
◇ soft-tissue swelling in a first joint, followed within three months by swelling in a second joint
◇ sterile turbid synovial fluid
◇ x-ray changes showing erosions

Therapy is aimed at relieving pain, maintaining or improving mobility, and minimizing disability. It may include medication, physical therapy, and patient education. Heat or cold, depending on which relieves pain, for fifteen to twenty minutes before exercise should reduce pain and stiffness.

NSAIDs

NSAIDs are the predominant drugs used in the treatment of arthritis, but they have many uses. Like salicylates, NSAIDs reduce fever and pain. They work to relieve inflammation and swelling, which in turn reduces pain. They take longer to reduce fever, but effects last longer. They are used for headache, menstrual cramps, backache, muscle aches, flu, fever, pain, and the inflammation of arthritis and rheumatism. They have similar side effects: GI upset, nausea, abdominal cramps, heartburn, indigestion, ringing in the ears, ulcer, jaundice, dizziness, and rash. These drugs are protein-bound; if they are displaced from protein by other drugs, such as aspirin, the result is decreased plasma concentration and increased clearance of NSAIDs. Concurrent use of the two should be discouraged, as the combination may lead to additive or synergistic toxicity rather than increased efficacy. Future research may disclose that agents that have slightly different mechanisms of action, as they do, lead to added efficacy, but at present, this theory requires further investigation.

NSAIDs inhibit PG synthesis in tissues, thereby preventing the sensitization of pain receptors to mediators of inflammation. Thus they generally act in the affected tissues and not centrally as do other pain killers. Any central actions they do exhibit are usually unwanted side effects with the exception of lowered body temperatures.

It is important to realize that while NSAIDs have similar mechanisms of action, there is considerable patient-to-patient variation in reaction. For this reason, no one NSAID should be considered superior to another. If one does not achieve the desired results, treatment with another NSAID would be warranted.

The primary side effect of NSAID therapy is gastrointestinal upset. One in five chronic NSAID users develops some type of GI gastropathy. The next most commonly occurring side effect is kidney damage. Acute renal failure, fluid retention, hypertension, hyperkalemia, interstitial nephritis, and papillary necrosis can all be attributed to NSAID use.

NSAIDs block PG synthesis. PGs perform three protective functions in the GI tract. They increase mucosal blood flow, increase mucus production, and decrease free acid production. To inhibit PG synthesis is to inhibit each of these three functions.

NSAIDs can interact with the following drugs.

◇ aspirin
◇ beta blockers
◇ Coumadin
◇ cyclosporin
◇ digoxin
◇ diuretics
◇ methotrexate
◇ oral hypoglycemics

Table 14.3 lists some common sense tips for NSAID users, and Table 14.4 presents the most-commonly used NSAIDs. All NSAIDs should be administered with food. Sufficient time, usually two to three weeks, must be allowed with one agent before changing to another. GI upset is the most common side effect. It is largely the result of inhibition of the protective effect of PGs on gastric mucosa and direct irritation of mucosal tissues. Concurrent H_2 administration with these agents may be indicated for use in selected patients. Several of these drugs have recently become OTC drugs, with the probability that others will follow.

CONVENTIONAL NSAIDs NSAID side effects include liver abnormalities, blood irregularities, rash, water retention, bone marrow depression, dry mouth, dizziness, and drowsiness. The only drugs with parenteral forms are indomethacin and ketorolac, for short-term use only.

Indocin (indomethacin) has been the prototype NSAID for comparison with other such drugs. It has more adverse effects than the newer agents. The drug is used in neonates to close the ductus arteriosus. Its patency is believed to be mediated by PGs. It normally constricts during the first day of life, resulting in functional closure. IV indomethacin promotes closure of the patent ductus arteriosus and alleviates the associated symptoms of cardiac failure in neonates. It should be administered over twenty to thirty minutes at a concentration of 0.5 to 1.0 mg/mL in preservative-free sterile water for injection. The IV formula should be reconstituted just before administration and any unused portion discarded. Because of the side effect profile, Indocin is not used as frequently as the other NSAIDs for arthritis. The primary use is in the treatment of gout.

Motrin for Children and **Advil (ibuprofen)** are liquid dosage forms and the first OTC analgesic for children since acetaminophen. They control fever well and can be alternated with Tylenol. The onset is slower than acetaminophen, but duration of action is

Table 14.3	Tips for NSAID Users
◇ Take with food.	◇ Use the lowest possible dose.
◇ Use antacids.	◇ Be aware of the side effects.
◇ Do not use gastric irritants such as alcohol.	◇ Take sufficient fluids.
◇ Stop the NSAID before any surgical procedure.	◇ If sensitive to aspirin, avoid it.

Table 14.4   Most-Commonly Used Drugs for Arthritis and Related Disorders

Generic Name	Brand Name	Dosage Form
Conventional NSAIDs		
diclofenac	Voltaren, Cataflam	solution, tablet, ophthalmic
diflunisal	Dolobid	tablet
etodolac	Lodine	tablet, capsule
fenoprofen	Nalfon	tablet, pulvule
flurbiprofen	Ansaid	tablet
	Ocufen	ophthalmic
ibuprofen	Motrin, Advil	tablet, liquid, chewable, drops
indomethacin	Indocin	capsule, IV, suppository
ketoprofen	Orudis, Oruvail	capsule
ketorolac	Toradol	tablet, IM, IV, ophthalmic
meclofenamate	Meclomen	capsule
mefenamic acid	Ponstel	capsule
nabumetone	Relafen	tablet
naproxen	Anaprox, Naprosyn	tablet
	Aleve	tablet, caplet
oxaprozin	Daypro	caplet
phenylbutazone	Butazolidin	tablet, capsule
piroxicam	Feldene	capsule
sulindac	Clinoril	tablet
tolmetin sodium	Tolectin	tablet, capsule
COX-2 Inhibitors		
celecoxib	Celebrex	capsule
rofecoxib	Vioxx	tablet
Other		
tramadol	Ultram	tablet

longer. That is why alternating these drugs works well. The adult formulations are also available OTC in strengths of 200 mg per tablet, caplet, or capsule. However, the patient can easily double up and attain the 400 mg, 600 mg, or 800 mg prescription formulation.

If the patient is taking agents such as OTCs, the physician should be notified if a fever lasts more than three days or pain longer than ten days. Because the NSAIDs work peripherally and opiates work primarily centrally, there is potentiation between them when they are combined. They are often combined with prescription drugs (e.g., Lortab). They often provide better analgesia than either type of agent alone, with lowered opiate requirement.

Ansaid and **Ocufen (flurbiprofen)** are used in treatment of arthritis and ocular inflammation. The ophthalmic preparation, Ocufen, is for management of postoperative inflammation. It may cause mild burning or stinging. It should be administered every thirty minutes, two hours prior to surgery. For best results Ansaid should be taken three to four times a day, not to exceed 300 mg per day. This drug is frequently prescribed for menstrual cramps, but this is an unapproved use.

Voltaren and **Cataflam (diclofenac)** can induce signs and symptoms of hepatotoxicity: nausea, fatigue, pruritus, jaundice, upper right-quadrant tenderness, and flulike symptoms. Therefore, regular liver function tests are important. The patient should report any blood in the stool to the prescriber. Cataflam has a more rapid onset of action than does the sodium salt Voltaren because it is absorbed in the stomach rather than the duodenum.

Lodine (etodolac) dosage should not exceed 1,200 mg per day. Patients should be told not to crush tablets and to report any blood in the stool to the prescriber. A

Warning

Voltaren could easily be mistaken for Ultram. Voltaren comes in 25 mg, 50 mg, and 75 mg, and Ultram in 50 mg. Watch out for those 50s.

black stool usually indicates blood of gastric origin. Bright red blood in the stool is usually from rectal origin and indicates hemorrhoids.

Toradol (ketorolac) is indicated for short-term use (less than 5 days) in moderate to severe pain. It acts peripherally to inhibit PG synthesis. It is useful in narcotic allergy. When injected, a dose of 30 mg provides the analgesia comparable to 12 mg of morphine or 100 mg of meperidine. Side effects include nausea, dyspepsia (abdominal discomfort, heartburn), GI pain, and drowsiness.

Clinoril (sulindac) is a renal-sparing drug metabolized in the liver. It is a prodrug that inhibits cyclooxygenase and is structurally similar to indomethacin. Both sulindac and indomethacin have more side effects than the newer agents.

Ponstel (mefenamic acid) should not be used for more than four to seven days because it can cause blood dyscrasias. It is used primarily for dysmenorrhea.

Relafen (nabumetone) should be taken in the morning with food in a dose of two tablets. Use the lowest effective dose for chronic treatment. As with other NSAIDs, aspirin and alcohol should be avoided since they may add to the irritant action of the drug in the stomach.

Feldene (piroxicam) has the advantage of once-a-day dosing. It is for acute or long-term therapy of arthritis. Therapeutic effects are evident early in treatment, and increased response progresses over several weeks. As with other NSAIDs, the patient needs to take the drug for at least two weeks before discontinuing it to allow time for the drug to reach its therapeutic effectiveness.

Butazolidin (phenylbutazone) is used only for ankylosing spondylitis, inflammation in arthritis, and acute gouty arthritis. It has a long half-life and is hard on the stomach. Response should be seen within two to three days. If there is no response within seven days, the drug should be discontinued.

COX-2 INHIBITORS A new class of NSAIDs called COX-2 inhibitors has emerged. While traditional NSAIDs nonselectively block both the COX-1 and COX-2 enzymes, COX-2 inhibitors block only the COX-2 enzyme, which is induced during inflammation. Inhibition of COX-2 alone has been shown to decrease pain with a much lower risk of adverse GI events. COX-2 inhibitors are prescribed for rheumatoid arthritis, osteoarthritis, menstrual cramps, and acute pain.

Celebrex (celecoxib) was the first COX-2 inhibitor to be FDA approved. Although GI upset is less than with the older NSAIDs, it remains the primary side effect. Fluid retention is another significant side effect with this drug. Celebrex has the potential for cross reactivity in patients who are allergic to sulfonamides. A "take with food" label should be attached when dispensing Celebrex.

Vioxx (rofecoxib) has a similar side effect profile to Celebrex. However, early evidence suggests that this drug will not impart cross reactivity in patients who are allergic to sulfonamides. Vioxx may be taken without regard to food.

OTHER DRUGS USED TO TREAT RHEUMATOID ARTHRITIS **Ultram (tramadol)** is a totally synthetic agent that acts centrally. It binds to opiate receptors and inhibits reuptake of norepinephrine and serotonin. It is used for moderate to severe pain. The most common side effects include dizziness, vertigo, nausea, constipation, and headache. There appears to be a low-abuse potential with this drug, and yet pain control seems to be equivalent to that with narcotics. Tramadol has a slow onset of action, but once it begins to act, it gives good control of pain.

Legatrin (acetaminophen-diphenhydramine) is a combination drug to alleviate leg cramps. It replaces quinine, which has been removed from the market for this indication. Tonic water contains quinine and, if it works, can replace some of the quinine for the patient who was using it for leg cramps.

Warning

Celebrex is easily confused with Cerebyx.

Warning

Ultram looks like Ultane, but since one is a gas, this should not be a big problem.

Disease-Modifying Antirheumatic Drugs

The existing treatments for rheumatoid arthritis are divided into two categories

1. agents that provide only symptomatic relief
2. agents that can potentially modify disease progression

The former category includes the NSAIDs and corticosteroids, previously discussed. The latter category includes a variety of agents that are collectively referred to as disease-modifying antirheumatic drugs (DMARDs). These drugs are considered to be second-line agents. Even though they may slow the progression of the disease, the side effects limit their use.

Chrysotherapy (gold therapy) has been used to treat these disorders because it interferes with leukocyte activity in the synovial fluid. It is used to reduce pain, improve movement, and reduce vascular problems. It may take several months to be effective. It is used when other treatments do not work. Gold is visible on an x-ray film.

Chrysotherapeutic agents (gold) have side effects of nausea, weakness, flushing, and fainting. Skin eruptions may develop, including rash, painful mouth ulcers, and exfoliative dermatitis; the last is a condition in which the top layer of skin falls away, a condition that may continue after discontinuing the drug. The blood must be monitored frequently for evidence of proteinuria, reduced number of white blood cells, and reduced hemoglobin concentration. Patients should definitely avoid the sun.

Newer therapeutic approaches to the treatment of rheumatoid arthritis focus on the use of novel biologic response modifiers with the ability to inhibit lymphocytes and cytokine activity.

Table 14.5 gives an overview of the most-commonly used DMARDs.

Cytoxan (cyclophosphamide) depresses the bone marrow, increasing the potential for infection. Other side effects are GI upset and ulcers, liver toxicity, reproductive organ failure, and hair loss. Patients must remain well hydrated during use of this drug. Without proper hydration, the drug can cause irreparable damage to the urinary bladder. The patient should force fluids up to 2 L per day.

Rheumatrex (methotrexate) is an antineoplastic agent used to treat metastasis, arthritic conditions, and psoriasis. It should be taken on an empty stomach. Side effects include nausea, vomiting, and hair loss. Exposure to sunlight should be avoided. For prolonged use, especially in rheumatoid arthritis (RA) and psoriasis, a baseline liver biopsy should be performed and repeated on a regular basis.

Table 14.5	Most-Commonly Used DMARDs	
Generic Name	**Brand Name**	**Dosage Form**
auranofin	Ridaura	capsule
aurothioglucose	Solganal	IM
azathioprine	Imuran	tablet, IV
cyclophosphamide	Cytoxan	tablet, IM, IV, SC
etanercept	Enbrel	SC
gold sodium thiomalate 50%	Myochrysine	IM
hydroxychloroquine	Plaquenil	tablet
infliximab	Remicade	IV
leflunomide	Arava	tablet
methotrexate	Rheumatrex	tablet, IM, IV
penicillamine	Cuprimine	capsule, tablet

Imuran (azathioprine) depresses bone marrow, thus increasing the potential for infection. Other side effects are liver toxicity and GI upset. Response in RA may not occur for up to three months.

Plaquenil (hydroxychloroquine) is used to suppress acute attacks of malaria and for treatment of systemic lupus and RA. It can cause corneal deposits, retinal changes, GI upset, and skin rash. The patient should always wear sunglasses in bright sunlight and watch for vision changes, ringing in the ears, or hearing loss.

Cuprimine (penicillamine) is a chelating agent used to treat lead, mercury, copper, and gold poisoning. It lowers the rheumatoid factor (RF) level and selectively inhibits T lymphocytes. Side effects are bone marrow depression (increased risk of infection), proteinuria, rash, and drug-induced autoimmune disease (lupus erythematosus). Cross-sensitivity with penicillin is possible. Loss of taste may occur. It should be taken on an empty stomach.

Enbrel (etanercept) is a biologically engineered protein that inhibits the action of tumor necrosis factor (TNF). (Growing evidence suggests that TNF plays a key role in the pathogenesis of rheumatoid arthritis.) Etanercept is the first biologically engineered product approved for the treatment of rheumatoid arthritis. This drug is indicated in the treatment of moderate to severe rheumatoid arthritis in patients who have experienced an inadequate response to one or more of the other arthritis drugs. Etanercept can be used in combination with methotrexate in patients who do not respond adequately to methotrexate alone. The drug is diluted with bateriostatic water prior to injection and must not be mixed with any other dilutent. The solution should be administered as soon as possible after reconstitution. Etanercept must be stored in the refrigerator. The prepared solution may be stored for up to six hours. The primary side effect is injection site reactions.

Remicade (infliximab) was initially approved for Crohn's disease and has been more recently approved for rheumatoid arthritis. See Chapter 11 for a full description of this drug.

Arava (leflunomide) is a pyrimidine synthesis inhibitor that interferes with the proliferation of lymphocytes. Leflunomide retards the progression of rheumatoid arthritis, reduces pain and joint swelling, and improves functional ability. Evidence suggests that this drug exhibits an additive effect when combined with methotrexate. Side effects of leflunomide include diarrhea, rash, and alopecia (hair loss). It is also associated with elevations in liver enzymes. In the event of overdose or toxicity, cholestyrmine should be administered. The tablets should be protected from light.

Drugs for Gouty Arthritis

Gouty arthritis usually affects single joints, causing deposits (tophi) in tissues, joint cartilage, ear lobe, and metatarsals. Typically the first joint affected is the great toe; it becomes painful, swollen, and red. The disease is related to the patient's metabolism of uric acid, which is normally excreted by the kidney. The affected patient overproduces or has improper excretion of uric acid, so aspirin is contraindicated as it competes with uric acid for kidney excretion. The condition is usually inherited.

Persons prone to gout should also avoid the following drugs, which could precipitate an attack.

- diuretics
- salicylates
- nicotinic acid
- ethanol
- cytotoxic agents

Table 14.6   Most-Commonly Used Drugs for Gouty Arthritis

Generic Name	Brand Name	Dosage Form
Acute Attacks		
colchicine	none	tablet, IM, IV, SC
Chronic Therapy		
allopurinol	Zyloprim	tablet
indomethacin	Indocin	capsule, IV, suppository
probenecid-colchicine	Col-Probenecid	tablet
sulfinpyrazone	Anturane	tablet, capsule

Table 14.6 presents the most-commonly used agents for gouty arthritis.

Colchicine is the drug of choice for acute attacks. It interferes with leukocytes, reducing their mobility and joint phagocytosis, and also reduces uric acid production. The oral dose is one to two tablets of 0.5 mg or 0.6 mg strength, then one tablet every hour (not more than ten to fifteen tablets) until relief of pain or GI side effects (nausea, vomiting, diarrhea) occur. The IV dose is 2 mg to 3 mg, diluted in 30 mL of normal saline and given slowly over five minutes; it may be repeated in six to eight hours. There is a high potential for phlebitis (inflammation of a vein).

Col-Probenecid (probenecid-colchicine) dissolves tophi deposits, reduces serum urate levels, and increases uric acid excretion in urine. It is not useful in acute attacks. Risk of kidney stone formation increases as more uric acid passes through the kidney. It is used in the treatment of chronic gouty arthritis complicated by frequent, recurrent acute attacks.

Indocin (indomethacin) is the NSAID most used for gouty arthritis.

Zyloprim (allopurinol) is a xanthine oxidase inhibitor used to prevent attacks of gouty arthritis. Uric acid forms primarily from metabolism of purine bases, guanine, and adenine. Side effects are rash and hepatotoxicity. The prescriber should monitor liver function and complete blood counts before initiating therapy and during therapy. Zyloprim should be used with caution in patients taking diuretics.

Anturane (sulfinpyrazone) prevents tubule reabsorption of uric acid in the kidney. It also has antithrombotic and antiplatelet activity. Side effects are rash and GI disorders. It should be taken with food or milk to avoid aggravation or reactivation of ulcers. It is used in treatment of chronic gouty arthritis.

Warning

Allopurinal can be mistaken for Apresoline especially if an error is made in dosing. Allopurinal comes in 100 mg, 300 mg, and 500 mg. Apresoline comes in 10 mg, 25 mg, and 50 mg.

Chapter Summary

Muscle Relaxants

- The side effects of muscle relaxants are sedation, reduced mental alertness, reduced motor abilities, and GI upset. Patients taking these drugs should avoid alcohol.
- Valium (diazepam), a benzodiazepine, is a highly effective muscle relaxer, but its addictive qualities restrict its use.
- Robaxin (methocarbamol) causes skeletal muscle relaxation by reducing transmission of impulses from the spinal cord to skeletal muscles.
- Norflex (orphenadrine) is an indirect skeletal muscle relaxant thought to work by central atropine-like effects. The tablet should be swallowed whole, not crushed or chewed.
- Soma (carisoprodol) is subject to much abuse. Once the drug is ingested, the molecules are cleaved to the major metabolite meprobamate, which is a controlled substance.
- Paraflex (chlorzoxazone) is for symptomatic treatment of muscle spasms and pain associated with acute musculoskeletal conditions. It acts on the spinal cord and subcortical levels by depressing polysynaptic reflexes.
- Flexeril (cyclobenzaprine) is centrally acting and pharmacologically related to tricyclic antidepressants. Onset is usually within one hour, and the drug should not be used more than two to three weeks.
- Lioresal (baclofen) is for treating reversible spasticity or spinal cord lesions. It is used in multiple sclerosis and sometimes for hiccups. It should be taken with food or milk.

Digestive Therapy for Herniated Disc

- Chymodiactin (chymopapain) is digestive therapy used to treat a herniated lumbar disc in patients not responsive to other conservative therapy.

Nonnarcotic Analgesics

- Analgesics are used for mild to moderate pain, inflammation, and fever. A widely accepted mechanism for many of their actions is their ability to inhibit the enzyme cyclooxygenase and thereby decrease the conversion of arachidonic acid to prostaglandins, thromboxane A_2, or prostacyclin.
- Somatic pain (from injury to skin, muscle, and bone) is dull and throbbing, while visceral pain (from the organs) is sharp and stabbing.
- Fever is a response by the body's regulating center (hypothalamus) to substances called endogenous pyrogens produced as a result of bacterial or viral infections. The subsequent release of PGs from the brain causes the body "thermostat" to reset at a higher temperature.
- Adverse GI effects may limit the use of nonnarcotic analgesics.
- Salicylates have analgesic (pain-relieving) and antipyretic (fever-reducing) properties.
- The primary analgesic actions are peripheral rather than central. The primary antipyretic action of salicylates is central and presumed to be in the hypothalamus.
- Salicylates are indicated for simple headache, arthritis, pain and fever with influenza, muscular aches and pains, menstrual cramps, and inflammation.

- Salicylates cause gastrointestinal ulceration. They should be avoided by patients with asthma, polyps, chronic sinusitis, bleeding ulcers, and hemophilia. They should not be taken after surgery or tooth extraction.
- For salicylates, more than 4 g per day can cause problems; 10 g can be lethal.
- Mild salicylate intoxication is characterized by ringing in the ears (tinnitus), dizziness, headache, and mental confusion.
- Acetaminophen acts centrally to cause antipyresis. It is an effective analgesic and antipyretic without the anti-inflammatory, antirheumatic, or uric acid excretory effects of aspirin.
- A patient with severe liver disease or alcoholism should not take acetaminophen.
- When the dose of acetaminophen is greater than 4 g per day, damage can occur to the liver; 10 g can be lethal.
- Depending on the reference source, the dosage for aspirin and acetaminophen damage and toxicity differ. For the purposes of this text, and to simplify matters, the pharmacy technician should definitely make the pharmacist aware if dosage of either drug exceeds 4 g per day.
- Alcohol can cause a problem with OTC analgesics, according to the FDA. For acetaminophen, it is liver toxicity; for ibuprofen, it is increased GI bleeding.

Drugs for Arthritis and Related Disorders

- The most common complaint from arthritis patients is persistent pain. Because cartilage has no nerves, pain originates from surrounding joint structures, such as bone, tendon, ligament, and muscle.
- Therapy for arthritis is aimed at relieving pain, maintaining or improving mobility, and minimizing disability. It may include medication, physical therapy, and patient education.
- Clinical trials have not shown the superiority of any of these agents over the others for the management of rheumatoid arthritis.
- NSAIDs are used for headache, menstrual cramps, backache, muscle aches, flu, fever, and the pain and inflammation of arthritis, rheumatism, and gouty arthritis.
- Side effects of NSAIDs are GI upset, nausea, abdominal cramps, heartburn, indigestion, ringing in the ears, ulcer, jaundice, dizziness, and rash.
- Concurrent use of NSAIDs and aspirin should be discouraged, as the combination may lead to additive or synergistic toxicity, rather than increased efficacy. However, some research indicates the use of the two agents with different mechanisms of action may be synergistic.
- Inadequate response or loss of response to one NSAID does not imply that the others would be ineffective. Usually after two to three weeks, if the patient is not responding to one NSAID, a change can be made to another one.
- All NSAIDs should be administered with food.
- Many patients will need to take an H_2 blocker, antacids, or Cytotec with NSAIDs.
- NSAIDs take longer to reduce fever than the other products, but the effect lasts longer.
- NSAIDs produce analgesia at lower doses and anti-inflammation at higher doses.
- NSAIDs inhibit PG synthesis in inflamed tissues, thereby preventing the sensitization of pain receptors to mediators of inflammation. Thus they generally act peripherally and not centrally as do other pain killers. There is considerable patient-to-patient variability. Gastropathy develops in one of five chronic NSAID users.

- PGs perform three protective functions in the GI tract: increase mucosal blood flow, increase mucus production, and decrease free acid production.
- Toradol has shown pain relief equal to narcotics. It is for short-term use only.
- Clinoril is the NSAID that can be given with lithium.
- Relafen should be taken in the morning with food; two tablets is the usual dose.
- Ultram is a nonnarcotic that acts centrally to bind opiate receptors. It is used for moderate to severe pain. Its onset is slow, but once it begins to act, pain control appears to be adequate compared with the narcotics. There appears to be very little abuse potential.
- Rheumatrex (methotrexate) should be taken on an empty stomach, and exposure to the sun should be avoided. Methotrexate is an antineoplastic agent commonly used to treat arthritic conditions.
- Plaquenil is an antimalarial drug also used to treat arthritis.
- DMARDs are disease-modifying antirheumatic drugs that are second-line agents for arthritis. Even though the drugs may slow progression of the disease, the side effect profiles limit the use of these drugs.
- Aspirin should not be given to a patient with gout; it competes with uric acid for kidney excretion.
- Colchicine is the drug frequently used for an acute gout attack.
- Diuretics, salicylates, nicotinic acid, ethanol, and cytotoxic drugs can precipitate a gout attack.
- Colchicine, probenecid, indomethacin, allopurinol, and sulfinpyrazone are all used for gout.

Drug Summary

The following drugs were discussed in this chapter. Each generic drug name is followed in parentheses by one or more brand names. An asterisk (*) indicates drugs frequently written using *either* brand *or* generic name. These need to be memorized.

Muscle Relaxants
baclofen (Lioresal)*
carisoprodol (Soma)*
chlorzoxazone (Paraflex, Parafon
    Forte DSC)*
cyclobenzaprine (Flexeril)*
dantrolene (Dantrium)
diazepam (Valium)*
metaxalone (Skelaxin)*
methocarbamol (Robaxin)*
orphenadrine (Norflex)

Digestive Therapy for Herniated Disc
chymopapain (Chymodiactin)

Salicylates
aspirin, acetylsalicylic acid
buffered aspirin (Bufferin, Ascriptin)
choline magnesium salicylate (Trilisate)
magnesium salicylate (Magan)
salsalate (Disalcid)*

Antipyretic Analgesic
acetaminophen (Tylenol)*

Nonsteroidal Anti-Inflammatory Drugs (NSAIDs)
celecoxib (Celebrex)
diclofenac (Voltaren, Cataflam)*
diflunisal (Dolobid)
etodolac (Lodine)*
fenoprofen (Nalfon)*
flurbiprofen (Ansaid, Ocufen)*
ibuprofen (Motrin, Motrin for Children,
    Advil)*
indomethacin (Indocin)*
ketoprofen (Orudis, Oruvail)*
ketorolac (Toradol)*

meclofenamate (Meclomen)*
mefenamic acid (Ponstel)*
nabumetone (Relafen)
naproxen (Anaprox, Aleve, Naprosyn)*
oxaprozin (Daypro)
phenylbutazone (Butazolidin)*
piroxicam (Feldene)*
rofecoxib (Vioxx)
sulindac (Clinoril)*
tolmetin sodium (Tolectin)*
tramadol (Ultram)

Miscellaneous
acetaminophen-diphenhydramine
    (Legatrin)
tramadol (Ultram)*

Disease-Modifying Antirheumatic Drugs (DMARDs)
auranofin (Ridaura)
aurothioglucose (Solganal)
azathioprine (Imuran)*
cyclophosphamide (Cytoxan)*
etanercept (Enbrel)
gold sodium thiomalate 50%
    (Myochrysine)
hydroxychloroquine (Plaquenil)*
infliximab (Remicade)
leflunomide (Arava)
methotrexate (Rheumatrex)*
penicillamine (Cuprimine)*

Drugs to Treat Gout
allopurinol (Zyloprim)*
colchicine
indomethacin (Indocin)*
probenecid-colchicine (Col-Probenecid)*
sulfinpyrazone (Anturane)*

Chapter Review

Pharmaceuticals and Body Functions

Select the best answer from the choices given.

1. Which drug, even though it is not a controlled substance, is subject to much abuse?
   a. Valium
   b. Flexeril
   c. Soma
   d. Robaxin

2. Which drug is digestive therapy for a herniated disc?
   a. Robaxin
   b. Flexeril
   c. Lioresal
   d. Chymodiactin

3. Which muscle relaxer is also used to prevent hyperthermia?
   a. Soma
   b. Dantrium
   c. Valium
   d. Robaxin

4. Which drug may turn urine black or brown?
   a. Valium
   b. Robaxin
   c. Norflex
   d. Soma

5. Which drug is sometimes used to control hiccups?
   a. Lioresal
   b. Skelaxin
   c. Flexeril
   d. Paraflex

6. Which sticker should be put on NSAIDs?
   a. Take with food.
   b. Avoid prolonged exposure to sunlight.
   c. Be sure to complete all medication.
   d. Keep refrigerated.

7. Mild salicylate intoxication is characterized by all except
   a. ringing in the ears.
   b. headache.
   c. dizziness.
   d. throbbing pain.

8. The problem with combining alcohol and acetaminophen is
   a. GI bleeding.
   b. liver toxicity.
   c. urinary tract infection.
   d. salicylate toxicity.

9. Centrally acting muscle relaxants do not
   a. directly relax muscles.
   b. depress CNS.
   c. reduce anxiety that increases muscle tone.
   d. cause sedation.

10. Which NSAID has an IM-IV dosage form?
    a. Ketorlac
    b. Piroxicam
    c. Sulindac
    d. Naproxen

The following statements are true or false. If the answer is false, rewrite the statement so it is true.

_____ 1. Clinical trials have shown the superiority of certain NSAIDs over others for the management of rheumatoid arthritis.

_____ 2. Salicylates can actually precipitate an attack of gout.

_____ 3. Relafen is used only in ankylosing spondylitis.

_____ 4. The only NSAIDs available in parenteral forms are Nalfon and Motrin.

_____ 5. The drug of choice for an acute gout attack is Anturane.

_____ 6. Voltaren is a nonnarcotic pain reliever that primarily acts centrally.

_____ 7. Criteria for rheumatoid arthritis are morning stiffness, joint tenderness or pain on motion, and presence of rheumatoid factor.

_____ 8. Salicylates are indicated for simple headache, arthritis, pain, and fever with flu.

_____ 9. An acceptable dose of Lodine would be 2,000 mg per day.

_____ 10. Two NSAIDs that come as ophthalmics are ketoprofen and indomethacin.

Diseases and Drug Therapies

1. List four ways to block normal muscle function.
2. Why is Soma such a potentially addictive substance?
3. Complete the chart by putting an X if the heading applies to the drug.

NSAIDs	Ophthalmic	OTC	IV
diclofenac			
etodolac			
fenoprofen			
flurbiprofen			
ibuprofen			
indomethacin			
ketoprofen			
ketorolac			
meclofenamate			
mefenamic acid			
nabumetone			
naproxen			
oxaprozin			
piroxicam			
salsalate			
sulindac			
tolmetin sodium			

4. Which of the drugs in the chart come in these forms?

   Suppository _____

   IM _____

5. Explain how Ultram works.
6. List the criteria for rheumatoid arthritis.

Dispensing Medications

1. List six classes of patients who come to the pharmacy needing an OTC analgesic for whom you would recommend use of acetaminophen.

2. What would you dispense? Give the brand name and route of administration.
   a. diclofenac: Instill one drop into the affected eye qid beginning 24 hours after cataract surgery and continuing 2 weeks.
   b. flurbiprofen: 100 mg tid #30
   c. indomethacin: 0.2 mg/kg over 20 to 30 minutes at 6 a.m. and 6 p.m.
   d. indomethacin: 50 mg rectally tid
   e. ketorolac: 30 mg q2h to q4h

3. How do you mix IV indomethacin?

Internet Research

Use the Internet to complete the following assignments.

1. OTC analgesics are used widely. Find a source of information that would be useful to a patient trying to select from among the commonly sold analgesics. Make a chart comparing aspirin, acetaminophen, and ibuprofen. List indications, contraindications, and side effects for each. List your Internet sources.

2. Locate information related to on-going clinical trials aimed at the development of new treatments for rheumatoid arthritis. Create a table listing at least three experimental therapies. Indicate the phase (one through three) of testing presently underway and where (institution and country) the trials are taking place. List your Internet sources.

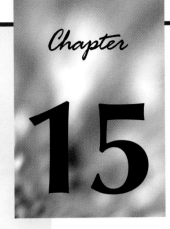

Hormones

Learning Objectives

- ◇ Explain the concept of hormones and how they regulate the body.
- ◇ Discuss thyroid replacement therapy.
- ◇ Discuss adrenal sex hormones and male dysfunction.
- ◇ Understand the concept of estrogen replacement therapy.
- ◇ Understand the formulation of oral contraceptives.
- ◇ Describe the diseases of the genital systems and how to avoid them.
- ◇ Discuss corticosteroids.
- ◇ Understand diabetes and the proper treatment and care of patients.
- ◇ Know the applications for growth hormone.

The endocrine system regulates a number of functions to keep the body in balance. The hormones that trigger the activity are also used in treatment to remedy defects. The pharmacologic agents used in these treatments include thyroid preparations, calcium, oral contraceptives, pregnancy tests, corticosteroids, antidiabetes therapy, and growth hormone.

THYROID HORMONES

The endocrine system maintains the body's homeostasis by regulating the physiologic functions involved in normal daily living and in stress. The thyroid produces hormones that stimulate various body tissues to increase their activity level. The affected tissue is called the target. Regulation of hormone synthesis is achieved via an intricate negative feedback mechanism involving the gland, the hypothalamic-pituitary axis, and autoregulation. Physiologic factors such as dopamine and stress are also known to influence the hypothalamic-pituitary axis and autoregulation. Figure 15.1 shows the regulation of hormone production and release.

The thyroid hormones, triiodothyronine (T_3) and thyroxine (T_4), are both stored as thyroglobulin, which the thyroid cells must break down before it can be released into the bloodstream. The feedback mechanism that controls the thyroid is the hypothalamic-pituitary axis, which produces thyroid stimulating hormone (TSH), which in turn stimulates the thyroid to produce T_3 and T_4. These hormones build up in circulating blood and slow the pituitary's activity in producing and releasing TSH. In response to rising levels of T_3 and T_4, the hypothalamic-pituitary axis produces less TSH. When a problem arises, measuring the amount of serum TSH can determine if the thyroid is functioning normally; if it is, another level of control may be involved. Important facts about this mechanism are: that there is peripheral conversion of some T_4 to T_3 by tissues; both T_3 and T_4 are highly protein-bound; activity comes from the free forms of T_3 and T_4; and T_3 is more potent than T_4.

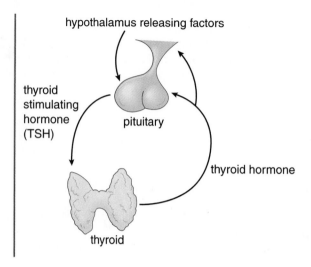

Figure 15.1

The Hypothalamic-Pituitary Axis

hypothalamus releasing factors

thyroid stimulating hormone (TSH)

pituitary

thyroid hormone

thyroid

Hypothyroidism

Hypothyroidism is a deficiency disease that causes cretinism in children. It is usually due to an iodine deficiency in the mother's diet during pregnancy. It results in severe mental retardation and is marked by a thick tongue, lethargy, lack of response to commands, and short stature. It can be corrected if treated within the first six months to the first year of life. In adults, symptoms include

- apathy
- constipation
- decreased heart rate
- depression
- dry skin, nails, and scalp
- easy fatiguing
- enlarged thyroid

- lowered voice pitch
- myxedema (distinct facial changes)
- puffy face
- reduced mental acuity
- swelling of eyelids
- tongue enlarged and thickened
- weight gain

The causes of hypothyroidism include inflammation of the thyroid gland, autoimmune destruction of the thyroid gland, or subacute (low-level) thyroiditis.

Thyroid replacement therapy is indicated for hypothyroid states and thyroid cancer. It should not be used to treat obesity. Drugs commonly used to treat hypothyroidism are listed in Table 15.1. Hypothyroid states cause increased sensitivity to numerous drugs. Correction may increase requirements for other drugs because of increases in the metabolism and conversion of drugs.

Table 15.1   **Most-Commonly Used Agents for Hypothyroidism**

Generic Name	Brand Name	Dosage Form
levothyroxine, T_4	Synthroid, Levothroid	tablet, injection
	Levoxyl	tablet
liothyronine, T_3	Cytomel	tablet
liotrix	Thyrolar	tablet
thyroid	Armour Thyroid	tablet

Synthroid, **Levothroid**, and **Levoxyl** (**levothyroxine, T_4**) in overdose can cause "too" rapid a correction and, therefore, a risk of cardiotoxicity and hyperthyroidism. Interactions are altered protein-binding of drugs, so the technician should check the patient profile for drugs currently being taken. Levothyroxine increases liver metabolism of phenytoin and phenobarbital.

For years pharmacists were told that there was no bioequivalent to Synthroid. It now appears that levothyroxine and Synthroid are therapeutically equivalent, even though they are not A/B rated. A study shows that switching products does not cause problems, but common sense says to try to keep patients on the same brand that achieved stabilization. It is never good to switch brands once a patient has become accustomed to one. All thyroid patients should get periodic TSH tests, definitely about six to eight weeks after a dose change. If a patient switches brands for any reason, the patient should be told that retesting is necessary.

Levothyroxine is recommended for chronic therapy. It can be very cardiotoxic, so the patient should immediately report any chest pain, increased pulse, palpitations, heat intolerance, or excessive sweating to the physician.

Cytomel (**liothyronine, T_3**) is more potent and less protein-bound than T_4. It is recommended for replacing supplemental therapy in hypothyroidism.

Thyrolar (**liotrix**) is supplied in a T_3 to T_4 ratio of four to one. It is difficult to stabilize the patient with this drug. Evaluation of the efficacy of therapy is based on iodine content, not hormone levels. The product has little advantage, so it is not often prescribed.

Hyperthyroidism

Hyperthyoridism, also called thyrotoxicosis or Grave's disease, is a disease marked by excessive secretion of thyroid hormones. Adults may have heart problems due to prolonged hyperactivity caused by the excessive hormone levels or by drug intake.

The causes of hyperthyroidism include

- thyroid nodules (Plummer's disease) or surgical removal of nodules
- excessive endogenous iodine from intake of thyroid hormones
- a tumor in the pituitary causing overproduction of TSH or a tumor causing excessive TSH releasing factor in the hypothalamus

Symptoms include

- decreased menses
- diarrhea
- exophthalmos (fat collects behind the eyeball, the lid does not close, lack of lubrication, with corneal ulceration)
- flushing of skin
- heat intolerance
- nervousness
- perspiration
- tachycardia
- weight loss

For children, the disease is managed with surgery and hormone replacement therapy. In adults, surgery is indicated for malignant lesions, esophageal obstruction, failure of thyroid therapy, or large multinodular goiter.

Thyroid storm presents with clinical features similar to thyrotoxicosis (Grave's disease) but the features are more exaggerated. Treatment includes IV fluids, antipyretics, cooling blankets, and sedation. Antithyroid drugs are given in large doses. It is a life-threatening medical emergency. It has a duration of seventy-two hours, although symptoms may persist for eight days.

Table 15.2 presents the most-commonly used agents for hyperthyroidism.

PTU (propylthiouracil) blocks synthesis of T_3 and T_4 and tissue conversion of T_4 to T_3. This drug is used for palliative treatment of hyperthyroidism, as adjunctive therapy to ameliorate hyperthyroidism in preparation for surgical treatment or ^{131}I therapy, and management of thyroid storm. The recommended dose should not be exceeded. The patient should notify the physician or pharmacist in the event of fever, sore throat, unusual bleeding or bruising, headache, or general malaise. If the patient is taking chronic therapy, the following monitoring parameters should be observed: CBC with differential, prothrombin time (PT), liver function tests, thyroid function tests (T_4, T_3, and TSH), and periodic blood cell counts. It is preferred over methimazole in thyroid storm because of its peripheral action.

Tapazole (methimazole) is used in the palliative treatment of hyperthyroidism to return the hyperthyroid patient to a normal metabolic state before thyroidectomy and to control thyrotoxic crisis that may accompany thyroidectomy. It is also used in preparation for radiation therapy involving the thyroid. The patient should be monitored for hypothyroidism, hyperthyroidism, T_3 and T_4 levels, CBC with differential, and liver function (baseline and as needed).

In preparation for thyroidectomy, both PTU and Tapazole inhibit synthesis of thyroid hormone and cause a euthyroid state, reducing surgical problems during thyroidectomy; as a result mortality in thyroidectomy is low.

Both drugs cause altered taste and mild alopecia. Bone marrow depression with fever, sore throat, and malaise can occur and be serious. An autoimmune reaction and a Coumadin-like anticoagulant reaction can occur.

Radioactive iodine, ^{131}I, is selectively absorbed by the thyroid tissue. It destroys thyroid cells. It is indicated for elderly and other patients. It should be used cautiously in children because of its carcinogenic potential and the hypothyroid effect on growth. An adverse effect can be hypothyroidism, and the patient must then receive thyroid hormones. Radiation burns may also injure tissue and last up to one year. It is used only when the patient is unresponsive to other therapy.

ADRENAL SEX HORMONES AND MALE IMPOTENCE

The adrenal sex hormones are controlled by the pituitary-releasing hormones, such as follicle-stimulating hormone (FSH) and luteinizing hormone (LH).

Androgens (male hormones) have a feedback control. They are produced in the hypothalamic-pituitary axis and circulate to the testes where they stimulate the

Table 15.2	Most-Commonly Used Agents for Hyperthyroidism		
Generic Name		**Brand Name**	**Dosage Form**
methimazole		Tapazole	tablet
propylthiouracil		PTU	tablet
radioactive iodine, ^{131}I			capsule, oral solution

Leydig cells to produce testosterone and release it into the blood. It then slows the activity of the hypothalamus in secreting the releasing factors. The male produces androgens in the testes, adrenals, and peripheral fat tissue. The female produces androgens in the ovaries, adrenals, and peripheral fat tissue. These hormones are replaced owing to hypogonadism in males, virilization (male characteristics), anabolic treatment (muscle building), and hematologic stimulation of erythropoiesis in renal failure. Administering androgens increases red blood cell production. Androgens are used to treat anemia, endometriosis (not the drug of choice), and breast cancer. The side effects are virilization, hirsutism (abnormal hairiness, especially in women), and acne. Hepatotoxicity and abnormally high levels of red blood cells are also problems.

Testosterone initiates sperm production and behavioral characteristics (e.g., normal aggressiveness), libido, and sexual potency. Testosterone is required during adulthood for the maintenance of libido, sexual potency, fertility (sperm production), muscle mass and strength, fat distribution, bone mass, erythropoiesis, prevention of baldness, and normal aggressive behavior.

Adverse effects from androgen therapy include acne, oily skin, gynecomastia (breast enlargement with or without tenderness), ankle edema, and priapism (frequent or prolonged, painful penile erections). Use of a low initial dosage in nonvirilized men (i.e., those lacking male secondary sex characteristics) mimics the natural increase in serum testosterone concentration during puberty. It produces virilization gradually, which minimizes adverse effects, especially priapism. Gynecomastia is the result of conversion of testosterone to estradiol (E_2) through peripheral pathways. Men with hepatic cirrhosis are predisposed to gynecomastia.

Preliminary data suggest that androgen therapy may decrease abdominal fat mass and increase muscle mass in elderly men.

Testosterone undergoes extensive first-pass metabolism in the gastrointestinal tract and liver after oral administration. To overcome this problem, various testosterone derivatives (e.g., fluoxymesterone and methyltestosterone) have been developed for oral administration. In the past, most men with hypogonadism received biweekly deep IM injections of testosterone. This therapy improves the patient's sense of well-being and increases libido and sexual potency within weeks or months.

Scrotal systems overcome some drawbacks associated with oral and IM administration. Applying a transdermal testosterone patch to the scrotal skin in the morning provides a serum testosterone concentration that mimics the natural circadian secretion of the hormone in young, healthy men. Because scrotal skin is as least five times more permeable to testosterone than skin at other sites, an inadequate serum testosterone concentration results if a scrotal system is applied to a nonscrotal area. To optimize contact, the scrotal skin should be dry-shaved before the system is applied. Many men prefer scrotal transdermal systems to IM testosterone injections because the patch avoids the pain and discomfort of injections and is easy to apply. Other patients find it embarrassing to explain the transdermal patch to their sex partners. Testosterone patches are classified as schedule III controlled substances because of the abuse potential as an anabolic steroid. Hepatotoxicity is also associated with the abuse of other androgens.

Impotence may have many causes, including testosterone deficiency, alcoholism, cigarette smoking, psychological factors, and medications. Table 15.3 lists drugs that may cause impotence. Alcohol is a primary reason for male dysfunction or impotence. Table 15.4 presents the most-commonly used agents for male impotence.

Androderm, Androgel, and **Testoderm (testosterone)** are transdermal systems. Androderm and Androgel are not applied to the genitals. Instead these are be applied to a fleshy area of the back, abdomen, upper arm, or thigh. In contrast, Testoderm is applied to the scrotum. The usual starting dosage for Androderm is two patches

Table 15.3   Drugs that May Cause Impotence

◇ alcohol (the most significant)	◇ H₂ blockers
◇ amphetamines	◇ haloperidol
◇ antihypertensives	◇ lithium
◇ corticosteroids	◇ opiates
◇ estrogens	◇ some antidepressants

Table 15.4   Most-Commonly Used Agents for Male Impotence

Generic Name	Brand Name	Dosage Form
alprostadil	Edex	injection
	Muse	suppository
	Caverject	injection kit
danazol	Danocrine, Cyclomen	capsule
methyltestosterone	Android, Testred	capsule
oxymetholone	Anadrol	tablet
papaverine	Pavabid	tablet, capsule, injection
sildenafil	Viagra	tablet
testosterone	Androderm (nonscrotal)	transdermal patch, IM
	Duratest	injection
	Testoderm (scrotal)	transdermal patch
	Androgel	gel

applied every evening (about every twenty-four hours). Patients should be cautioned to not use the same site more than once every seven days. The system may be worn while taking a shower or bath. Virilization of the female sex partners is unlikely because the occlusive outer film prevents the partner from coming in contact with the drug. These drugs increase libido and sexual potency and also improve the patient's sense of well-being.

Androgel should be applied once daily, preferably in the morning, to clean, dry, intact skin. The application site should be allowed to dry before dressing. Hands should be washed with soap and water after handling this drug.

Alprostadil is available in three forms to treat impotence. **Edex** is a penile injection. **Muse** (medicated urethral system for erection) is a urethral suppository for impotence. It is a small plastic applicator that inserts a micropellet of alprostadil into the urethra. It works quickly, usually within ten minutes. The side effects are penile pain and urethral burning. High doses can cause hypotension and dizziness. It can also affect the female partner, causing vaginal burning and itching. It should be refrigerated unless it is going to be used within fourteen days. **Caverject** is the first drug specifically approved for impotence. It comes as a kit containing six syringes and single-dose vials of freeze-dried powder for reconstitution and administration. The vials should be refrigerated until dispensed, but they may be kept at room temperature for up to three months.

Viagra (sildenafil), the first oral therapy for impotence, enhances the relaxant effect of nitric oxide released in response to sexual stimulation. This allows an erection to occur naturally. It should be taken one hour before sexual activity. Its interaction with nitrates is potentially lethal. Other interactions to watch for are erythromycin and antifungals. It can cause temporary vision disturbances, headache, and indigestion.

FEMALE HORMONES

Progestins

Progestins are a component in oral contraceptives and are used to treat dysfunctional uterine bleeding, endometriosis, as well as endometrial and breast cancer. Progestins emulate progesterone effects, which are generally opposite to those of estrogen. They are used primarily in birth control pills and to prevent uterine cancer in the post-menopausal woman taking estrogen replacement therapy. Progestins, like estrogen, inhibit luteinizing hormone secretion through a negative feedback on the hypothalamic anterior pituitary axis. This is one of the mechanisms by which they prevent conception. Progestins also alter cervical mucus from a watery, nonviscous secretion to a viscous, cellular secretion that provides a physical barrier to sperm penetration. Furthermore, progestational stimulation early in the ovarian cycle causes premature development of endometrial glands and involution. A second mechanism of action impairs implantation of a fertilized egg. The estrogen component of the birth control preparation stimulates stromal development, and the resulting endometrium is unsuitable for implantation. Ovulation is not suppressed and fertilization can occur, but the egg is "aborted." Progestins are sometimes used alone for birth control.

Progestins are used to treat menstrual dysfunction such as irregular cycles, protracted uterine bleeding, dysmenorrhea, amenorrhea, and endometriosis. Table 15.5 lists the most-commonly used progestins. It is believed that poorly cycling estrogens may promote hypertrophy of the endometrium. Adding a progestin has lowered incidence of endometrial hyperplasia. Progestins alone do not promote menstrual bleeding, but in patients who either have endogenous estrogen or are treated first with estrogen, the cyclic treatment with progestin helps to restore normal cycling. Evidence indicates that oral birth control pills protect against ovarian cancer.

Norplant (levonorgestrel) comes in matchstick-sized, flexible, closed capsules filled with levonorgestrel. The capsules are implanted under local anesthesia through a single incision in the subcutaneous tissue of the upper arm, where the hormone is released and easily diffused into the bloodstream. The implants maintain their effectiveness for as long as five years and must be removed surgically, by the end of the fifth year of use.

Many side effects associated with oral contraceptives or progestational agents are similar to pregnancy symptoms. The effects generally attributed to the progestational component include weight gain, depression, fatigue, acne, and hirsutism.

Estrogen

The hypothalamic pituitary axis releases FSH to the ovary, where it stimulates estrogen production for one to fourteen days and progesterone for fourteen to twenty-eight days.

Table 15.5	Most-Commonly Used Progestins	
Generic Name	**Brand Name**	**Dosage Form**
hydroxyprogesterone	Hylutin, Gesterol	IM
levonorgestrel	Norplant	implant
medroxyprogesterone	Amen, Provera, Cycrin	tablet
	Depo-Provera	IM

Both hormones build up in the bloodstream and reduce the activity of the hypothalamus in producing and releasing the gonadotropic-releasing factor (GRF).

Estrogens are formed from androgenic precursors and are the growth hormones of reproductive tissue in females. In addition, they share some actions of androgens on the skeleton and other tissues. Estrogen suppresses FSH secretion, which blocks follicular development and ovulation. Progesterone suppresses luteinizing hormone secretion, preventing ovulation. Estrogen produces endometrial growth, increased cervical mucus, cornification (thickening and maturing) of vaginal mucosa, growth of breast tissue (ducts and fat deposit), increased epiphyseal closure, sodium retention, carbohydrate metabolism, and calcium utilization.

Estrogen is used for birth control formulations, relief of menopausal symptoms, reduction of osteoporosis in combination with other drugs (e.g., Fosamax and calcium), gonadal failure, and prostatic cancer. Symptoms of estrogen deficiency are irregular bleeding and irregular cycles. "Hot flashes" start in the face and move down over the body; they are related to the rate of estrogen decline. Atrophic vulvovaginitis is characterized by excessive vaginal dryness, dyspareunia (painful intercourse), and infections because fewer lactobacilli are present due to reduced estrogen level. Estrogen depletion leads to reduced glycogen to be metabolized, with raised pH and loss of natural protection, causing urethral and bladder atrophy. A certain amount of depression is related to menopause.

Estrogen replacement therapy (ERT) relieves symptoms of estrogen deficiency. Menopause occurs with the cessation of menses for one year, with a change in site, amount, and pattern of estrogen production (reduced rate). The climacteric is characterized by gradual loss of ovarian function and irregular bleeding before termination of menses. With decreased estrogen production at menopause, estrogen-responsive tissues atrophy. The menopausal symptoms may include vasomotor instability (hot flashes), drying and atrophy of the vaginal mucosa, insomnia, irritability, and other mood changes.

As ovarian function declines with age and androstenedione from the adrenal cortex becomes the primary source of estrogen, estrone is the dominant circulating estrogen. Because the naturally occurring concentration of androstenedione and the efficiency of its conversion may vary considerably among persons, ERT is often provided to ease the transition into menopause. Estrogen is also effective in preventing bone loss, lowering cholesterol levels, improving color and turgor of skin, and improving mental functions. Table 15.6 presents the most-commonly used estrogens.

When dispensing estrogen, the technician should check with the patient to see if she has had a hysterectomy; if she has not, a progesterone prescription should accompany the estrogen. It is especially important to remind patients on any form of estrogen, whether it is birth control pills or ERT, that smoking is associated with greater morbidity, especially in patients over thirty-five years of age.

The adverse effects of estrogens are nausea, vomiting, bloating, weight gain, breast tenderness, and breakthrough bleeding. Other side effects (hypercoagulability, thrombophlebitis, and faster clotting) are related to dose and nicotine use. Glucose intolerance can also be a side effect, so diabetics often need to increase their diabetes medication when taking estrogen. The weight gain is probably due to fluid retention, and often a diuretic is needed. The blood loss during menstrual periods is less, as is the fluid accumulation the week before onset. The risks of breast cancer associated with estrogen are minimal but may be slightly increased in some women who take estrogen long term. During reproductive life, lipid levels are reduced. Menopause increases lipids. Estrogen is contraindicated in patients with migraines, mild hypertension, a history of thrombosis, endometriosis, and chronic mastitis. Some practitioners do not give estrogen if the patient has had breast cancer or it runs in the family. Patients taking ERT should not smoke; estrogen plus nicotine

Table 15.6   Most-Commonly Used Estrogens

Generic Name	Brand Name	Dosage Form
conjugated estrogen	Premarin	tablet, cream, IM, IV
conjugated estrogen-medroxyprogesterone	Prempro, Premphase	tablet
diethylstilbestrol	Stilphostrol	tablet, IM
estradiol	Estrace	tablet, transdermal, cream, IM
	Estraderm	IM, tablet, transdermal system
	Vivelle, Climara	transdermal system
estradiol-norgestimate	Ortho-Prefest	tablet
estradiol-norethindrone acetate	Activella	tablet
estropipate	Ogen	tablet, cream
ethinyl estradiol	Estinyl	tablet
ethinyl estradiol-norethindrone acetate	Femhrt	tablet

increases the risk of blood clots, which increases risk of deep vein thrombosis. In most women, the benefits in reducing bone loss and cardiovascular disease as a result of estrogen therapy far outweigh the small risk of breast cancer.

Combination therapies for the treatment of ERT can provide some special benefits. For example, **Prempro (conjugated estrogen-medroxyprogesterone)** provides both estrogen replacement as well as progesterone to prevent uterine cancer with only one prescription. **Femhrt (ethinyl estradiol-norethindrone acetate)** and **Ortho-Prefest (estradiol-norgestimate)**, which are also prescribed as birth control pills, provide many health benefits (e.g., prevention of bone loss, lowered risk of ovarian and endometrial cancer) in addition to estrogen replacement. In order to prevent pregnancy, however, these drugs use higher levels of estrogen than other ERT therapies.

Contraceptives

Prescription contraceptives, typically oral contraceptives (OCs), are among the most-frequently prescribed agents. For these products to be optimally effective with the lowest frequency of side effects, patients should be well informed as to their proper use.

The advantages of OCs include ease of use, high efficacy rate, and relative safety. Most OCs prescribed today are a steroidal combination of estrogen and progestin. These combination pills suppress ovulation by interfering with production of the hormones that regulate the menstrual cycle. They also alter the cervical mucus to prevent penetration of sperm and change the composition of the endometrium to inhibit implantation. Some progestin-only forms of "the pill" are also available, and their mechanism relies on the effects of progestin on the cervical mucus and endometrium.

Combination OCs provide both estrogen and progestin in the same pill for each of twenty-one consecutive days. Progestin-only OCs are usually taken once a day, every day, without a pill-free interval. In addition to preventing pregnancy, oral contraceptives have several noncontraceptive benefits. Many women taking the pill experience more regular menstrual cycles, reduced menstrual flow, and less-severe menstrual pain and cramps. Epidemiologic evidence shows that OCs may protect against ovarian and endometrial cancer, benign breast disease, ectopic pregnancy, fibroadenomas, and ovarian cysts. They may also reduce the risk of pelvic inflammatory disease.

The most serious adverse effect of OCs is development of cardiovascular complications, such as heart attack, stroke, or other forms of thromboembolic disease. The

OCs available contain much lower amounts of estrogen and progestin than those first introduced in the 1960s, and the frequency of adverse cardiovascular effects has been reduced.

Table 15.7 presents the most-commonly used contraceptive agents. Most OCs available today contain norethindrone, ethynodiol, or levonorgestrel as the progestin. The classic side effects associated with birth control pills (nausea, weight gain, and breast tenderness) result from the levels of these progestins necessary for effectiveness. Other complaints include fluid retention, chloasma (skin discoloration), and irregular vaginal bleeding. They probably should not be prescribed to women who have hypertension, diabetes mellitus, or elevated cholesterol levels. However, pregnancy could be more of a health risk for these individuals than the side effects of the pills, so they often are prescribed. Women who smoke are at increased risk for thromboembolic complications, and those who are prescribed oral contraceptives should not smoke. The combination of nicotine and estrogen tends to cause blood to clot.

Achieving proper hormonal balance in OCs is the key to taking them successfully. There are various combinations of estrogen and progestin, often with the same name. For example, **Ortho Novum** comes in 7/7/7 and 1/35 formulations. Patient tolerance and symptoms help the clinician make the decision as to which formulation to prescribe. An excess of estrogen causes nausea, bloating, migraine headaches, edema, and hypertension. With insufficient estrogen, the patient experiences early or midcycle breakthrough bleeding and increased spotting. With an excess of progestin, the patient has increased appetite and weight gain. Acne and depression can also occur. With a deficiency of progestin, there is late breakthrough bleeding or cessation of menses altogether. Examples of the combinations are intermediate-potency estrogen with high-potency progestin, intermediate-potency of both, high potency of both, and low potency of both.

Tricycling is the practice of taking three twenty-one-day cycles of OCs without a pill-free interval. Evidence suggests that because the OC suppresses endometrial thickening, menstrual cycles (i.e., the cyclic sloughing off of this layer) can be safely

Table 15.7	Most-Commonly Used Contraceptive Agents		
Generic Name		**Brand Name**	**Dosage Form**
Biphasic			
ethinyl estradiol-ethynodiol diacetate		Demulen	tablet
ethinyl estradiol-levonorgestrel		Levlen, Tri-Levlen, Triphasil	tablet
ethinyl estradiol-norethindrone		Genora, Loestrin, Ortho Novum, Ovcon	tablet
ethinyl estradiol-norgestrel		Lo/Ovral, Ovral	tablet
mestranol-norethindrone		Genora 1/50	tablet
Progestin			
norgestrel		Ovrette	tablet
Parenteral			
estradiol cypionate-medroxyprogesterone		Lunelle	injection
medroxyprogesterone		Depo-Provera	tablet, injection
Implant			
levonorgestrel		Norplant	capsule

extended to three months. The benefits of tricylcing include less menstrual pain and lower incidences of pre-menstrual syndrome (PMS), headaches, and endometriosis.

Patients prescribed an OC should be instructed to take the tablet at the same time every day; taking the medication at bedtime reduces the possibility of nausea or chloasma (discoloration of the skin).

Lunelle (estradiol cypionate-medroxyprogesterone) is an injectable contraceptive. It is given once a month. It acts more like an oral contraceptive than Depo-Provera because it has an estrogen component. Patients tend to have irregular periods or none. It may take up to thirteen months after the last injection before normal fertility resumes. Since many state practice acts now permit pharmacists to give injections, these may be given in the pharmacy.

OCs interact with many drugs. The drug classes are the important element to watch in this list. If OCs interact with any drug in a class, there is an excellent chance it will react with all the drugs in that class. The technician should search the patient profile carefully for any of these drugs, as outlined in Table 15.8.

Home Pregnancy Tests

Detecting a pregnancy early allows the mother to make informed lifestyle decisions and seek out the appropriate healthcare resources for an optimal outcome. Critical organ

Table 15.8	Oral Contraception Interactions	
Class	**Drugs**	**Type of Interaction**
antibiotics	erythromycin, griseofulvin, penicillins, rifampin, tetracyclines	may decrease OC effectiveness, interference with enterohepatic cycling and recycling of estrogen, which can cause a fluctuation in hormone levels
anticonvulsants	Tegretol, Felbatol, phenobarbital, Dilantin, Mysoline	decreases OC action due to increased metabolism of hormones
antifungals	Diflucan, Sporanox, Nizoral	may decrease OC action (see antibiotics)
benzodiazepines	Xanax, Librium, Valium, Dalmane, Halcion	metabolism of benzodiazepines that undergo oxidation may be decreased, increasing CNS effects
bronchodilator	theophylline	theophylline metabolism may be decreased, increasing side effects
corticosteroids	hydrocortisone, methylprednisolone, prednisolone, prednisone	effects may be increased owing to inhibition of metabolism by OC
lipid-lowering agents	Atromid-S	metabolism of clofibrate may be increased, decreasing OC effect
tricyclic antidepressants	Elavil, Tofranil	TCA metabolism may be decreased, increasing the side effects

systems develop during the first month of embryogenesis; these systems are affected by the mother's diet (e.g., vitamins, caffeine), environment (e.g., smoking), medications, and consumption of alcoholic beverages. Early confirmation of pregnancy allows for earlier prenatal care, earlier detection of an ectopic pregnancy (a potentially life-threatening condition), and more time for counseling and consideration of alternatives.

Pregnancy tests are based on detecting the hormone human chorionic gonadotropin (HCG), a glycoprotein produced by trophoblastic cells and the placenta. Because HCG levels can be measured as early as six to eight days after conception, a woman may test for pregnancy after the first day of a missed menstrual period (depending on the test used). All currently marketed tests detect HCG with mono-clonal antibodies (MCAs) specific for the hormone. A chromogen-reactive enzyme linked to one of the antibodies changes color in the presence of HCG, indicating pregnancy. MCA tests give results in one to five minutes. These tests differ in the time and number of steps required to complete the test, the clarity of instructions, and the ease with which the test results can be determined. Consumers generally achieve better than ninety-five percent accuracy with home pregnancy tests.

False-negative results can be due to chilled urine, chilled test reagents, diluted urine, or high-dose pancreatic enzyme replacement. False-positive results can be due to collecting the urine in a waxed paper cup, undetected or recent abortion, or elevated levels of HCG (e.g., in tumor).

The steps in the procedure for using the kit properly are as follows.

1. Check the expiration date.
2. Read the instructions twice.
3. Wait the recommended number of days after the menstrual period.
4. Collect the sample from the first morning urine.
5. Collect urine in a clean container; do not use a plastic cup.
6. If the test cannot be done immediately, refrigerate the urine. Be sure to set the urine out twenty to thirty minutes before the test is performed.
7. If the test is positive, make an appointment to see a doctor.
8. If the test is negative, wait three to five days. If menstruation does not start, perform the test again. If the second test is negative and menstruation has not started, see a doctor.

DRUGS FOR BONE DISEASES

Reduction or weakening of the bone mass increases the risk of bone fracture. The condition is called osteoporosis, and it occurs faster in women after age fifty than in men. The reduction is accelerated and more severe in women who have had early hysterectomy. Estrogen helps get calcium into the bone. If the body is producing less estrogen, then these patients need to take calcium and vitamin D along with estrogen.

Bone is a living tissue continuously being replaced as a result of activity of osteo-clasts (cells that resorb bone) and osteoblasts (cells that form bone). The opposing activities of osteoclasts and osteoblasts are balanced in normal, healthy bone. Many risk factors for osteoporosis (e.g., gender, race, and heredity) cannot be changed, but certain lifestyle risk factors (e.g., low calcium intake, cigarette smoking, alcohol abuse, and lack of weight-bearing exercise) can be modified. Modification of osteoporosis risk factors benefits all patients, regardless of gender, age, or type of osteoporosis.

Weight-bearing exercise contributes to developing and maintaining bone mass, provided that calcium intake is adequate. Walking, jogging, weight lifting, and dancing are examples of weight-bearing exercise. Elderly persons may benefit from careful exercise because it improves muscle function and agility, which reduces the risk of falls.

Hormone replacement therapy (HRT), with or without progestin, is recommended for most postmenopausal women at risk of osteoporosis. Table 15.9 lists the most-commonly used agents for prevention and treatment of bone diseases. HRT reduces the rate of bone loss in women with estrogen deficiency. In women with established osteoporosis, HRT maintains or increases bone density at all skeletal sites and decreases the risk of hip fracture. Use of estrogen alone increases the risk of endometrial hyperplasia and cancer. Women with an intact uterus should receive progestin with the estrogen. Women who have undergone hysterectomy may take estrogen alone. A small increase in the risk of breast cancer among postmenopausal women has been associated with long-term HRT. Nevertheless, many clinicians believe the benefits of HRT outweigh the risks in a majority of women.

Fosamax (alendronate) is the only bisphosphonate approved by the FDA for treating osteoporosis. Bisphosphonates inhibit bone resorption by osteoclasts. They prevent bone loss associated with estrogen deficiency and partially reverse bone loss in women with postmenopausal osteoporosis. Fosamax binds to hydroxyapatite to inhibit bone osteoclastic reabsorption. In addition to its indication for preventing osteoporosis, alendronate is used in hypercalcemia of malignancy and in Paget's disease of unknown cause affecting the middle-aged and elderly, which results in excess bone destruction and unorganized bone repair.

Alendronate must be taken at least thirty minutes before the first food, beverage, or medication of the day with plain water only. It should be taken with six to eight ounces of water to avoid esophageal burning. Waiting more than thirty minutes before eating will improve absorption. The patient should avoid lying down for at least thirty minutes after taking this drug.

Didronel (etidronate) is indicated for treating Paget's disease, hypercalcemia, and ossification due to spinal cord injury; it is not often used for osteoporosis. Patients must maintain adequate intake of calcium and vitamin D. The drug should be taken on an empty stomach. Serum calcium and phosphorus should be monitored, as well as levels of creatinine and blood urea nitrogen (BUN).

Actonel (risedronate) is a biphosphate which inhibits bone resorption by actions on osteoclasts or on osteoclast precursors. It should be used only for Paget's disease since the dose is inappropriate for osteoporosis.

Miacalcin (calcitonin-salmon) in nasal spray form should be reserved for women who refuse or cannot tolerate ERT or in whom ERT is contraindicated. The spray should be applied to a different nostril each day. The medication may be used at any time of day. The pump must be activated before the first dose. Most adverse effects are local, involving the nose.

Table 15.9	**Most-Commonly Used Agents for Bone Diseases**	
Generic Name	**Brand Name**	**Dosage Form**
alendronate	Fosamax	tablet
calcitonin-salmon	Miacalcin	nasal spray, IM, SC
calcium	Tums, Caltrate	tablet
	Os-Cal	tablet, chewable
	Titralac	tablet, suspension
	Viactiv	chewable
etidronate	Didronel	tablet, IV
raloxifene	Evista	tablet
risedronate	Actonel	tablet

Evista (raloxifene) is a selective estrogen receptor modulator which acts, like estrogen, to prevent bone loss and improve lipid profiles. Because Evista actually inhibits some estrogen receptors, this drug has the potential to block some estrogen effects such as those associated with an increased risk of breast and uterine cancer.

Tums, Caltrate, Os-Cal, and Titralac (calcium) should be taken daily. The recommended dose is 1,000 to 1,500 mg plus dietary supplements. This treatment prevents a negative calcium balance that may contribute to osteoporosis. Calcium carbonate is probably better absorbed when taken orally. Tums is an inexpensive way to get one's daily supply of calcium. Viactiv is an excellent way to get calcium. Three of these soft, milk chocolate, calcium chews can provide 1,500 mg.

DRUGS FOR SEXUALLY TRANSMITTED DISEASES

Most genital system diseases are transmitted by sexual activity and are, therefore, called sexually transmitted diseases (STDs). Figure 15.2 shows the structural anatomy of the male and female genital systems.

Gonorrhea

Gonorrhea is the most commonly reported STD. It is caused by *Neisseria gonorrhoeae* and was described by the Greek physician Galen in 150 A.D. About one million cases are reported each year; of these, sixty percent are in the fifteen- to twenty-four-year age

Figure 15.2

Genital System Anatomy
(a) Female
(b) Male

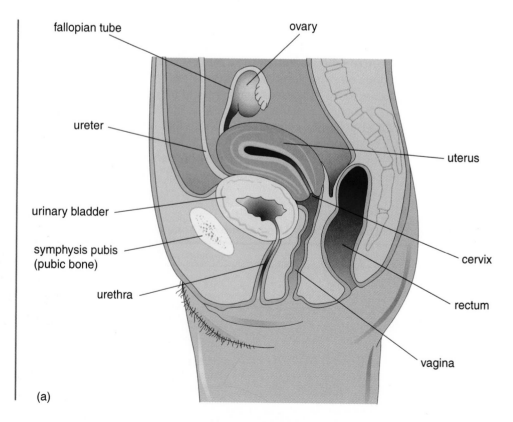

(a)

group. The organism attaches to mucosal cells in the oropharyngeal area, eye, joints, rectum, and male and female genitalia. Infection sets up inflammation, with leukocytes moving into the area and pus production. Incubation takes a few days, but less than a week. Males have painful urination and pus discharge. Complications can cause urethral scarring with partial blockage. Blockage of the ductus deferens results in sterility. The female disease is more insidious. It may cause abdominal pain due to extensive infection of the uterus, cervix, fallopian tubes, and ovaries (pelvic inflammatory disease [PID]).

Scarring may block fallopian tubes to ovum movement, which may cause ectopic pregnancy or sterility if blockage is total. Untreated disease in either sex could cause systemic infection involving the heart, meninges, eyes, pharynx, and joints (arthritis). Eye infections occur most often in newborns and can result in blindness. In most states, erythromycin or silver nitrate solution is applied to eyes of newborns. If the mother is known to be infected, the infant is given penicillin IM.

Gonorrhea infection can be acquired at any point of sexual contact, including pharynx and anus. Immunity to reinfection does not result from recovery; reinfection is possible. Penicillin has been effective for years, although higher doses are now needed because the organism has developed some resistance. **Rocephin (ceftriaxone)** is used frequently, especially in penicillinase-producing bacteria. **Spectinomycin** is an alternate drug in cases of resistance. Another microorganism often found with gonorrhea is *Chlamydia trachomatis*; **tetracycline** is often used to control this organism.

Syphilis

Syphilis first appeared in Europe in the fifteenth century and is due to *Treponema pallidum*. A long incubation time allows tracing and treating sexual partners before

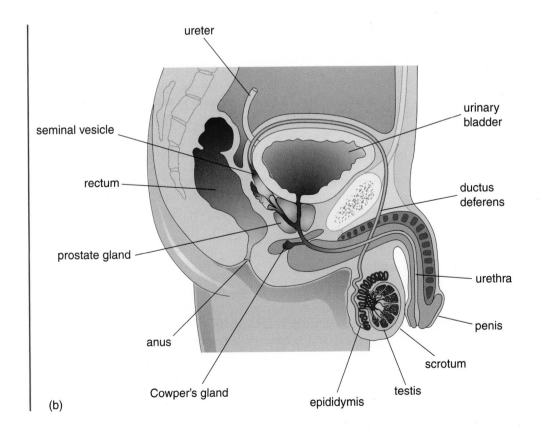

(b)

symptoms are apparent. Incubation averages three weeks (two weeks to several months). The course develops in three stages.

PRIMARY-STAGE INFECTION A primary-stage infection produces a small, hard-based chancre (sore) at the site of infection. Usually, the lesion heals in a few weeks and is painless. Females may be unaware of the infection if the chancre is on the cervix. In males, the chancre may be in the urethra. Fluids from the sore are highly infectious. Bacteria enter the bloodstream and lymphatic system.

SECONDARY-STAGE INFECTION A secondary-stage infection produces skin rashes, patchy hair loss, malaise, and mild fever. Lesions on mucous membranes contain organisms and are highly infectious. Symptoms subside after a few weeks, and the disease becomes latent. After two to four years of latency, the disease is usually no longer infectious.

TERTIARY-STAGE INFECTION A tertiary-stage infection occurs usually after an interval of at least ten years. Lesions appear as a rubbery mass of tissue in many organs and sometimes the skin. There may be extensive damage, including deafness, blindness, CNS lesions, or perforation of the roof of the mouth resulting from a hyperimmune reaction to the remaining spirochetes. Because symptoms in the first two stages are not disabling, patients often enter the latent period without receiving medical attention.

Congenital Syphilis

Congenital syphilis crosses the placenta into the fetus. Neurologic damage to the fetus results if pregnancy occurs during the tertiary stage. Pregnancy during the primary or secondary stage is likely to produce a stillborn child. **Penn G (benzathine)** is the drug most often used to treat this infection.

Nongonococcal Urethritis (NGU)

Nongonococcal urethritis (NGU) may be caused by catheters or chemical agents; forty percent of the cases are acquired sexually. Symptoms are often mild in males, but serious in females.

Lymphogranuloma Venereum

Lymphogranuloma venereum is a disease caused by *Chlamydia trachomatis* that often occurs with gonorrhea. Symptoms are mild or absent, but the disease can cause sterility or infect infant eyes during birth. It can be treated with **Doryx (doxycycline)**.

Genital Herpes

Genital herpes is caused by the herpes simplex virus. Lesions appear after about a week of incubation and cause a burning sensation. Vesicles develop, with infectious fluid, and then heal in about two weeks. The virus goes into a latent period in nerve cells and reappears in response to emotional stress, menstruation, illness, or scratching of the infected area. A pregnant mother may deliver by cesarean section to avoid the infant contracting the virus in the birth canal. If infection occurs in the uterus, birth defects may occur. **Zovirax (acyclovir)** and **Valtrex (valacyclovir)** are used in this disease state.

Candidiasis

Candidiasis is a yeast-like fungal disease caused by *Candida albicans*, usually as an opportunistic overgrowth. It causes itching and a thick, yellow, cheesy discharge. **Nizoral (ketoconazole)** and **Diflucan (fluconazole)** are frequently used.

Vaginitis

Vaginitis due to infection with *Gardnerella vaginitis* results from interaction between the organism and an anaerobic bacteria in the vagina, neither of which alone can produce the disease. It is characterized by a frothy discharge with fishy odor and a vaginal pH of five to six. **Metronidazole**, for patient and partner, is used to treat this. Vaginitis may also be caused by *Trichomonas vaginalis*, an organism normally found in both sexes. It causes an infection if vaginal acidity is disturbed. Leukocytes infiltrate the site and result in profuse, yellowish or light cream-colored discharge with a disagreeable odor. It causes irritation and itching. Vaginitis may also be caused by *Haemophilus vaginalis*, which interferes with microbial folic acid synthesis and growth via inhibition of para-aminobenzoic acid (PABA) synthesis. Metronidazole, for patient and partner, is frequently used.

Agents for Sexually Transmitted Diseases

Table 15.10 presents the most-commonly used agents for sexually transmitted diseases.

Bicillin L-A is used to treat syphilis. Penicillin is especially effective during the primary stage; it is the only agent active against growing bacteria. It **(penicillin G benzathine)** is effective for about two weeks; however, it is in low concentration. It is appropriate treatment as the spirochete grows slowly.

Tetracycline and **erythromycin** are both effective against *Chlamydia*.

Flagyl (metronidazole) and **Sultrin** or **Trysul (triple sulfa)** are used to treat *Gardnerella vaginitis* (formerly called *Haemophilus vaginalis*) infections. It is important that the patient complete the full course of treatment with triple sulfa.

Zovirax (acyclovir) is often used to treat genital herpes. It interferes with the DNA synthesis of the virus and lessens severity, shortens healing time, and lessens frequency of attacks.

Table 15.10	Most-Commonly Used Agents for Sexually Transmitted Diseases	
Generic Name	**Brand Name**	**Dosage Form**
acyclovir	Zovirax	capsule, suspension, ointment
ceftriaxone	Rocephin	IM, IV
clotrimazole	GyneLotrimin, Lotrimin	cream, lotion, solution, tablet, troche
doxycycline	Doryx	capsule, tablet, IM, IV, syrup
erythromycin	numerous (many salts)	
fluconazole	Diflucan	tablet
ketoconazole	Nizoral	tablet, cream, shampoo
metronidazole	Flagyl	capsule, tablet, gel, injection, powder
miconazole	Monistat	cream, lotion, powder, spray, suppository, injection
penicillin G benzathine	Bicillin L-A	IM
tetracycline	Achromycin	capsule, tablet, ointment, suspension, solution
tioconazole	Vagistat	cream
triple sulfa	Sultrin	tablet
	Trysul	cream
valacyclovir	Valtrex	capsule

Monistat (miconazole) and **GyneLotrimin (clotrimazole)** are used to treat *Candida albicans* infections.

CORTICOSTEROIDS

The adrenal glands are located on the top of the kidneys. The medulla on the inner portion produces catecholamines; the cortex on the outer produces glucocortico-steroids. They control glucose level, mineral balance, and sexual regulation. The medulla functions like the sympathetic nervous system.

The cortex produces glucocorticoids, primarily cortisol, responsible for gluconeogenesis, protein catabolism, anti-inflammatory reactions, stimulation of fat deposition, and sodium and water retention (steroids are necessary for mineral retention).

Steroid production begins in the hypothalamic-pituitary axis. The hypothalamus produces corticotropin releasing factor (CRF) which stimulates the pituitary to produce adrenocorticotropic hormone (ACTH), which enters the bloodstream and travels to the adrenal cortex, where cortisol is released into the blood and slows the action of the hypothalamus in producing and releasing CRF. Steroid production follows a circadian rhythm. Figure 15.3 shows that it peaks in the morning, and the low point occurs around midnight.

When the corticosteroid cortisol was isolated, a milestone in medicine was reached. Results of clinical trials in rheumatoid arthritis were dramatic, and soon cortisone was found to cause symptomatic improvement in an amazing number of disease states. Further research led to developing other corticosteroids that had greater anti-inflammatory potency and less effect on renal sodium reabsorption. This is true of prednisone, methylprednisolone, triamcinolone, and dexamethasone. These drugs are used as anti-inflammatory or immunosuppressive agents in treating a variety of diseases, including those of hematologic, allergic, inflammatory, neoplastic, and autoimmune origin.

Addison's disease is a life-threatening deficiency of glucocorticoids and mineralo-corticoids which is treated with daily administration of corticosteroid. Long-term use of corticosteroids may have several side effects. If steroids are stopped suddenly, however, the glands may stop working completely, so it is important to taper off the dosage. The symptoms include

◇ debilitating weakness (may have respiratory failure)
◇ weight loss

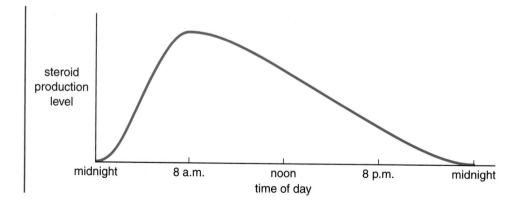

Figure 15.3

Steroid Production

- hyperpigmentation of skin, both labial and oral (bronze color produced by excessive melanin production)
- reduced blood pressure
- low levels of serum sodium and glucose
- hyperkalemia

Cushing's disease is caused by an overproduction of steroid; it can also result from excessive administration of corticosteroids over an extended period. Patients have a protruding abdomen and fat over the shoulder blades. Fat distribution may not go away even with cessation of the drug.

Corticosteroids are available in many dosage forms: tablets, syrups, injections, inhalants, nose drops, IV, creams, and lotions, to name a few. They play a significant role in treating asthma, rashes, and skin disorders. Hydrocortisone is produced by the adrenal cortex at a rate of approximately 20 mg per day. Equivalencies indicate how much or how little of each hormone it would take to equal the effect of 20 mg of hydrocortisone. Table 15.11 lists corticosteroid preparations in relation to the average daily secretion of hydrocortisone.

The major reason for using corticosteroids is to inhibit inflammation. Corticosteroids cause leukocytes to be sluggish; lessen the ability of these cells to destroy infection; decrease fever, redness, and swelling; and may cause an infection to spread. When taking a patient off steroids it is important to always taper the dose.

A patient taking a corticosteroid within the last twelve to eighteen months who is going into a stressful situation (e.g., surgery or tooth extraction) may need steroid supplementation.

Corticosteroids are often packed in dose packs. For example, the Medrol dose pack contains twenty-one 4 mg tablets. On the first day, the patient takes a loading dose and then decreases the dose each day thereafter. Package directions are self-explanatory. Corticosteroids come in every dosage form—cream, ointment, lotion, oral solution, tablet, suppository, IM, and IV.

Table 15.12 lists the adverse effects of glucocorticoids. Caution should be used in patients with diabetes mellitus, uncontrolled hypertension, tendency to congestive heart failure, severe infection or altered immunity, or peptic ulcer disease with active gastrointestinal bleeding. Glucocorticoids can cause hypothalamic-pituitary axis suppression related to the dose and duration. If given for a week or longer, there is a risk of adrenal insufficiency. If this happens, the corticosteroid should be tapered off and discontinued.

Table 15.11	Equivalency of Corticosteroid Preparations in Relation to the Average Daily Secretion of Hydrocortisone (20 mg)		
Corticosteroid	**Brand Name**	**Equivalency (mg)**	**Anti-Inflammatory Potency**
betamethasone	Diprolene	0.6	25.0
cortisone	Cortone	25.0	0.8
dexamethasone	Decadron	0.75	30.0
hydrocortisone	many	20.0	1.5
methylprednisolone	Medrol, Solu-Medrol	4.0	5.0
prednisolone	Pediapred	5.0	4.0
prednisone	Deltasone	5.0	3.0
triamcinolone	Aristocort	4.0	5.0

Table 15.12   Adverse Effects of Glucocorticoids Related to Dose and Duration

Type of Effect	Side Effect
cardiovascular	hypertension due to sodium retention
dermatologic	impaired wound healing
	striae and thinning of skin (thin facial skin; veins may be visible)
	petechiae and purpura
gastrointestinal	precipitation of peptic ulcer disease (irritating to the gastrointestinal tract)
	pancreatitis
immune system	infections
	suppression of skin test (reduces inflammation)
	reduces WBC function (suppresses WBCs in bone marrow)
	increases susceptibility to infections
metabolic	redistribution of fat deposits (truncal obesity, moon facies, buffalo hump)
	acne, hirsutism, menstrual irregularities
	growth suppression (children)
	hyperglycemia (diabetogenic)
	hypokalemia
	sodium and water retention leading to swelling and edema
musculoskeletal	osteoporosis, vertebral compression (bone reabsorption)
	spontaneous fractures
	aseptic necrosis of bone (death of bone, generally in the heads of long bones)
neuropsychiatric	alterations in mood and/or schizophrenic tendencies
	rebound of psychosis when drug is discontinued
	manic-depressive, suicidal, or schizophrenic tendencies
ophthalmic	cataracts due to precipitation with long-term use
	increased intraocular pressure, thus a potential for glaucoma

Corticosteroids are usually given in the morning in order to minimize the hypo-thalamic-pituitary axis suppression and side effects and to better mimic the natural circadian body rhythm. Frequently there is every-other-day dosing.

Steroid withdrawal can cause anorexia, nausea, and vomiting; mylagia and arthralgia; lethargy, headache, and sluggishness; weight loss; postural hypotension; fever; and depression.

HYPOGLYCEMIC AGENTS

The pancreas produces digestive enzymes that are deposited in the small intestine. Scattered throughout the pancreas are islets of specialized cells (islets of Langerhans). The two types of cells are alpha (produce glucagon, which raises blood sugar levels) and beta (produce insulin, which lowers blood glucose levels). Insulin helps cells burn glucose for energy, combines with membrane receptors to allow glucose uptake, enhances transport and incorporation of amino acids into protein, affects ion transport into tissues (increases transport), and inhibits fat breakdown.

One of every twenty-nine Americans has diabetes (lack of insulin). Diabetes is the third leading cause of death in the United States. There are fourteen million diabetics, but only seven million are diagnosed. All major organ systems can be damaged by diabetes. Over time, diabetes can destroy the eyesight, the kidneys, and the peripheral circulation. The results are blindness, need for dialysis, and lost limbs. Hypoglycemia is more dangerous acutely, but long-term hyperglycemia, if uncontrolled, is devastating. The normal blood glucose level is 100 mg/dL; if it is too high, glucose will spill into the urine. Levels consistently above 140 to 160 mg/dL are associated with long-term effects of diabetes.

Types of Diabetes

Type I diabetes most commonly occurs in children and young adults, but it may occur at any age. The average age of diagnosis is eleven or twelve years. These patients are insulin-dependent and have no ability to produce insulin. They may produce antibodies to islet cells (autoimmune response). This group comprises five to ten percent of the diabetic population.

Type II diabetes affects eighty to ninety percent of diabetic patients. They have a relative insulin insufficiency (impaired insulin secretion), often with insulin resistance. The peripheral target tissues are resistant to insulin produced. Glucose is not absorbed because cells do not respond to insulin. Most type II diabetics are overweight, and the best treatment is to lose weight. Most patients are over forty years of age, and there are more females than males affected.

Gestational diabetes occurs during pregnancy. The onset is during the second and third trimesters. It increases risk of fetal morbidity and death. Diabetes develops in thirty to forty percent of these mothers in five to ten years. It can be treated with diet, exercise, and insulin. Oral contraceptives raise blood glucose levels, especially in these women. It is debatable whether they should use this type of birth control.

Secondary diabetes is caused by drugs. Some of these drugs are OCs, beta blockers, diuretics, calcium channel blockers, glucocorticoids, and phenytoin.

Symptoms of diabetes include

- increased urination (polyuria) and nocturia (excessive urination at night)
- thirst
- hunger
- weight loss, easy fatigability, irritability, nausea, and ketoacidosis (ketonuria)
- vomiting
- visual changes
- glycosuria (presence of glucose in the urine)
- numbness and tingling
- slow wound healing (hyperglycemia inhibits activity of neutrophils, a type of WBC)
- frequent infections

Long-term complications of diabetes can destroy the quality of life. The following conditions can result from diabetes.

- Retinopathy is the leading cause of blindness in the United States. The vessels become damaged, resulting in insufficient blood supply; rupture causes loss of sight.
- Neuropathy is the result of a lack of blood flow to nerves, leaving them unable to function. Symptoms are dull aching to sharp stabbing pains.
- Vascular problems lead to atherosclerosis of peripheral coronary and cerebrovascular vessels. The decreased blood flow causes neuropathy and slows healing, especially in the feet and legs. Non-healing wounds can lead to amputation.
- Dermatologic involvement, often expressed as boils, acne, or fungal infections.
- Nephropathy or kidney damage occurs in 10–21% of diabetics and is the primary cause of end stage renal disease.

Lack of Insulin

A lack of insulin results in a conversion from glucose oxidation and metabolism to lipid oxidation and metabolism. The liver will over produce glucose in an effort to meet cellular energy needs, although excess glucose may already be in circulation. The term gluconeogenesis means the formation of new glucose and refers to the conversion of protein (amino acids) and fatty acids into immediate energy sources.

Fatty acids are oxidized into ketones (B-hydroxybutric acid, acetoacetic acid, and acetone). Without insulin, more ketones will be produced than can be either oxidized or excreted in the urine or eliminated by respiration. The ketones are stong acids that cause body pH to drop.

Hyperosmolar coma occurs in the type II diabetic, usually an elderly person with some kidney dysfunction. Plasma glucose is above 600 mg/dL of blood, whereas normal fasting glucose is 80–120 mg/dL of blood.

Lack of insulin leads to loss of water and glucose through the kidney and decreased kidney function. Reducing fluid intake further exacerbates the problem. Coma, kidney shutdown, thrombosis, vascular collapse, lactic acidosis, and death can occur. Replacing fluid is the highest priority, usually starting with hypotonic saline and followed by isotonic solutions.

Treating Diabetes

The goal of treatment is to approximate nondiabetic physiology as closely as possible. The treatment consists of diet, exercise, and medications. Blood glucose monitoring is very important for prevention of both acute and long-term complications and to guide treatment for reaching target fasting blood glucose goals. Because diabetics cannot use glucose; they metabolize fat, but lack energy for the liver to metabolize by-products of the fat. These by-products are ketones, which present through an odor on the breath. It is a fruity, acetone smell and may be mistaken for alcohol.

The stepwise approach for type II diabetes is

1. lifestyle changes
2. oral monotherapy
3. combination oral therapy
4. oral drug plus insulin
5. insulin only

Diabetes should be controlled to maintain fasting blood glucose levels between 80–120mg/dL to avoid long-term complications. Type I diabetics must have insulin. Type II diabetics may be able to control the disease through diet and exercise alone, but often have to add a drug and eventually may need insulin.

Patient education is an important feature of therapy. Acutely, hypoglycemia is more dangerous, but chronically, the long-term effects of diabetes can be devastating. If diabetes goes unchecked, the diabetic runs the risk of developing complications. Blindness often results from damage to the small blood vessels of the eyes.

Treatment guidelines for the patient are

- patient education
- attention to diet
- increased physical activity
- compliance with the medication regimen
- ability to recognize hypoglycemia
- setting individual goals
- monitoring progress at home through blood glucose testing
- monitoring progress at the doctor's office through measurement of glycosylated hemoglobin
- daily foot inspections
- prompt treatment of all infections
- blood pressure control
- control of hyperlipidemia

Diet is very important. Eating about the same amount of food on a consistent schedule every day makes it easier to keep insulin and food working together. Exercise is equally important. The diabetic should exercise regularly unless the blood glucose level is above 240 mg/dL or below 100 mg/dL. It is best to exercise about the same time each day.

Diabetic ulcers (open wounds which are typically slow to heal) are the leading cause of foot and leg amputation and the leading reason for hospital admissions among diabetics.

Diabetics must also take very good care of their feet which are particularly vulnerable to infections. These patients should be instructed to avoid the use of OTC foot products, unless directed by the physician. They should be instructed to moisturize their feet daily as a means to prevent the skin from cracking. They should also keep nails trimmed to avoid ingrown toenails.

Regranex (becaplermin gel) is a recombinant human platelet derived growth factor which speeds the healing of lower extremity diabetic ulcers. Some studies have shown that Regranex, which acts locally and has very little systemic effect, can actually increase the incidence of complete healing in the treatment of diabetic foot ulcer. If the wound does not decrease by thirty percent in ten weeks or heal in twenty weeks use of this drug should be reassessed.

When buying any food or OTC drug, the diabetic should always read the list of ingredients on the label. Many of these preparations could contain sugars. Some sugarless OTC products are listed in Table 15.13.

Insulin

Brittle diabetes is very difficult to control. Insulin needs may vary every six to eight hours. Normal fasting levels range from 80–100 mg/dL.

Human insulin is composed of two protein chains. Chain A has twenty-one amino acids and is acidic. Chain B has thirty amino acids and is basic. The two protein chains are joined by disulfide linking. Insulin is a protein that is enzymatically degraded in the GI tract, so it cannot be given orally. Insulin is administered subcutaneously.

Insulins are classified based on the time of pharmacological action as rapid acting, short acting, intermediate acting, and long acting. Most diabetic patients require a combination of shorter-acting insulin to cover post-meal glucose elevations and longer-acting insulin to provide basal levels throughout the day.

Regular insulin has a strong attraction between its own molecules. Insulin molecules clump together in groups of six. These clumps are called hexamers. Clumping delays absorption as the clumps slowly dissociate (break up). Absorption is delayed thirty to sixty minutes.

Warning

It is very easy to grab the wrong insulin in the refrigerator. Always double check insulins. They look exactly alike.

Table 15.13	Sugarless OTC Products	
Drug Type	**Brand**
analgesics	Panadol, Tempra
antacid	Di Gel liquid, Maalox, Mylanta, Phosphagel, Riopan, Titralac
antidiarrheal	Pepto-Bismol
cough drops	Cepastat, Nice
cough syrups	Codimal DM, Naldecon, Novahistine, Robitussin, Tavist
laxatives	Correctol, Fiberall, Konsyl

Short-acting insulins differ in action due to replacing an amino acid or changing positions of amino acids on a chain. Modifying the structure of the insulin molecule prevents hexamer formation. The result is faster onset of action (fifteen to thirty minutes) and shorter time to peak action for a dose (thirty to ninety minutes), but also makes duration of action shorter.

Table 15.14 lists the types of insulin available and the duration of action for each type.

Insulin has adverse effects of which every diabetic should be aware. There is risk of hypoglycemia due to excessive dosage, inappropriate timing of meals, or exercise. If a patient is experiencing hypoglycemia, this could be due to several factors: skipping or not finishing meals, too much exercise, a poorly adjusted medication regimen, or certain drugs (anabolic steroids, beta blockers, disopyramide, ethanol, pentamidine, salicylates, sulfonamides, phenobarbital, and quinine). There can be lipoatrophy from decreased subcutaneous fat at injection site (depression), therefore, injections sites should be rotated frequently. Also, more insulin may be required during stress, infection, and pregnancy.

When mixing two insulins, regular insulin should be drawn up first. Regular and Lente do not mix, but regular and NPH are stable. Glargine should not be mixed with any other insulin. Insulin should not be injected into an area that will receive a rigorous workout. The injection sites should be rotated. Figure 15.4 illustrates the method of rotating insulin administration sites. Insulin enters blood best from the abdomen, then the arms and legs, and last the buttocks.

Signs and symptoms of hypoglycemia, are

- thirst
- hunger
- nervousness
- sweating
- palpitations
- headache
- double vision
- confusion
- weakness
- visual disturbances
- numbness and tingling in mouth and lips

Treatment of hypoglycemia (blood glucose < 70 mg/dL) necessitates giving the patient additional sugars. Milk or sugars in any form (fruit juices, soft drinks, or candy) are highly effective. Diabetics should carry candy with them at all times. Glucose tablets are available, and Type I diabetics should have a Glucagon kit. It requires a prescription.

Humalog (lispro) is a rapid onset insulin which allows patients to inject it immediately before or after meals. In this way, the dose can be adjusted depending on the amounts and types of foods eaten. In addition, blood glucose can be tested and then the drug can be dosed accordingly.

Table 15.14   Insulin's Duration of Action

Type	Duration of Action
regular	5 to 6 hours (starts working in 30 minutes)
NPH	10 to 16 hours
Lente	12 to 18 hours
Ultralente	18 to 20 hours
Humalog, NovoLog	1 hour (works in 15 minutes, gone in about 1 hour; more closely mimics natural insulin release)
Lantus	24 hours (no peak of action)

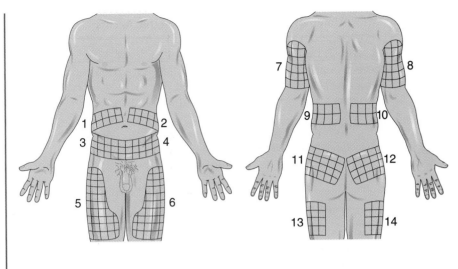

NovoLog (insulin aspart) is a rapid-acting insulin analog. It is similar to Humalog. Each dose should be injected before meals. A longer-acting insulin to maintain glucose may be needed because it is so short acting. It is made by substituting one of insulin's amino acids with aspartic acid. Humalog uses lysine.

Lantus (insulin glargine) is a synthetic, long acting insulin which differs from human insulin by only three amino acids. It is associated with less nocturnal hypoglcemia and weight gain than conventional insulin. Lantus precipitates when injected in subcutaneous tissue. The precipitate causes the insulin to be absorbed slowly with a relatively constant blood level over twenty-four hours. There is no noticeable peak in action and it more closely approximates physiologic insulin release.

Oral Hypoglycemic Agents

Oral hypoglycemic agents cause the pancreas to release stored insulin. They are not effective in Type I diabetes, because there is no insulin available for the body to release. Table 15.15 presents the most-commonly used oral hypoglycemic agents.

FIRST-GENERATION SULFONYLUREAS First-generation sulfonylureas increase insulin release. They are older drugs with more side effects than more recent agents.

SECOND-GENERATION SULFONYLUREAS Glucotrol and Glucotrol XL (glipizide) are taken with breakfast. If Glucotrol is switched to the XL form, it should be given in the same total daily dose. This drug promotes release of insulin from beta cells of the pancreas, increases insulin sensitivity at peripheral sites, and lowers blood glucose concentration.

DiaBeta, Glynase, and Micronase (glyburide) are supplied in micronized dosage forms. They are an adjunct to diet and exercise in management of diabetes.

Amaryl (glimepiride) causes a lesser degree of hypoglycemia than glyburide. It should be taken with breakfast or the first main meal.

ENZYME INHIBITORS Precose (acarbose) inhibits intestinal wall enzymes that convert saccharides into glucose, thereby lowering postprandial hyperglycemia. For "hypoglycemia" while taking this drug, the patient should use oral glucose tablets, since

Table 15.15   Most-Commonly Used Oral Hypoglycemic Agents

Generic Name	Brand Name	Dosage Form
First-Generation Sulfonylureas		
acetohexamide	Dymelor	tablet
chlorpropamide	Diabinese	tablet
tolazamide	Tolinase	tablet
tolbutamide	Orinase	tablet
Second-Generation Sulfonylureas		
glimepiride	Amaryl	tablet
glipizide	Glucotrol, Glucotrol XL	tablet
glyburide	DiaBeta, Glynase, Micronase	tablet
Enzyme Inhibitors		
acarbose	Precose	tablet
miglitol	Glyset	tablet
Biguanide		
metformin	Glucophage	tablet
Glitazones		
pioglitazone	Actos	tablet
rosiglitazone	Avandia	tablet

Warning

Acetazolamide looks like acetohexamide.

Warning

Chlorpropamide is similar to chlor-promazine.

sucrose and other sugars are inhibited in the conversion. The primary side effects of acarbose are abdominal pain, diarrhea, and flatulence (gas), which may be due to undigested carbohydrates undergoing digestion by bacteria in the large bowel. The drug is contraindicated in the presence of cirrhosis, inflammatory bowel disease, colon ulceration, and intestinal obstruction.

Glyset (miglitol), like Precose, reduces hyperglycemia by slowing carbohydrate absorption in the small intestine. Side effects are similar to Precose. Glyset is indicated in the treatment of type II diabetes and is prescribed both as a first-line monotherapy or in combination with other medications.

BIGUANIDE **Glucophage (metformin)** decreases intestinal absorption of glucose and improves insulin sensitivity. This drug rarely causes hypoglycemia and has a favorable effect on serum lipids. It should be used with caution in patients with liver, heart, or lung disease. The dose should be increased over several weeks, and it should be taken with food. The drug is withheld for eighteen hours before testing with iodinated material. It interacts with cimetidine, vitamin B_{12}, and folic acid. It is synergistic with sulfonylureas. Side effects are nausea, metallic aftertaste, and weight loss. The best candidates are overweight diabetics with a high lipid profile. The drug decreases triglyceride levels and blood pressure. Lactic acidosis is a rare, but possible, sequela.

GLITAZONES **Actos (pioglitazone)** lowers blood glucose by improving cellular response to insulin. Its activity thus depends on the presence of insulin. Liver enzymes should be carefully monitored for elevated enzyme levels every two months for the first twelve months. Side effects due to increased plasma volume include elevated HDL levels, lowered triglyceride levels, weight gain, anemia, and edema. Actos may be taken without regard to food. Patients taking this drug must avoid alcohol.

Avandia (rosiglitazone) increases insulin sensitivity in muscle and adipose tissues. It is indicated in the treatment of hyperglycemia and is prescribed alone or as an adjunct to metformin. The side effects of Avandia are similar to those listed for Actos. Avandia can be taken without regard to food.

GROWTH HORMONE

From childhood to adulthood, growth hormone (GH) is a fundamental part of the process of metabolism. Measurements of height and weight over time serve as an index of physical and emotional health. Growth failure is a well-recognized disorder of childhood. In many children a deficiency of endogenous growth hormone causes growth retardation, which may be treated with exogenous hormone replacement.

Some causes of growth delay are malnutrition, systemic illness, endocrine deficiency, psychosocial stress, or a combination of these. Growth rates vary by sex and age throughout childhood. Endocrine function greatly affects growth and development in childhood. Thyroxine, cortisol, insulin, and GH all affect skeletal and somatic growth. Other factors include family growth patterns, genetic disorders, extreme stress, and chronic disease.

Nonendocrine-related disorders include intrauterine growth retardation, chromosomal defects, abnormal growth of cartilage or bone, poor nutrition, and a variety of systemic diseases. Some patients show a variation from normal growth (constitutional growth delay); these patients include those who are small for their age and those who have delay in skeletal growth, in onset of puberty, and in adolescent development. They begin their growth spurt after other children and continue to grow when their peers have stopped. Another type of growth delay is family or genetically related (short stature). These patients are shorter than their peers, but are comparable in height with other family members and grow at a parallel rate. Puberty occurs at the expected time and progresses as usual. However, adult height is short (less than 5'4" for men and less than 4'11" for women).

Growth hormone deficiency occurs in one in 5,000 children in a male-female ratio of four to one. Among the known causes are intracranial infection (from TB and meningitis), skull fracture, radiation, and cancer.

GH is released in response to growth hormone releasing factor (GHRF), a mixture of peptides from the pituitary gland. The major component is the peptide somatropin. The pituitary releases GH in response to stimulation by GHRF, which is secreted by the hypothalamus. GH release occurs irregularly throughout the day and during sleep stages III and IV. It is inhibited by glucocorticoids, obesity, depression, progesterone, hypokalemia, and altered thyroid function. GH stimulates the growth of skeletal muscle and connective tissue. It increases the rate of protein synthesis and fatty acid mobilization from adipose tissue and decreases the rate of glucose use.

The younger the patient at the time of treatment, the greater is the height that may be achieved with GH replacement. Bone age and the extent of epiphyseal fusion at the time of treatment also influence the eventual response to GH. Little response is seen after ages fifteen to sixteen years in boys or fourteen to fifteen years in girls. About eighty percent to ninety percent of patients who receive GH experience "catch-up" growth. Maximal increases in growth velocity occur within the first six to twelve months of therapy, with a decline in response after that. GH therapy should be continued throughout childhood and adolescence to avoid slowing of growth velocity. When epiphyseal closure has occurred, little further response can be expected. Treatment duration usually varies from two to ten years. GH has not been effective in families of short stature; growth retardation associated with psychosocial dwarfism; steroid-induced short stature; Down's syndrome; bone and cartilage disorders; or renal, GI, or cardiac disease.

Originally, supplies of **somatropin** were taken from the pituitary of human cadavers, requiring twenty to thirty cadavers to obtain sufficient hormone to treat one patient. Today the drug is supplied through recombinant DNA technology. Genetic material from the human cell is inserted into microorganisms, the organism reproduces with the genes, and this produces the hormone. The hormone is recovered, purified, and packaged. This process is illustrated in Chapter 17.

Table 15.16 presents the most-commonly used growth-promotion agents.

One problem with growth-promotion agents is antibody formation. As many as thirty to eighty percent of treated patients may develop antibodies. Antibody formed within the first three months may affect growth; a later formed antibody does not. Less than one percent of treated patients have antibody-induced altered growth.

Hypothyroidism has been observed in less than five percent of treated patients. However, thyroid supplementation is unnecessary unless the patient has thyroid deficiency during treatment. It appears to be more a conversion of thyroxine or thyroid-controlling hormone change rather than a true deficiency. Glucose intolerance may develop. Transient immune changes may reduce beta-lymphocyte numbers with variations in T helper and T suppressor numbers also. There may be some pain and pruritus at the injection site. In adults, acromegaly may occur, or diabetes mellitus, hypertension, or atherosclerosis may develop.

Table 15.16 Most-Commonly Used Growth-Promotion Agents

Generic Name	Brand Name	Dosage Form
somatrem	Protropin	IM, SC
somatropin	Humatrope	IM, SC

Chapter Summary

Thyroid Hormones

- The endocrine system maintains the body's homeostasis by regulating physiologic functions involved in normal daily living and stress.
- Regulation of hormone synthesis is achieved via an intricate negative feedback mechanism involving the gland, the hypothalamic-pituitary axis, and autoregulation. Glands produce hormones that stimulate various body tissues to increase the level of activity. The affected tissue is called the target.
- Thyroid replacement activity should not be used to treat obesity.
- Hypothyroidism is treated with Synthroid, Levoxine, Cytomel, and Thyrolar.
- Hyperthyroidism is treated with PTU and Tapazole; both drugs cause altered taste and mild alopecia.

Adrenal Sex Hormones and Male Impotence

- Testosterone undergoes extensive first-pass metabolism in the gastrointestinal tract and liver after oral administration. To overcome this problem, various testosterone derivatives have been developed, as well as other dosage forms.
- Testosterone substances are classified as schedule III.
- Impotence may have many causes, including testosterone deficiency, alcoholism, cigarette smoking, medications, and psychological factors.
- The following drugs may cause impotence: alcohol, amphetamines, antidepressants, antihypertensives, corticosteroids, estrogens, haloperidol, H_2 blockers, lithium, and opiates.
- Alcohol is a primary reason for male dysfunction.
- The testosterone patch not only increases libido and sexual potency, but also improves the patient's sense of well-being.

Female Hormones

- Progestins are used primarily in birth control pills and to prevent uterine cancer in the postmenopausal woman on estrogen replacement therapy.
- The side effects of progestin are weight gain, depression, fatigue, acne, and hirsutism.
- ERT prevents bone loss, lowers cholesterol, improves color and turgor of skin, and improves mental functions.
- The adverse effects of estrogen are nausea, fluid retention, breast tenderness, vomiting, weight gain, and breakthrough bleeding. Hypercoagulability is also attributed to estrogen use, especially if combined with nicotine.
- The advantages of oral contraceptives include ease of use, high efficacy rate, and relative safety. Most are a combination of estrogen and progestin. They suppress ovulation by interfering with the production of hormones that regulate the menstrual cycle. They also alter the cervical mucus to prevent penetration of sperm and change the composition of the endometrium to inhibit implantation. The progestin-only pills rely on the effects of the progestin on the cervical mucus and endometrium.
- Many women taking "the pill" experience more regular menstrual cycles, reduced menstrual flow, and less severe menstrual pain and cramps. There is evidence that oral contraceptives may protect against ovarian and endometrial

cancer, benign breast disease, ectopic pregnancy, fibroadenomas, and ovarian cysts. This may also reduce the risk of pelvic inflammatory disease.

◇ Some studies indicate that birth control pills should not be prescribed to women who have hypertension, diabetes mellitus, or elevated cholesterol. Women should not smoke while on "the pill."

◇ "The pill" should be taken at the same time every day. Taking it at bedtime reduces the possibility of nausea and skin discoloration.

◇ Lunelle is an injectable contraceptive that in many states may be administered in the pharmacy by the pharmacist.

◇ Oral contraceptives can interact with the following classes of drugs: antibiotics, anticonvulsants, antifungals, benzodiazepines, bronchodilators, corticosteroids, lipid-lower agents, and TCAs.

◇ Pregnancy tests are based on detecting the hormone HCG.

Drugs for Bone Diseases

◇ Lifestyle changes to decrease bone loss are related to calcium intake, cigarette smoking, alcohol abuse, and weight-bearing exercises.

◇ Fosamax is approved by the FDA for the treatment of osteoporosis. It should be taken thirty minutes before the first meal of the day with a full glass of water, and the patient must not lie down for thirty minutes after taking it and should not take food before thirty minutes. It is 100- to 150-fold more potent as an inhibitor of bone resorption than is etidronate.

◇ Miacalcin should be reserved for women who refuse or cannot tolerate ERT or in whom ERT is contraindicated.

◇ Tums is an inexpensive way to get one's daily supply of calcium. It prevents a negative calcium balance, a factor in osteoporosis.

Drugs for Sexually Transmitted Diseases

◇ Most diseases of the genital system are transmitted by sexual activity and are, therefore, called sexually transmitted diseases (STDs). Gonorrhea is the most commonly reported STD.

Corticosteroids

◇ Corticosteroids are used as anti-inflammatories and immunosuppressants and in treating diseases of hematologic, allergic, neoplastic, and autoimmune origin.

◇ The major reason for using corticosteroids is to inhibit inflammation.

◇ Addison's disease is a deficiency of steroids; Cushing's disease is an overproduction or excessive administration of steroids over an extended period.

◇ Corticosteroids have adverse effects with metabolic, cardiovascular, gastrointestinal, immunologic, dermatologic, musculoskeletal, ophthalmic, and neuropsychiatric implications. They should be used with great caution in diabetes, hypertension, CHF, severe infections, and PUD. HPA axis suppression is dose-related. If possible, patients should take the dose in the morning to minimize HPA axis suppression and side effects. This more closely mimics the body's release of corticosteroids—circadian rhythm.

Hypoglycemic Agents

- Scattered throughout the pancreas are islets of specialized cells. Alpha cells produce glucagon, which raises blood sugar; beta cells produce insulin and lower blood sugar levels.
- The four types of diabetes are type I, type II, gestational, and secondary.
- Type I diabetics must have insulin. Type II may be able to control the disease through diet and exercise, but often have to add a drug or even insulin. Gestational diabetes usually returns to normal after the baby's birth, but the mother is at high risk of developing type II diabetes. Secondary (drug-induced) diabetes can return to normal when the drug is discontinued.
- Short-term hypoglycemia is more dangerous, but long-term hyperglycemia has devastating complications. Retinopathy, neuropathy, nephropathy, and vascular and dermatologic complications can affect the quality and length of life.
- Insulin does not require a prescription, but needles and syringes may.
- Humalog is a rapid onset insulin which allows patients to inject it immediately before or after meals.
- Lantus (insulin glargine) is a long acting insulin which provides a constant concentration level over twenty-four hours. It more closely approximates physiological insulin release.

Growth Hormone

- Measurement of height and weight over time serves as an index of physical and emotional health. A deficiency of growth hormone causes growth failure.
- Once epiphyseal closure has occurred, little further response to GH treatment can be expected.
- Somatropin is supplied through recombinant DNA technology.

Drug Summary

The following drugs were discussed in this chapter. Each generic drug name is followed in parentheses by one or more brand names. An asterisk (*) indicates drugs frequently written using *either* brand *or* generic name. These need to be memorized.

Thyroid Preparations
levothyroxine, T_4 (Synthroid, Levothroid, Lovoxyl)*
liothyronine, T_3 (Cytomel)
liotrix (Thyrolar)
methimazole (Tapazole)
propylthiouracil (PTU)
radioactive iodine, ^{131}I
thyroid (Armour Thyroid)

Drugs to Treat Male Impotence
alprostadil (Edex, Muse, Caverject)
danazol (Danocrine, Cyclomen)
methyltestosterone (Android, Testred)
oxymetholone (Anadrol)
papaverine (Pavabid)
sildenafil (Viagra)
testosterone (Androderm, Duratest, Testoderm, Androgel)*

Progestins
hydroxyprogesterone (Hylutin, Gesterol)
levonorgestrel (Norplant)
medroxyprogesterone (Amen, Provera, Depo-Provera, Cycrin)*

Estrogens
conjugated estrogen (Premarin)
conjugated estrogen-medroxyproges-terone (Prempro, Premphase)
diethylstilbestrol (Stilphostrol)
estradiol (Estrace, Estraderm, Vivelle, Climara)
estradiol-norgestimate (Ortho-Prefest)
estradiol-northidrone acetate (Activella)
estropipate (Ogen)
ethinyl estradiol (Estinyl)
ethinyl estradiol-norethindrone acetate (Femhrt)

Contraceptives
Biphasic
ethinyl estradiol-ethynodiol diacetate (Demulen)

ethinyl estradiol-levonorgestrel (Levlen, Tri-Levlen, Triphasil)
ethinyl estradiol-norethindrone (Genora, Loestrin, Ortho Novum, Ovcom)
ethinyl estradiol-norgestrel (Lo/Ovral, Ovral)
mestranol-norethindrone (Genora 1/50)
Progestin
norgestrel (Ovrette)
Parenteral
estradiol cypionate-medroxyproges-terone (Lunelle)
medroxyprogesterone (Depo-Provera)
Implant
levonorgestrel (Norplant)

Agents for Bone Diseases
alendronate (Fosamax)
calcitonin-salmon (Miacalcin)
calcium (Tums, Caltrate, Os-Cal, Titralac, Viactiv)
etidronate (Didronel)
raloxifene (Evista)
risedronate (Actonel)

Agents for Sexually Transmitted Diseases
acyclovir (Zovirax)
ceftriaxone (Rocephin)
clotrimazole (GyneLotrimin, Lotrimin)
doxycycline (Doryx)
erythromycin
fluconazole (Diflucan)
ketoconazole (Nizoral)
metronidazole (Flagyl)
miconazole (Monistat)
penicillin G benzathine (Bicillin L-A)
tetracycline (Achromycin)
tioconazole (Vagistat)
triple sulfa (Sultrin, Trysul)
valacyclovir (Valtrex)

Corticosteroids
betamethasone (Diprolene)
cortisone (Cortone)
dexamethasone (Decadron)*
hydrocortisone (many)
methylprednisolone (Medrol, Solu-Medrol)*
prednisolone (Pediapred)*
prednisone (Deltasone)*
triamcinolone (Aristocort)*

Platelet-Derived Growth Factor
becalpermin gel (Regranex)

Insulins
Humulin
insulin glargine (Lantus)
insulin aspart (Norvolog)
lispro (Humalog)
Novolin

Oral Hypoglycemics
First-Generation Sulfonylureas
acetohexamide (Dymelor)
chlorpropamide (Diabinese)
tolazamide (Tolinase)
tolbutamide (Orinase)
Second-Generation Sulfonylureas
glimepiride (Amaryl)
glipizide (Glucotrol, Glucotrol XL)
glyburide (DiaBeta, Glynase, Micronase)
Enzyme Inhibitors
acarbose (Precose)
miglitol (Glyset)
Biguanide
metformin (Glucophage)
Glitazones
pioglitazone (Actos)
rosiglitazone (Avandia)

Growth Hormones
somatropin (Humatrope)*
somatrem (Protropin)

Chapter Review

Pharmaceuticals and Body Functions

Select the best answer from the choices given.

1. The thyroid hormones T_3 and T_4 are both formed from
    a. serotonin.
    b. thyroglobulin.
    c. acetylcholine.
    d. norepinephrine.

2. The most frequently prescribed thyroid agent is
    a. Synthroid.
    b. Thyrolar.
    c. Cytomel.
    d. All of the above

3. Hydrocortisone has the same activity as
    a. cortisol.
    b. prednisolone.
    c. prednisone.
    d. methylprednisolone.

4. Oral contraceptives may interact with all the listed drugs except
    a. antifungals.
    b. antibiotics.
    c. NSAIDs.
    d. TCAs.

5. All the listed drugs can cause secondary diabetes, except
    a. beta blockers.
    b. birth control pills.
    c. glucocorticoids.
    d. NSAIDs.

6. Which drug decreases intestinal enzyme conversion of sugars into glucose?
    a. Glucophage
    b. Regranex
    c. Precose
    d. Glucotrol

7. For which type of diabetes is insulin always indicated?
    a. Type I
    b. Type II
    c. Gestational
    d. All of the above

8. The steroid with the most anti-inflammatory potency is
   a. hydrocortisone.
   b. prednisone.
   c. dexamethasone.
   d. triamcinolone.

9. Which drug is for osteoporosis?
   a. Fosamax
   b. Glucophage
   c. Flagyl
   d. Protropin

10. Most diseases of the genital system are transmitted by
    a. using public bathrooms.
    b. not going to the bathroom when one really needs to.
    c. uncleanliness.
    d. sexual activity.

The following statements are true or false. If the answer is false, rewrite the statement so it is true.

_____ 1. Steroids are frequently dosed every other day to avoid HPA axis involvement.

_____ 2. Treatment of the diabetic includes diet, exercise, and medication.

_____ 3. Caution should be used in treating patients with corticosteroids if they have diabetes, severe infection, or PUD.

_____ 4. There is considerable evidence that oral birth control pills protect against ovarian cancer.

_____ 5. Pregnancy tests are based on detecting the hormone HPA.

_____ 6. Steroid levels are highest at 7 to 8 p.m.

_____ 7. The major reason for using corticosteroids is to inhibit inflammation.

_____ 8. The risk of hyperglycemia is more important acutely, and of hypoglycemia, long term.

_____ 9. Androgens do not have a feedback control.

_____ 10. Androderm is a system that should be applied to the scrotum.

Diseases and Drug Therapies

1. List the positive effects and side effects of estrogen.
2. List the symptoms of diabetes.
3. List the conditions in which estrogen is contraindicated.
4. List and identify the differences in the thyroid medications.
5. What are some causes for growth delay?

Match the following adjectives with the listed drugs.
   a. first generation
   b. second generation
   c. enzyme inhibitor
   d. biguanide

   1. Glucophage   _____
   2. Precose   _____
   3. glyburide   _____
   4. chlorpropamide   _____
   5. Tolinase   _____

Match the following two diseases with the listed symptoms.
   a. Addison's disease
   b. Cushing's disease

   1. deficiency of glucocorticoids _____
   2. overproduction or excessive administration of steroids over an
       extended period _____
   3. buffalo hump _____
   4. round, puffy face _____
   5. weakness (respiratory failure) _____

Dispensing Medications

   1. Mrs. Jones is picking up the following prescription. What definite instructions
       should she be given?

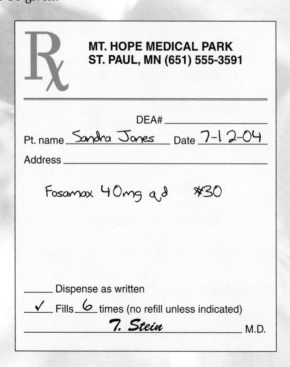

MT. HOPE MEDICAL PARK
ST. PAUL, MN (651) 555-3591

DEA# _____
Pt. name _Sandra Jones_   Date _7-12-04_
Address _____

Fosamax 40mg qd   #30

____ Dispense as written
_✓_ Fills _6_ times (no refill unless indicated)
            7. Stein _____ M.D.

2. Betty Sue Jones brings in the following prescriptions. Identify the problem areas.

```
  R     MT. HOPE MEDICAL PARK
   x     ST. PAUL, MN (651) 555-3591
  _____

                 DEA#_____
  Pt. name Brenda O'Donnell  Date 7-16-04
  Address _____

     DiabeTa 5 mg q am      #30
     Inderal 5 mg q d       #30
     Medrol dose pack — Take as directed
     Premarin 2.5 mg q d  #30


  _____ Dispense as written
    ✓  Fills 6 times (no refill unless indicated)
          T. Stein              ___ M.D.
```

3. Mary Lee delivered an eleven-pound boy. She is doing well and is ready to return to work. She has a UTI and brings in the following prescription. Check her profile and identify the problem areas.

```
  R     MT. HOPE MEDICAL PARK
   x     ST. PAUL, MN (651) 555-3591
  _____

                 DEA#_____
  Pt. name Angela Kamps  Date 12-6-04
  Address _____

     Macrodantin q 6 hours  100mg
            Take with food        #28
     Pyridium tid  100 mg      #10
     Ovral q d    #28


  _____ Dispense as written        (Ovral only)
    ✓  Fills 12 times (no refill unless indicated)
          T. Stein              ___ M.D.
```

Patient Profile

Patient name __Angela Kamps__
Address __7243 Sandpiper Cove__
Age __28__   Sex __F__   Race __Cau__   Height __5'6"__   Weight __130__
Allergies __none__

DIAGNOSES

__gestational dibetes__

MEDICATIONS

Date	No.	Prescriber	Drug and Strength	Quantity	Sig	Refills
6/04	103	T. Stein	Prenatal vitamins	30	qd	6
10/04	1002	T. Stein	Humalog	2	prn	prn

Internet Research

Use the Internet to complete the following activities.

1. Osteoporosis is the most common bone disease affecting the Western world. Use the Internet to find out who is at risk for this disease and how it is diagnosed? Who should be screened? List your Internet sources.
2. Patient education is an important part of managing diabetes. Find three Internet sites that help address this need. Create a table comparing and contrasting the sites. For each site list its strengths and weakness in two separate columns.

Topicals, Ophthalmics, and Otics

16

Learning Objectives

- ◇ Describe the skin as an organ.
- ◇ Understand the physiology of the skin.
- ◇ Recognize the classes of antiseptics and disinfectants.
- ◇ Identify the parasites that infest the skin.
- ◇ Know the topical drugs and the conditions they treat.
- ◇ Explain the action of the topical corticosteroids and their application.
- ◇ Recognize the ophthalmic and otic agents and their uses.

These classes of drugs range from mild agents to stronger forms of antibiotics, antiseptics, disinfectants, and corticosteroids. They treat a variety of conditions, such as skin disorders, allergic and inflammatory reactions, infections, infestations, glaucoma, conjunctivitis, and otalgia.

STRUCTURE AND FUNCTION OF SKIN

The skin is a major organ that accounts for ten percent of body weight. It is equipped to deal with microbiologic, chemical, and physical assaults on the body. It is an important source of sensory input and is the main organ involved in temperature regulation. Correction of skin defects may be indicated even when there is no hazard to health because of the mental attitude of the affected person or of society.

Figure 16.1 illustrates the anatomy of the skin. Epidermis is the top layer of the skin and is derived from embryonic ectoderm. It continually forms new cells in a basal layer and produces nails, hair, and glands. Pressure or friction on any part of the body stimulates skin growth, resulting in a thickening called a callus. Melanocytes are interspersed, often slightly below the basal layer, with cytoplasmic processes extending between the epidermal cells. These cells produce melanin.

Dermis is composed of connective tissue with upward projections into the epidermis. It is supplied with capillaries and sensory nerve terminals that do not penetrate the epidermis. The dermis contains smooth muscle in hair follicles (arrector pili), in sheets of the areola of the nipple, and in the scrotum, which causes wrinkled skin.

Eccrine (sweat) glands are simple tube glands; they are numerous on the palms and soles and secrete fluids rich in glycogen, some mucopolysaccharides, and urea. Their function is to regulate temperature.

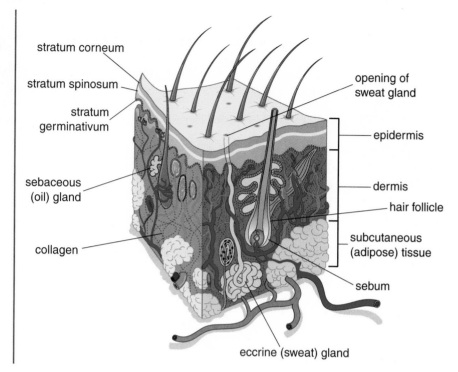

Figure 16.1

Anatomy of the Skin

stratum corneum

stratum spinosum

stratum germinativum

sebaceous (oil) gland

collagen

opening of sweat gland

epidermis

dermis

hair follicle

subcutaneous (adipose) tissue

sebum

eccrine (sweat) gland

Apocrine (sweat) glands are found primarily in the axillary, perineal, and genital regions. Their secretions contain protein, carbohydrates, and lipids. These glands become active at adolescence. Body odor arises from bacterial decomposition of constituents of apocrine sweat. The secretions of modified apocrine glands in the skin of the external ear canal, together with squamous cells and dust, make up cerumen (earwax), which has antibacterial and antifungal activity.

DISORDERS OF THE SKIN AND AGENTS TO TREAT THEM

Skin disorders may present as a variety of conditions. Diagnosis of abnormalities may be revealed by characteristics such as size, color, shape, location of the problem, and other symptoms that are either present or absent. A biopsy may be taken for microscopic examination which could further expose the exact nature and extent of the skin problem. Such conditions may be confined to the skin or reveal disease processes affecting the entire body.

Disorders of the Sebaceous Glands

Seborrhea is a skin condition caused by excessive secretion, which gives the skin an oily appearance, especially in areas where glands are most active. This condition can fluctuate in severity as a result of stress.

Acne vulgaris results from increased glandular activity at puberty, when glands enlarge and become more productive. Acne usually resolves in early adulthood, but chronic forms or severe exacerbations may last into adult life. Lesions are most common on the head and neck. They begin when the terminal of a sebaceous duct becomes plugged, forming a blackhead. It is characterized by elevated sebum secretion. The gland and hair follicle become engorged with sebum to form a papule. If contents of the papule become infected, it turns into a pustule surrounded by an inflamed area. Most cases respond to ultraviolet light. Maintaining free-flowing sebum is the aim of treatment. Washing with soap and water also has a drying effect. Systemic treatment with antibiotics (tetracycline and, to a lesser extent, erythromycin or clindamycin) has been helpful in moderate to severe acne. Treatment may have to be continued for long periods. **Retin-A (retinoic acid)** is a topical approved for treatment of this disorder.

Pruritus

Pruritus (itching) is associated with a number of skin disorders, such as urticaria (rash), infections, or irritation from powder. Topically applied baths may contain starch, sodium bicarbonate, magnesium sulfate (Epsom salts), colloidal oatmeal, or potassium permanganate. Camphor in liniments and ointments has a cooling, antipruritic effect. Several systemic diseases cause itching, among them, liver disease, uremia, Hodgkin's disease, diabetes, thyroid disorders, pregnancy, senility, and psychological and psychiatric disorders. Antihistamines are often used to relieve itching.

Ultraviolet Radiation and Phototoxicity

Reaction to ultraviolet radiation can be suppressed by anti-inflammatory drugs, steroidal and nonsteroidal. For severe sunburn, corticosteroids are usually used. Aspirin can reduce irritation, pain, and edema. With prolonged exposure, the skin undergoes hypermelanization and hyperkeratosis. Fair-skinned persons are more likely to have atrophy and scaling of the epidermis than dark-skinned persons. Skin cancer is more prevalent in lightly pigmented persons than in those with dark skin. Tumors grow more often in exposed than in covered or shaded areas of the body.

There are several categories of skin cancer.

- Basal cell carcinoma is slow growing, usually forming polyps, and rarely metastasizing.
- Squamous cell carcinoma grows more rapidly, and cells tend to keratinize; metastasis is uncommon.
- Keratoacanthoma is an epithelial tumor that first grows rapidly, but usually regresses and heals.
- Melanoma forms from melanocytes and is highly malignant. Sunburn greatly increases the risk of this skin disorder.
- Actinic keratosis is a precancerous condition resulting from overexposure to sunlight.

Phototoxicity is an excessive response to solar radiation in the presence of a sensitizing agent. Topical agents causing phototoxicity are found in medications, suntan preparations, scents, cosmetics, certain dyes, and industrial products. Systemically administered drugs, such as sulfonylureas, sulfonamides, thiazide diuretics, phenothiazines, chlordiazepoxide, tetracycline antibiotics, and antifungal agents, can all cause photosensitivity. To block this, sunscreens that protect against UV-A and UV-B rays should be applied; they should contain a combination of oxybenzone and aminobenzoic acid or combinations of other agents that block both UV-A and UV-B rays. The UV-A spectrum is sometimes referred to as the suntanning region, and UV-B as the sunburn region. Drugs that can cause photosensitivity are listed in Table 16.1.

Table 16.1   **Drugs That Cause Photosensitivity**

Drug Class	Drug Example	
	Generic	*Brand*
ACE inhibitors	all agents	
antibiotics	azithromycin	Zithromax
	tetracyclines	
	griseofulvin	Fulvicin, Grisactin
	sulfas	
	quinolones	
antidepressants	clomipramine	Anafranil
	maprotiline	Ludiomil
	sertraline	Zoloft
	tricyclic antidepressants (TCAs)	
antihistamines	cyproheptadine	Periactin
	diphenhydramine	Benadryl
antipsychotics	haloperidol	Haldol
	phenothiazines	
cardiovascular drugs	amiodarone	Cordarone
	diltiazem	Cardizem
	disopyramide	Norpace
	lovastatin	Mevacor
	nifedipine	Procardia
	pravastatin	Pravachol
	quinidine	Quinaglute
	simvastatin	Zocor
	sotalol	Betapace
chemotherapeutic agents	dacarbazine	DTIC
	fluorouracil, 5-FU	Adrucil
	methotrexate	Mexate, Rheumatrex
	procarbazine	Matulane, Natulan
	vinblastine	Velban, Velbe
diuretics	acetazolamide	Diamox
	furosemide	Lasix
	metolazone	Zaroxolyn
	thiazides	
hypoglycemics	sulfonylureas	
NSAIDs	all agents	

Allergic and Inflammatory Reactions

Eczema is a hot, itchy, red, oozing condition characteristic of an acute stage of inflammation.

Contact dermatitis is an inflammatory reaction produced by contact with an irritating agent.

Atopic dermatitis is a chronic pruritic eruption of unknown etiology; allergic, hereditary, and psychogenic factors appear to be involved. It is treated with **Zonalon (doxepin)**, a topical tricyclic antidepressant (TCA) with a strong antihistaminic effect.

Viral Infections

Herpes zoster (shingles) is caused by the same virus as chicken pox. The distribution is usually unilateral and confined to one or more dermatomes. Vesicles appear with erythema and edema. Pain in the area may precede the outbreak and linger afterward. The virus resides in dorsal root ganglions until immunity wanes. Treatment is palliative (affords relief but does not cure).

Warts are virally caused epidermal tumors. Remission is due to developing immunity. The virus may lie dormant and later cause reinfection. Genital warts are transmitted by sexual contact. Warts can be removed by surgery or destroyed by local freezing. Some OTC products may be effective if the wart is small. Most agents contain salicylic acid as an active ingredient.

Fungal Infections

Ringworm is caused by a microscopic fungus that infects the horny (scaly) layer of skin or the nails. Infection of the skin spreads outward as the center heals, leaving a ring. It responds to topical antifungal agents. All forms can be controlled by oral antifungal **Fulvicin (griseofulvin)**, which accumulates in keratin. Topical **Lotrimin (clotrimazole)** or **Lamisil (terbinafine)** is used to treat this condition.

Candidiasis is a fungal infection usually causing lesions in the mouth (thrush) and vagina. It may be treated with agents such as clotrimazole and miconazole. Swish and swallow nystatin is frequently used if the mouth is involved.

Pulse dosing is a good way to administer antifungals for finger and toenail infections; it is effective, but less expensive than other forms. Pulse dosing was explained in Chapter 5.

Common Agents for Skin Diseases and Disorders

Table 16.2 presents the most-commonly used agents for skin diseases and disorders.

PSORIASIS Psoriasis produces patches of red, scaly skin, slightly raised with defined margins, usually on elbows and knees, but any part of the body may be affected. Tendency to these lesions is genetically determined, but usually they do not occur until adulthood. Attacks are precipitated by illness, injury, or emotional stress.

Rheumatrex (methotrexate) is used in oral or injectable forms to treat psoriasis. It may inhibit normal cell growth of bone marrow tissues.

Dovonex (calcipotriene) is a topical treatment for psoriasis. It is a synthetic analogue of vitamin D that regulates skin cell production and proliferation. It should not be used on the face because the face is especially sensitive to the skin irritation, stinging, redness, and peeling caused by this drug. The patient should wash his or her hands after each application. Watch that patients do not use more than 100 g of ointment per week because absorption of the vitamin D might cause serum calcium levels to get too high.

DANDRUFF Dandruff is shedding of scales from the scalp that is more rapid than in other parts of the body. When entrapped by hair, these scales become more noticeable. Dandruff is more a cosmetic than a medical problem. If one product does not work, the patient should switch to one with a different mechanism of action. **Selsun Blue (selenium sulfide)** has a direct antimitotic effect on epidermal cells. If used daily, dandruff should be controlled. **Head and Shoulders (pyrithione zinc)** is strongly bound to both hair and the external skin layers. It appears to work more slowly than other products. Used daily, it should control dandruff.

ACNE VULGARIS AND WRINKLES **Retin-A (tretinoin, retinoic acid, or vitamin A acid)** is used to treat acne vulgaris, photo-damaged skin, and some skin cancers. It removes keratinocytes in the sebaceous follicle. It loosens the horny cells at the mouth of the ducts, causing easy sloughing and sebum discharge. In normal skin it may cause a mild inflammatory reaction. The sloughing action allows new tissue to form that does not have the wrinkled appearance of older tissue. The hands should

Table 16.2   **Most-Commonly Used Agents for Skin Diseases and Disorders**

Generic Name	Brand Name	Dosage Form
Psoriasis		
calcipotriene	Dovonex	cream, ointment
coal tar	Tegrin	shampoo
methotrexate	Rheumatrex	tablet, IM, IV
Dandruff		
pyrithione zinc	Head and Shoulders	shampoo
selenium sulfide	Selsun Blue	shampoo
Acne Vulgaris		
adapalene	Differin	gel
azelaic acid	Azelex	cream
furfuryladenine	Kinerase	cream
tretinoin (retinoic acid,	Retin-A	capsule, cream, gel, lotion
vitamin A acid)	Renova	cream
Actinic Keratoses		
aminolevulinic acid	Levulan	solution
fluorouracil	Efudex	cream, solution
masoprocol	Actinex	cream
Atopic Dermatitis		
doxepin	Zonalon	cream
Fungi		
amphotericin B	Fungizone	cream, lotion, ointment, injection
	Abelcet	injection
butenafine	Mentax	cream
clotrimazole	Lotrimin, FemCare, Mycelex	cream, lotion, vaginal, troche
econazole	Spectazole	cream
griseofulvin	Fulvicin	tablet, capsule, oral suspension
miconazole	Monistat	cream, vaginal, IV, spray
nystatin	Mycolog II, Mycostatin, Nilstat	cream, ointment, oral suspension, tablet, troche
oxiconazole	Oxistat	cream, lotion
sulconazole	Exelderm	cream, solution
terbinafine	Lamisil	cream
tolnaftate	Tinactin	liquid, powder, cream, solution
Other Skin Conditions		
decosanol	Abreva	cream
mequinol-tretinoin	Solage	solution

be thoroughly washed after each application. The patient should avoid the sun and should not exceed the prescribed dose, as severe irritation can result. **Renova** is a lower dosage form used to eliminate wrinkles. It comes in only one strength in an emollient cream base that is more moisturizing than Retin-A. It does help to reduce some effects of too much sun exposure, fine wrinkles, rough skin, and brown spots. If the drug is discontinued, the wrinkles reappear.

Kinerase (furfuryladenine) is a plant-derived growth hormone, thought to delay the aging of skin cells. It is supplied in the form of a cosmetic cream and is indicated for the treatment of wrinkles, brown spots, and skin roughness. Kinerase is an alternative to Renova and Retin-A because it causes less skin irritation. Kinerase must be used for three to six months to be fully effective.

Differin (adapalene) is an acne treatment less likely to cause skin irritation than Retin-A because it is water-based, and Retin-A contains alcohol. It is applied at night or as a sunscreen during the day.

Azelex (azelaic acid) is a topical treatment for mild to moderate inflammatory acne vulgaris. After the skin is washed and patted dry, a thin film of cream should be gently rubbed into the affected area twice daily. Hands should be washed after each application. Improvement usually occurs within four weeks.

ACTINIC KERATOSES **Actinex (masoprocol)** is an antiproliferative agent for skin cancers. The area should be washed and dried, and the cream gently massaged into the skin. It should be used for twenty-eight days. It causes transient local burning.

Efudex (fluorouracil) is used topically for management of multiple actinic keratoses and superficial basal cell carcinomas. Efudex is an antimetabolite. Procedures for proper handling and disposal of antineoplastic drugs should be followed when working with this drug. Nausea, vomiting, and hair loss sometimes occur. Direct sunlight should be avoided. The drug may cause permanent sterility.

Levulan (aminolevulinic acid) is a topical compound indicated for the treatment of actinic keratosis. Levulan undergoes a photodynamic reaction upon exposure to light of the appropriate wavelength. This drug must be applied by a health professional and followed by a blue light treatment. It is important that the drug's application be limited to the lesion. Levulan must be used immediately after compounding. Patients undergoing photodynamic treatment must be instructed to avoid sunlight and tanning beds during the course of their treatment.

ATOPIC DERMATITIS **Zonalon (doxepin)** is prescribed for itching because it has strong antihistaminic effects. A thin film should be applied four times a day with at least three- to four-hour intervals between applications. It is a stronger histamine blocker than diphenhydramine or hydroxyzine. Sunlight and alcohol should be avoided. It may cause drug interactions just like oral doxepin. Patients can get significant absorption, especially if they are using it on a fairly large area.

FUNGI **Mentax (butenafine)** is used to treat athlete's foot, ringworm, and jock itch. It is applied once daily for four weeks. After the last application, the drug may maintain its effect for an additional four weeks.

Lotrimin (clotrimazole) is an OTC drug and the preferred drug to treat ringworm.

Lamisil (terbinafine) is a topical cream that inhibits biosynthesis of fungal membrane sterols. For athlete's foot, it should be applied twice daily, for ringworm four times daily, and for jock itch four times daily. The treatment course takes only one week, as opposed to four weeks for other antifungals. Systemic absorption is also low.

Tinactin (tolnaftate) is an OTC drug recommended for treating jock itch. It is not recommended for nail infections and should not be used around the eyes. Side effects are pruritus, contact dermatitis, irritation, and stinging. If skin irritation develops, infection worsens, or there is no improvement within ten days, the patient should consult a physician.

OTHER SKIN CONDITIONS **Abreva (decosanol)** is an OTC topical indicated for the treatment of cold sores. It blocks the virus from invading the body's cells and is most effective when administered at the first sign of an outbreak. Abreva must be applied five times a day.

Solage (mequinol-tretinoin) is a vitamin A derivative that competitively inhibits the formation of melanin precursors. The drug is prescribed for the treatment of freckles. Mequinol is a substrate for the enzyme tyrosinase. The mechanism of depigmentation for both drugs is unknown. Photosensitizing drugs and sunlight must be avoided when using this drug. Patients should also be instructed not to bathe or shower for at least six hours following application. They should also be instructed not to apply make-up until at least thirty minutes have passed. The application of Solage may induce minor stinging or burning. Some freckles may reappear after the drug is discontinued. Solage is highly flammable and therefore should be kept away from open flames or high temperatures.

Antiseptics and Disinfectants

Chemicals have long been used to control suppuration (formation or discharge of pus), to control the spread of disease, and to preserve food. Investigators such as Koch and Pasteur showed that infection and putrefaction were due to microorganisms. However, it was only after Lister developed techniques for antiseptic surgery and the control of postoperative sepsis that physicians began to appreciate the importance of disinfecting the skin of the patient undergoing surgery, the hands of the surgeon, the instruments, and the operation theater.

A variety of agents are used as antiseptics and disinfectants, and they have specific actions. These are listed in Table 16.3.

The most desirable property of a germicide is its ability to destroy microorganisms rapidly and completely. Many agents that rapidly destroy organisms also may be too toxic if applied to human or animal tissue cells. No single germicide is equally effective against all types of organisms. Esthetic factors, such as odor, taste, and staining quality, may influence antiseptic selection. If a germicide is used in or around the mouth, bad odor or taste may reduce patient compliance. Patients may also object to materials that stain the oral mucosa, skin, or clothing.

Antiseptics and disinfectants have two uses. They are used to disinfect instruments and to treat accessible infections in the oral cavity and on body surfaces. The ideal antiseptic must possess the ability to destroy all forms of infectious organisms without being toxic or inducing sensitization of human tissues. It should be capable of penetrating tissues and of acting in the presence of body fluids (i.e., serum, pus, and mucus). It should be soluble in water, stable, noncorrosive, and inexpensive. No agent meets all these requirements. If an antiseptic is being used to clean instruments or used in a clean room to maintain sterility, it is always best to use two separate ones with different mechanisms of action. Table 16.4 lists the most-commonly used antiseptics and disinfectants.

Heavy-metal compounds inhibit microorganisms in concentrations as low as one part per million. These ions have strong affinity for proteins. Activity is reduced in the presence of organic matter (mucus). These compounds are irritating and astringent (constricting or drawing together). They do not consistently kill bacteria. With improved chemicals, they are not frequently used.

Table 16.3	Actions of Antiseptics and Disinfectants
Agent	**Action**
antiseptic	a substance that inhibits growth and development of microorganisms, but does not necessarily kill them
disinfectant	a chemical applied to objects to free them from pathogenic organisms or render them inert
fungicide	anything that destroys fungi
germicide	anything that destroys bacteria, but not necessarily spores
preservative	an agent that prevents decomposition by either chemical or physical means
sporicide	anything that destroys spores
sanitizer	an agent that reduces the number of bacterial contaminants to a safe level

Table 16.4   Most-Used Antiseptics and Disinfectants

Generic Name	Brand Name	Dosage Form
alcohol	Isopropyl	liquid disinfectant
chlorhexidine	Hibiclens	liquid antiseptic
hexachlorophene	pHisoHex	liquid antiseptic
providone-iodine	Betadine	solution, antiseptic, cream, douche, aerosol, foam, gel, ointment, shampoo, suppository
sodium hypochlorite	Clorox	liquid disinfectant
Heavy Metal Compounds		
silver nitrate		ointment, solution
zinc oxide	Desitin	cream
Other Agents		
benzalkonium chloride	Zephiran	solution
carbamide peroxide	Gly-Oxide	solution
clove oil	Eugenol	oil
hydrogen peroxide		solution

Alcohol is supplied as 70% ethyl and isopropyl alcohols; it spreads well, dries slowly, and does not extract cutaneous fats. It is inexpensive. It primarily removes bacteria, but can kill some. It denatures proteins and produces a marked stinging reaction when applied to cuts or abrasions. To be effective, alcohol must dry and be left on for at least two minutes.

Clorox (sodium hypochlorite) disinfects and deodorizes by killing most germs and their odors. It is a common laundry and household product used in cleaning and stain removal.

pHisoHex (hexachlorophene) is a surgical scrub and bacteriostatic skin cleanser that is especially effective if gram-positive infection is present. It should not be left on the skin for long periods of time.

Hibiclens (chlorhexidine) is a skin cleanser for surgical scrub, skin wounds, germicidal hand rinse, and antibacterial dental rinse. It is active against gram-positive and gram-negative organisms and yeast.

Betadine (povidone-iodine) is an aqueous solution that does not stain and causes little discomfort when applied to an open wound. It is among the most effective disinfectants available. It has a broad microbicidal spectrum against bacteria, fungi, viruses, protozoa, and yeasts.

Silver nitrate has traditionally been used in the eyes of newborns to prevent gonococcal infection. It has been replaced by erythromycin ointment. The primary use for this chemical is in compounding topicals used in wound healing.

Zinc oxide is a mild antiseptic and astringent used for some conjunctival and skin diseases. It is the main ingredient in calamine lotion. The oxide salt, a zinc salt, is combined with a petrolatum and lanolin base for the use of diaper rash and other minor skin irritations.

Eugenol (clove oil) is an antiseptic with sedative properties on exposed dentin. Mixed with zinc oxide or zinc acetate, it has dental applications in temporary fillings and cements and in periodontal and intra-alveolar packs.

Zephiran (benzalkonium chloride) is used as a preoperative skin disinfectant and for storing instruments and hospital utensils.

Hydrogen peroxide is a strongly disinfecting, cleansing, and bleaching agent. It is used to prepare dental surfaces before filling and to clean wounds. The release of oxygen provides the antiseptic action.

Gly-Oxide (carbamide peroxide) releases oxygen on contact with oral tissues and reduces inflammation, inhibits odor-forming bacteria, and relieves pain in periodontal pockets, oral ulcers, and dental sores. It also emulsifies and disperses earwax.

Infections and Topical Antibiotics

Skin infections are common, and most can be managed with nonprescription topical antimicrobial products. Sometimes, however, a prescription drug may be needed. The severity of a skin infection depends on the extent of involvement of the skin and its structures. There can be drainage, swelling, fever, and malaise.

COMMON SKIN INFECTIONS Impetigo is a superficial, but highly contagious, skin infection, common in early childhood, particularly in warm, humid climates where hygiene is poor. It is due to *Staphylococcus* or *Streptococcus* and forms bullae and encrustations. If streptococcal, the infection could become systemic and may cause kidney damage. It is uncommon in adults, but may be seen particularly in elderly and immunocompromised patients. Lesions initially are small red spots that rapidly evolve into vesicles filled with fluid. Exposed parts of the body, such as the face and hands, are affected. In several days the vesicles break, become crusted, and are surrounded by a zone of erythema. Fever and other symptoms usually are not present. Impetigo is treated with Bactroban cream or ointment. For disseminated involvement with multiple lesions, systemic therapy with an antibiotic is recommended.

Erysipelas, a form of cellulitis, involves a progressively rapid spread of infection through the superficial layers of the skin. Facial involvement may assume a butterfly distribution. It is characterized by redness and warmth, local pain, edematous plaque with sharply established borders, chills, malaise, and fever. It usually responds well to oral antibiotics. However, if systemic toxicity (high fever with elevated WBC) results, parenteral antibiotics should be given.

Folliculitis is inflammation of the hair follicle by a minute, red, pustulated nodule without involvement of surrounding tissues. There is little pain. It commonly occurs in men on the bearded part of the face.

Furunculus (boil) is a staphylococcal infection of a sebaceous gland and the associated hair follicle. The follicular infection is more extensive and deeper than in folliculitis. It begins with itching, local tenderness, and erythema, followed by swelling, marked local pain, and pus formation within the lesion. Carbuncles are coalescent masses of infected follicles with deeper penetration than furuncles. Pain, erythema, swelling, purulent drainage, fever, and systemic toxicity are common.

Burns are especially difficult to treat. The use of effective topical antimicrobial agents has been associated with reduction in mortality. **Silvadene (silver sulfadiazine)** is a cream that is extensively used. It works on the bacterial cell wall and cell membrane. The drug will frequently darken in the jar or after being applied to skin, but this color change does not interfere with the antimicrobial properties of the drug. Hypersensitivity to this drug is rare and it is painless upon application. **Sulfamylon (mafenide acetate)** is more effective than Silvadene against some bacteria and has better penetration. The problem with this drug is pain upon application. Infections can occur despite adequate topical treatment. Routine use of prophylactic antibiotics is recommended.

TOPICAL ANTIBIOTICS Table 16.5 presents the most-commonly used topical antibiotics.

Triple Antibiotic (bacitracin-neomycin-polymixin B) is used to prevent or treat minor skin infections.

Table 16.5	Most-Commonly Used Topical Antibiotics	
Generic Name	**Brand Name**	**Dosage Form**
bacitracin-neomycin-polymixin B	Triple Antibiotic	ointment
clindamycin	Cleocin T	gel, lotion, solution, cream
erythromycin	T-Stat	gel, swab
	ATS, EryDerm	solution
mafenide acetate	Sulfamylon	cream
metronidazole	Metro-Gel	gel
mupirocin	Bactroban	ointment
neomycin-polymixin B	Neosporin	ointment
silver sulfadiazine	Silvadene	cream
tetracycline	Topicycline	solution

Cleocin T (clindamycin) is considered to be an effective topical antibiotic for acne.

Topicycline (tetracycline) is rarely prescribed because it photoxidizes to produce a visible yellow tinting and has a relative lack of efficacy, although the oral form is effective for skin problems.

Bactroban (mupirocin) is a topical treatment for impetigo due to *Staphylococcus aureus*, *S. pyogenes*, and *Streptococcus*. It should not be applied to the eye; use should be discontinued if rash, itching, or irritation occurs or no improvement results within five days.

Topical Corticosteroids

Topical corticosteroids should be applied as a very thin film and used sparingly. They may be absorbed to significant levels in systemic circulation because they can penetrate the skin; thus they have the ability to suppress the hypothalamus-pituitary axis. Local effects can be skin eruptions, burning sensation, atropic striae (streaks and lines), and petechiae (minute red spots due to escape of a small amount of blood). In the last few years the 0.5% and the 1.0% hydrocortisone have become available OTC. Both strengths can be effective and are the drugs of choice for poison ivy. They are also effective in cases of severe diaper rash. However, the 1.0% form should be reserved for adults; children's tender skin can easily be penetrated by the drug, therefore there is a greater potential for adverse effects.

It is the general consensus that creams are prescribed more often by physicians than ointments. Dermatologists, however, prescribe ointments more often than creams because they are usually treating more troublesome skin problems. Creams and ointments should not be considered interchangeable. As a general rule, a dry skin problem is treated with an ointment, and a wet, oozing lesion is treated with a cream. Substituting a cream for an ointment on a dermatologist's prescription could result in treatment failure.

Warning

Creams and ointments should not be considered interchangeable.

Corticosteroids applied to inflamed skin suppress the immune response, thereby relieving the redness, swelling, and itching. Topical products vary greatly in potency and delivery system (vehicle). The same drug can be found in different classes of potency. As a rule, ointment formulations are more potent than creams; gels are somewhere in between. Exceptions occur when manufacturers alter the vehicle of a cream or gel to enhance penetration, thereby delivering more drug to the lower layer of skin. These alterations result in superpotent topical steroids that are class I. Table 16.6 lists the two strongest classes of the superpotent topicals.

Most superpotent topical steroids have restrictions limiting their use to two consecutive weeks of treatment and/or a maximum of 45 g to 50 g in any one week due to systemic absorption. Exceptions are diflorasone diacetate, 0.05% ointment (Psorcon), which has no two-week or grams-per-week restrictions. Psorcon is also the only superpotent topical steroid approved for use under occlusive dressings when enhanced penetration is required.

Pediculicides and Scabicides

Human lice and scabies are external parasites. They use the human body as a host. Lice spend their entire life cycle on a host's skin surface, hair, and clothing fibers. Scabies may spend part of their life cycle on the skin surface with the remainder in burrows in the host's skin.

HUMAN LICE Human lice are found in every climate (arctic to tropics) and may infest persons of any walk of life. Human lice belong to an insect group called Anoplura (sucking).

Head lice infestation is one of the most common contagious diseases in the United States. Children are the age group at the greatest risk because they play in close contact and often share possessions. Head lice are easily identified and treated. Adults usually have a sense of shame and revulsion because of the many myths associated with head lice, including the common false belief that only people who exercise poor hygiene get them.

The causal agent is *Pediculus humanus capitis* (Figure 16.2), although on rare occasions the pubic (crab) louse can be found on the scalp. The head louse is not generally believed to transmit any viral or bacterial diseases. They feed on blood from the scalp, which produces the intense pruritus. A female louse has a life span of forty days, during which she lays about ten eggs (nits) per day. These nits are cemented to hair shafts close to the scalp and take advantage of body heat, which helps them to hatch in about eight days. The nits are best seen by shining a bright light on the scalp. They appear white and look like dandruff. They cannot be shaken off. Head lice are transmitted by direct contact.

Table 16.6	Superpotent Topical Steroid Classes		
Generic Name	**Brand Name**	**Dosage Form**	**Percent**
Class I			
betamethasone	Diprolene	gel, ointment	0.05
clobetasol	Temovate	cream, ointment	0.05
diflorasone	Psorcon	ointment	0.05
halobetasol	Ultravate	cream, ointment	0.05
Class II			
amcinonide	Cyclocort	ointment	0.10
mometasone	Elocon	ointment	0.10
halcinonide	Halog	cream	0.10
betamethasone	Diprolene	cream	0.05
betamethasone	Diprosone	ointment	0.05
diflorasone	Florone	ointment	0.05
desoximetasone	Topicort	gel	0.05
diflorasone	Psorcon	cream	0.05
fluocinonide	Lidex	cream, ointment	0.05
desoximetasone	Topicort	cream, ointment	0.25

Figure 16.2

Human Head Louse
(a) Adult on Hair
(b) Nit on Hair Shaft

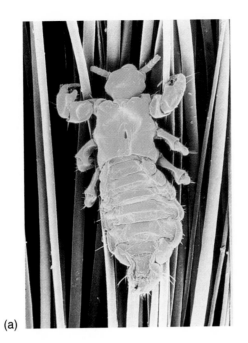

(a)

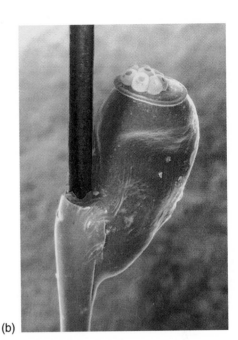

(b)

There are three types of human lice. Body lice are 2 mm to 4 mm long and are found most often in clothing and moist areas of the body (waistline, armpits). Head lice are 1 mm to 2 mm long and are found on the scalp and hair, but not on the eyebrows or lashes. Pubic lice, or crab lice are 0.8 mm to 1.2 mm long and are found in the pubic area.

The louse has three body parts, one pair of eyes, and one pair of antennae. The body consists of the head, the thorax (covered with lateral plates), and the segmented abdomen.

Lice live up to forty-five days, but many die because of scratching, combing, or disease. Injured or weak lice fall off the host. Human blood is the only source of nourishment; lice feed about five times a day for thirty-five to forty-five minutes. Adult lice and nymphs are active travelers, which explains their rapid passage from host to host. Lice are spread by direct contact with the infested person's head, body, or personal items (hats, hair brushes, combs, bedding). The symptoms are scratching not due to dermatitis.

Body lice do not always necessitate treatment. Body lice are heat-sensitive (hot water washing or putting in the clothes dryer eliminates adults and eggs). Treatment is to remove clothing, bathe the patient, and put on clean bedding and clothes.

Pubic lice are transmitted by sexual contact and should be treated. Table 16.7 presents the most-commonly used agents for lice.

Table 16.7   Most-Commonly Used Agents for Lice

Generic Name	Brand Name	Dosage Form
lindane	Kwell, G-well, Scabene	shampoo, cream, lotion
permethrin	Nix, Elimite	cream rinse
pyrethrins-piperonyl butoxide	Rid, A-200	spray, shampoo

Kwell, **G-well**, and **Scabera (lindane)** are used for treating head and pubic lice. It is directly absorbed by parasites and ova through the exoskeleton; it stimulates their nervous system, causing seizures and death of the parasites. This drug requires a prescription and is for topical use only. Very specific instructions come with the product. Clothing and bedding should be washed in hot water or dry-cleaned. Combs and brushes may be washed with lindane shampoo, then thoroughly rinsed with water. This drug should be a second line to an OTC medication. It can cause neurotoxicity. These preparations can be irritating to eyes, mucous membranes, and skin. Overuse may cause dermatitis.

Instructions to the patient vary with the type of lice.

- ◇ **Body Lice** Shower or bathe and apply 20 g to 30 g of cream or lotion to whole body from neck down, then wash off in twenty-four hours. Repeat in one week.
- ◇ **Head Lice** Massage two ounces or less into premoistened hair for four minutes, and rinse out. Repeat in one week; this is important to eliminate the eggs.
- ◇ **Pubic Lice** Apply thin layer extended to thighs, trunk, axillary regions (infestation may resemble dermatitis, is very itchy; corticosteroids make it worse). Wash off within twenty-four hours. Repeat in one week.

For both head and pubic lice it is important to comb hair with a clean, fine-toothed comb to clear nits.

Rid and **A-200 (pyrethrins-piperonyl butoxide)**, extracted from chrysanthemums, is an OTC drug usually used for head lice. The mechanism of action involves disruption of the louse's neuronal transmission and is similar to the action of DDT. Comparison with lindane indicates comparable efficacy, but less toxicity. The drug must be applied to premoistened hair and scalp for ten minutes and rinsed off; treatment is repeated in one week. Patients sensitive to ragweed may be sensitive to impurities in pyrethrins (hay fever).

Nix and **Elimite (permethrin)** is at least as effective as lindane, with the advantage that it produces virtually no CNS effects. A 1% concentration is the drug of choice for treating head lice. It has residual action lasting up to fourteen days that continues to kill any lice hatched after the initial application. It is available as an OTC drug.

SCABIES Scabies are white, eyeless, translucent, small, oval, flattened mites (Figure 16.3). The body is marked by wrinkle-like transverse corrugations with brown spines and bristles on the dorsal surface. Eight legs extend from the ventral surface. The female is 0.33 mm long; the male is even smaller.

Figure 16.3

Scabie

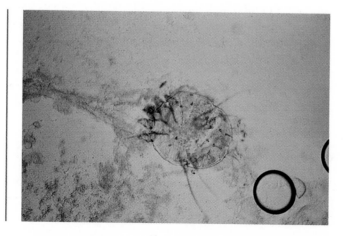

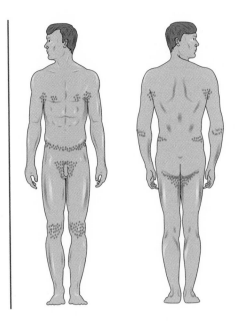

Figure 16.4

Sites of Scabies Infestation

Fertilization occurs on the skin surface. The female burrows into the epidermis, but seldom goes deep enough to enter living tissue. As the female burrows, she secretes substances that disintegrate the skin, which is then digested, and then sucks the intercellular fluid. No blood is consumed, as capillaries are below the epidermis. The deposited fecal pellets probably cause the intense itch.

Scabies infestation has been attributed to poor hygiene and population mobility. Major infestations occur in thirty-year cycles and are more common in urban areas of poor hygiene and overcrowding. Scabies are most often transmitted by close contact with infested individuals, sharing a bed (with or without sexual contact), dancing, or even holding hands. When infected, the patient has an intense itching that worsens at night after the bed is warmed by body heat. This intense itch may be due to increased activity, feeding, and excretion of the scabies. Lesions appear as very small, wavy, threadlike, slightly elevated, grayish-white burrows most often in the finger webs. Burrows usually are from 1 mm to 10 mm long. Figure 16.4 shows the common sites of scabies infestation.

Some of the products used for lice infestation are effective for treating scabies. The common treatment consists of a 25% benzyl benzoate cream or lotion that is spread over the entire skin from the neck down at bedtime. The application should be repeated in the morning. Re-treatment is rarely needed. Persistent inflammation and itching may be due to scratching, contact dermatitis, or a secondary infection rather than the mite infestation. Additional applications could cause dermatitis. A 5% to 10% sulfur ointment should be used for infants under two years of age. This is preferred because of potential absorption of gamma benzene hexachloride with neurological toxicity.

OPHTHALMICS

Ophthalmics and otics can easily be confused. They often have similar names and sometimes are stocked next to each other on the shelves. Table 16.8 presents the most-commonly used ophthalmic agents.

Table 16.8   **Most-Commonly Used Ophthalmic Agents**

Generic Name	Brand Name	Dosage Form
Antibiotics		
bacitracin	AK-Tracin	ointment
bacitracin-neomycin-polymixin B	AK-Spore	ointment
chloramphenicol	Chloroptic	solution
ciprofloxacin	Ciloxan	solution
gentamicin	Gentak	solution
norfloxacin	Chibroxin	solution
ofloxacin	Ocuflox	solution
sulfacetamide sodium	AK-Sulf, Bleph-10	ointment, solution
Corticosteroids		
bacitracin-neomycin-polymixin B-hydrocortisone	AK-Spore H.C.	ointment
sulfacetamide-prednisolone	Blephamide	ointment, solution, suspension
loteprednol	Alrex, Lotemax	solution
neomycin-polymyxin B-dexamethasone	AK-Trol, Dexacidin, Maxitrol	solution
tobramycin-dexamethasone	TobraDex	ointment, solution
Antifungal		
natamycin	Natacyn	suspension
Decongestant		
naphazoline	AK Con, Naphcon, Vasocon A	solution
Antivirals		
idoxuridine	Herplex	solution
fomivirsen sodium	Vitravene	solution
trifluridine	Viroptic	solution
vidarabine	Vira-A	ointment
Corticosteroids		
dexamethasone	AK-Dex	ointment
fluorometholone	FML Forte	ointment, suspension
Mast Cell Stabilizer		
cromolyn sodium	Crolom	solution
Antihistamines		
ketotifen	Zaditor	solution
pemirolast	Alamast	solution
NSAIDs		
diclofenac	Voltaren	solution
flurbiprofen	Ocufen	solution
ketorolac	Acular	solution
suprofen	Profenal	solution

Warning

Confusing AK-Spore and AK-Spore H.C. could easily create a dispensing error.

Glaucoma

Glaucoma is the most-commonly occurring eye disease. Drug treatment cannot cure, but can control glaucoma. It is a chronic disorder characterized by abnormally high internal eye pressure that destroys the optic nerve and causes partial to complete loss of vision. Increased intraocular pressure is due to an imbalance between production and drainage of the liquid (aqueous humor) in the front portion of the eye; obstruction to normal drainage is the main mechanism.

There are three types of glaucoma. In open-angle glaucoma, the angle of the anterior chamber remains open, but filtration is gradually diminished because of the tissues of the angle. It is usually treated with drops, but many of these medications have systemic effects. Narrow-angle glaucoma is characterized by a shallow anterior chamber and a narrow-angle in which filtration is compromised as a result of the iris blocking the angle. It is acute and treated as soon as possible by laser iridotomy. The open-angle and narrow-angle glaucoma occur in individuals with heredity predisposition. Secondary glaucoma is characterized by increased intraocular pressure due to disease or injury to the eye.

The goals of treatment are prompt reduction of intraocular pressure in narrow-angle closure glaucoma and stabilization of eye status in preparation for corrective surgery; gradual reduction and long-term normalization of intraocular pressure in chronic, simple, open-angle glaucoma; and prevention of optic nerve damage and preservation of vision in all cases. Patients should be instructed to avoid OTC drugs for cold remedies, appetite suppressants, antimotion sickness, and sleep aids.

Table 16.9 presents the most-commonly used agents for glaucoma.

Alphagan (brimonidine) is a selective alpha$_2$ agonist that lowers intraocular pressure by reducing fluid production in the eye and increasing the outflow. Sometimes the effectiveness will diminish with time.

Iopidine (apraclonidine) is an alpha adrenergic agonist that reduces intraocular pressure, possibly by decreasing aqueous humor production. Systemic effects are uncommon.

Xalatan (latanoprost) is a prostaglandin (PG) that reduces intraocular pressure by slowing the production of aqueous humor and increasing drainage of fluid from the eye. It is approved only for patients who cannot tolerate current treatment. It has an unusual side effect: it causes light-colored eyes to turn brown by increasing the pigment in the iris. It should be stored in the refrigerator. However, it is stable at room temperature for six weeks.

Azopt (brinzolamide) inhibits carbonic anhydrase, decreasing aqueous humor secretion and resulting in a decrease in intraocular pressure. If more than one eye drop is prescribed, they should be administered at least ten minutes apart. Concomitant use of oral carbonic anhydrase inhibitors, i.e., acetazolamide, could result in additive effects and toxicity.

Table 16.9	**Most-Commonly Used Agents for Glaucoma**		
Generic Name		**Brand Name**	**Dosage Form**
Eyedrops or Inserts			
apraclonidine		Iopidine	solution
betaxolol		Betoptic	solution, suspension
brimonidine		Alphagan	solution
brinzolamide		Azopt	solution
carbachol		Isopto Carbachol	solution
dipivefrin		Propine	solution
dorzolamide		Trusopt	solution
echothiophate iodide		Phospholine Iodide	powder
latanoprost		Xalatan	solution
pilocarpine		Isopto Carpine	solution
		Ocuserts	insert
timolol		Timoptic	solution
Oral Agent			
acetazolamide		Diamox	capsule, tablet, injection

Trusopt (dorzolamide) is a reversible inhibitor of carbonic anhydrase. The drug produces an increase of renal excretion, thereby decreasing aqueous humor. Trusopt also inhibits carbonic anhydrase in the CNS. Most patients complain of a bitter taste after administration. The patient should be instructed to discontinue the use of the drug if any eye lid or ocular reactions, such as conjunctivitis, occur. Ocular solutions can easily become contaminated by bacteria and can cause serious damage to the eye. Thus, the patient should be told to avoid allowing the tip of the dropper to touch any part of the eye.

Diamox (acetazolamide), a carbonic anhydrase inhibitor, is the oral agent used to treat glaucoma. It is also used for altitude sickness. It inhibits the conversion of carbon dioxide to bicarbonate, increasing oxygenation.

Conjunctivitis

Conjunctivitis (pink eye) is another common eye disorder. It is evidenced by many signs and symptoms including increased tearing, itching, chemosis (conjunctival swelling), and hyperemia (redness). Treatments include topical vasoconstrictors, cromolyn sodium, antihistamines, corticosteroids, antibiotics, and antivirals.

Alrex and **Lotemax (loteprednol)** are ophthalmic corticosteriods prescribed to relieve signs and symptoms of seasonal allergic conjunctivitis. They are also prescribed for the treatment of postoperative inflammation following ocular surgery. Loteprednol is less likely to increase intraocular pressure because it converts to an inactive metabolite in the eye. Patients should be reevaluated if symptoms fail to improve after two days of treatment. A "shake well before using" sticker should be placed on the bottle. Altrex is a 0.2% solution and Lotemax is a 0.5% solution.

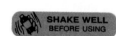

Alamast (pemirolast) is a mast cell stabilizer that inhibits chemotaxis of eosinophils into the ocular tissue and block their release of mediators. Alamast is also believed to prevent the calcium influx into mast cells that occurs following antigen stimulation. Decreased itching may occur within a few days; however, four weeks of treatment is generally required for complete remission. Patients who wear soft contact lenses should be instructed to allow for at least ten minutes between the administration of Alamast and the insertion of their lenses.

Zaditor (ketotifen) is a H_1 blocker indicated for the treatment of conjunctivitis. This drug must not be used to treat contact lens-related irritation. Contact lens wearers should allow for ten minutes between the administration of the eye drops and the insertion of their lenses. Care should be taken not to contaminate the dropper or bottle.

Vitravene (fomivirsen sodium) is an intravitreal injection used for the treatment of CMV retinitis. The drug blocks the replication of the CMV virus by binding to the mRNA of the affected cells. Because its mechanism of action differs from other antiviral agents, vitravene may be effective against viral isolates which have developed resistance to ganciclovir, foscarnet, or cidofir. Vitravene should only be used once other treatments have failed because of its side effects. Uveitis (inflammation of the iris, ciliary body, and choroid) is a frequent, occurrence with the use of this drug. It will also increase intraocular pressure. It is administered by intravitreal injection following the application of standard topical and/or local anesthetics and antibiotics.

OTICS

Earache (otalgia) is usually treated with a prescription drug. The only OTC medications are earwax (cerumen) solvents and a product to dry water in the ear canal after swimming. Wax dissolvers are used to emulsify and disperse excessive buildup

RNA is treated with reverse transcriptase enzyme. The result is a single-stranded DNA called complementary DNA (cDNA). The cDNA then serves as the template for DNA polymerase enzyme to add the second strand. This newly formed DNA (gene) is now added to the vector (plasmid) that has been cut with restriction endonucleases. Solutions of DNA and plasmids are mixed in the presence of ligases. A commonly used vector is a virus called a bacteriophage.

After the virus DNA is mixed with newly formed plasmids, virus, and plasmids are coated with a protein to form a new virus particle. The phage virus is then mixed with bacterial cells. The virus enters some of the cells and replicates. The culture is incubated for a time. Infected cells are destroyed (ruptured), and the viral DNA is harvested. The viral DNA is then chemically treated to expose the recombinant DNA. This is done by splitting the DNA into two single strands. The probe selectively identifies the recombinant DNA portion. The culture showing the correct probe identification is selected to receive the recombinant gene. Once the desired protein coding has been identified, control signals must be added that convert DNA into RNA. Control signals differ from one organism to another and are not copied into RNA. Bacterial cells do not read human controls. Promoters start protein production; terminators stop protein production (Figure 17.2). The receiving host cell must produce these controls for the inserted recombinant DNA.

The environment of the host cell is critical for the proper folding of the protein. Some proteins are modified by the host cell with the addition of sugars and realignment of the chains themselves. Without the modifications and proper folding, the protein does not work therapeutically, and the human body rejects it by forming antibodies. Once the proper recombinant gene has been identified, duplication can proceed. The organism is put into an appropriate growth medium and allowed to ferment. Cell division occurs many times over (thousands to millions to billions), resulting in a high concentration of product, and, therefore, producing large quantities of the desired protein. Protein is then harvested, purified, and packaged. Figure 17.3 illustrates this process.

The disadvantages of protein extraction from plasma include limited sources, small quantities of protein, and unsure purity.

Economic Challenges

The high cost of these products may require pharmacoeconomic analysis. To appreciate the value of these drugs, more studies are needed to report pharmacoeconomic

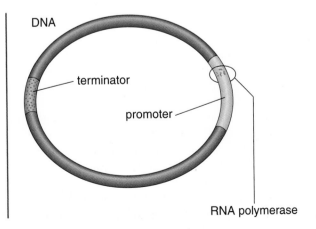

Figure 17.2

Promoter and Terminator Controls in a Cell
They are produced on a plasmid that is carrying the desired human gene.

DNA

terminator

promoter

RNA polymerase

Figure 17.3

Production of Protein Through Recombinant DNA Technology

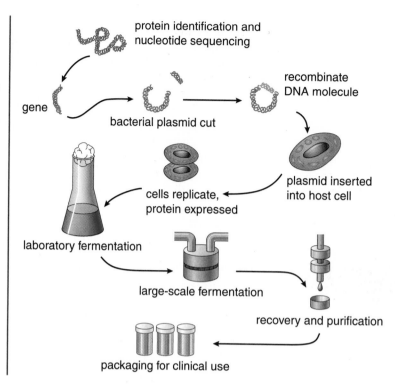

protein identification and nucleotide sequencing

gene

bacterial plasmid cut

recombinate DNA molecule

plasmid inserted into host cell

cells replicate, protein expressed

laboratory fermentation

large-scale fermentation

recovery and purification

packaging for clinical use

outcomes (i.e., cost-effectiveness, cost-benefit ratio, cost-minimization, cost-utility ratio, and cost of illness). In many hospitals the standard of practice supports the combination of antibiotic therapy and hospitalization for four to fourteen days if neutropenia develops. If the patient does not experience neutropenia, the economic impact in terms of cost savings is significant. The hospital stay for bone marrow transplant patients was reduced by six days with granulocyte-macrophage colony-stimulating factor (GM-CSF). This saves patients more in hospital costs than the cost of the GM-CSF itself.

Recombinant DNA Agents

Table 17.1 presents the most-commonly used agents for recombinant DNA procedures.

COLONY-STIMULATING FACTORS   Colony-stimulating factors (CSFs) have potential clinical implications, including decreasing the period of severe neutropenia after cytotoxic chemotherapy or marrow transplantation, treatment of aplastic anemia, and treatment of other immunodeficiency states associated with cytopenia. These agents are expensive, complex, chemical entities with unique therapeutic indications that necessitate specific storage and preparation, utilization review standards, and outcome monitoring.

   Neupogen (filgrastim) increases granulocyte production by acting on hematopoietic cells by binding to specific cell surface receptors and stimulating proliferation, differentiation, commitment, and some end-cell functional activation. This agent is produced by *Escherichia coli* organisms into which the human granulocyte colony-stimulating factor (G-CSF) gene has been inserted. (G-CSF is a synonym

Warning

Neupogen and Epogen are often confused.

Table 17.1

Table 17.1   Most-Commonly Used Agents for Recombinant DNA Procedures

Generic Name	Brand Name	Dosage Form
Colony-Stimulating Factors (CSFs)		
erythropoietin, epoetin alpha	Epogen, Procrit	IV, SC
filgrastim	Neupogen	IV, SC
sargramostim	Prokine, Leukine	IV, SC
Biological-Response Modifiers		
aldesleukin	Proleukin, Interleukin-2	IV
interferon alfa-2a	Roferon	IM, IV, SC
interferon alfa-2b	Intron	IM, IV, SC
interferon beta-1a	Avonex	IM
interferon beta-1b	Betaseron	SC
Human Growth Hormones		
somatrem	Protropin	IM, SC
somatropin	Humatrope, Nutropin	IM, SC
Fibrinolytic Agent		
alteplase	Activase	IV
Secretion-Thinning Enzyme		
dornase	Pulmozyme	inhalation
Hematologic Agent		
antihemophilic factor, factor VIII	Hemofil M	IV
Fusion Protein		
denileukin	Ontak	IV

for filgrastim.) CBC and platelet count should be obtained before beginning therapy with filgrastim. The agent should not be used in the period from twenty-four hours before to twenty-four hours after chemotherapy because of the potential sensitivity of rapidly dividing cells to cytotoxic chemotherapy. It is incompatible with normal saline and should be mixed in 5% dextrose. Also, when administering IV, it is best not to flush the lines with normal saline. Five percent dextrose flushes should be used instead of normal saline prior to administering a second drug and/or heparinizing the catheter.

G-CSF can potentially act as a growth factor for any tumor type, particularly myeloid malignancies. Tumors may have surface receptors for G-CSF. Side effects are generally mild and dose-related. The most common are fever, alopecia, nausea, vomiting, and bone pain. Mucositis or diarrhea may also occur. A transient increase in neutrophil count is typically seen one to two days after initiation of therapy.

Prokine and **Leukine (sargramostim)** have been demonstrated to accelerate myeloid engraftment in autologous bone marrow transplantation, to decrease duration of antibiotic administration, to reduce the incidence of infections, and to shorten hospital stays. There has been no difference in relapse rate of survival. The drug stimulates proliferation and differentiation of neutrophils, eosinophils, monocytes, and macrophages. The WBC increases in seven to fourteen days, but returns to normal within one week after discontinuance of the drug. The drug is given daily for up to thirty days or until the absolute neutrophilic count (ANC) has reached 1,000/mm for three consecutive days. A CBC with differential is recommended twice a week. Sargramostim is given SC or IV. When given by IV infusion, it must run at least two hours. It should not be mixed with dextrose. Reconstitute with sterile water. Direct the water at the side of the vial and gently swirl to avoid foaming during dissolution. Do not shake. Use only normal saline for infusion. It has a first-

Warning

Leukine, Leukeran, and leucovorin can be mixed up.

dose effect of fever, hypotension, tachycardia, rigors, flushing, nausea, vomiting, and dyspnea. Alopecia, nausea, vomiting, bone pain, myalgia, and mucositis can all be longer-lasting side effects.

Epogen and **Procrit (erythropoietin)** mimic naturally occurring erythropoietin, which is produced by the kidneys. It stimulates the division and differentiation of bone marrow cells to produce red blood cells. Hematocrit should be monitored at least twice daily during the initiation of therapy and during any dosage adjustment; the dose should be withheld if the hematocrit exceeds 36%. Frequent blood tests are necessary to determine the correct dose. The following clinical evaluations should precede treatment and then be continued daily during treatment: CBC, differential, and platelet counts; blood chemistries (electrolytes); renal and hepatic function tests; and chest x-rays. Close monitoring of blood pressure is also recommended. Most patients also require supplemental iron therapy. Erythropoietin is used in anemia associated with end-stage renal disease and other anemias unresponsive to the usual treatment modality. Do not shake. Vigorous shaking may denature the glycoprotein, rendering it biologically inactive.

BIOLOGICAL-RESPONSE MODIFIERS Biological response modifiers alter the expression and response to surface antigens and enhance immune cell activities. They modify the biological responses of the body to attack and kill the invading organism.

Betaseron (interferon beta-1b) and **Avonex (interferon beta-1a)** reduce cytokines and increase the activity of T-suppressor cells. They reduce the frequency of clinical exacerbations in ambulatory patients with relapsing multiple sclerosis (MS). Flulike symptoms of myalgia, fever, chills, malaise, fatigue, and sweating are common following initiation of therapy.

Roferon (interferon alfa-2a) is FDA-approved for hairy cell leukemia and AIDS-related Kaposi's sarcoma. Chemo precautions should be observed when dispensing and using this drug. Usually within four to six hours the patient experiences chills, fever, malaise, fatigue, tiredness, and dizziness. WBCs are suppressed in seven to ten days, but recover within twenty-one days. Other longer-lasting side effects are weight loss, metallic taste, nausea, vomiting, and abdominal cramps.

Intron (interferon alfa-2b) is used for hairy cell leukemia, AIDS-related Kaposi's sarcoma, and chronic hepatitis C and B. Baseline chest x-ray films, electrocardiogram (ECG), CBC with differential, liver function tests, electrolyte levels, platelets, and weight should be monitored. Changes in mental status are common with patients on this drug. The physician should be informed of any persistent or severe sore throat, fever, fatigue, or unusual bleeding or bruising. The patient should be cautioned not to change brands of interferons, since they are not interchangeable.

Proleukin (aldesleukin) is synthesized using *E. coli*. It promotes proliferation, differentiation, and recruitment of T and B cells, natural killer (NK) cells, and thymocytes. It can stimulate lymphokine-activated killer (LAK) cells that have the ability to lyse cells resistant to NK cells. Orders should be written in million international units (million IU). Treatment consists of two five-day treatment cycles separated by a rest period of nine days.

HUMAN GROWTH HORMONES Human growth hormones stimulate growth of linear bone, skeletal muscle, and organs. They also stimulate erythropoietin which increases red blood cell mass. Human growth hormone stimulates growth in children, where, for whatever reason, an insufficient endogenous hormone has prevented normal development in stature.

Humatrope and **Nutropin (somatropin)** are used for long-term treatment of growth failure from lack of adequate endogenous growth hormone secretion. Nutropin is used in children with growth failure associated with chronic renal insufficiency up to the time of renal transplantation. These agents should be used cautiously in patients with diabetes. Somatropin stimulates growth of linear bone, skeletal muscle, and organs and increases RBC mass by stimulating erythropoietin. It exerts both insulin-like (hypoglycemia) and diabetogenic (hyperglycemia) effects. SC or IM routes are used. The drug should not be shaken.

Protropin (somatrem) and Humatrope and Nutropin (somatropin) are approved for long-term growth delay and short stature in children who lack adequate and endogenous growth hormone secretion. Growth hormone is supplied in powdered form accompanied by diluent for reconstitution. It should be refrigerated. Somatrem is given as an SC injection every day, or three times a week at about twice the usual daily dose. Sodium retention and increased blood glucose level are both side effects, but are minimal with proper follow-up. The dose is adjusted according to dose response.

FIBRINOLYTIC AGENT Fibrinolytic agents are referred to as clot busters. They lyse thrombi that are already formed. Heparin and Coumadin (warfarin) prevent clot formation, but fibrinolytic products will break up the clot once it is formed.

Activase (alteplase) is a tissue plasminogen activator. It is an enzyme that catalyzes the conversion of tissue plasminogen to plasmin in the presence of fibrin. Fibrin specificity produces local fibrinolysis in the area of recent clot formation, with limited systemic proteolysis. In patients with myocardial infarction (MI) this allows reperfusion of ischemic cardiac muscle and improved left ventricular function, with a decreased incidence of congestive heart failure (CHF) after MI. Heparin is usually given during or after alteplase. It is also used in acute ischemic strokes once bleeding has been ruled out. It must be given within three hours of onset of symptoms.

SECRETION-THINNING ENZYME Deoxyribonuclease (DNA) enzyme is produced by recombinant DNA, gene technology. It cleaves DNA, reducing mucus viscosity.

Pulmozyme (dornase) is used in managing cystic fibrosis. The hallmark of this disease is the presence of purulent airway secretions composed primarily of highly polymerized DNA. The principal source of this DNA is the nuclei of degenerating neutrophils which are present in large concentrations of lung secretions. When this DNA is cleaved, mucus viscosity is reduced and airflow in the lung is improved. Thus the risk of bacterial infection is decreased.

HEMATOLOGIC AGENT A hematologic agent is a replacement plasma protein necessary for blood coagulation and not produced in the hemophilic. Hemofil M (antihemophilic factor, factor VIII) is recombinant therapy to supply antihemophilic factor to patients not producing factor VIII. A plastic syringe is used as the solution may stick to glass. Refrigerate before reconstitution. It should not be refrigerated after reconstitution, and it should be administered within three hours.

FUSION PROTEIN A fusion protein is a combination of a toxic portion of an exogenous protein in combination with a naturally occurring protein, such as interleukin-2. Specific (malignant) cells are targeted, bound, and thus are prevented from making their protein. As a result, the cells die. Ontak (denileukin) is a recombinant DNA-derived cytotoxic protein that is composed of amino acid sequences for diptheria toxin fragments followed by the sequences for interleukin-2. It is a fusion protein that is designed to direct the cytocidal action of diptheria toxin to the malignant lymphoid cells which express the interleukin-2 (IL-2) receptor. The drug interacts with the IL-2 receptor on the cell surface and inhibits cellular protein synthesis, resulting in death to the malignant cell within hours.

Ontak is indicated for the treatment of patients with persistent or recurrent cutaneous T-cell lymphomas (CTCLs) whose malignant cells express the CD25 component.

CTCL is a general term for a group of low-grade non-Hodgkin's lymphomas which involves the manifestation of malignant T cells. These lymphomas present initially in the form of skin lesions, which typically progress through three phases—patch, plaque, and tumor. Ontak, which received accelerated approval by FDA, is the first drug indicated for this disorder. Its predominant side effect is a flu-like syndrome.

Ontak is supplied as a solution. It must remain frozen during storage. Before preparing the dose, the solution must be brought to room temperature. Do not heat the vials. Preparations should be administered within six hours of thawing. The solution must never be heated. It must not be shaken vigorously but can be mixed by swirling gently. The concentration must be at least 15 µg/mL during all steps in the preparation of the infusion. This can best be accomplished by withdrawing the calculated dose from the vials and injecting it into an empty IV infusion bag. For each 1 mL of the solution from the vial, no more than 9 mL of sterile saline without preservative should be added to the IV bag. The diluted solution should be prepared in soft IV bags as the drug may be adsorbed onto glass when it is in its diluted state. This drug should not be physically mixed with other drugs, nor should it come into contact with other drugs within the IV line.

IMMUNE SYSTEM

Small lymphocytes are cells with a dense nucleus surrounded by a thin layer of cytoplasm containing a few mitochondria, ribosomes, and other organelles. These cells are in a resting state to serve as a repository of genetically derived information about recognition of antigens. Any one lymphocyte normally has one gene capable of expression committed to that antigen. When activated by that antigen it recognizes, it divides and proliferates to produce a clone.

T cells respond directly to antigens to form clones. T cells are stimulated by only certain antigens, viruses, acid-fast bacilli, fungi, foreign cells, and neoplastic cells.

B cells require the cooperation of a T cell before they can form a clone in response to antigens. B cells are stimulated by a wider range of antigens. B-cell or T-cell antigen recognition involves combination of the antigen with an antibody-like component on the cell membrane receptor. Clones of T and B cells also produce a population of small lymphocytes termed memory cells, which are specifically committed to recognizing the particular antigen and react rapidly (more so than in the initial response) in mounting responses.

Macrophages process the antigen and transfer the antigenic determinants to the lymphocytes. In the process of phagocytosis, the macrophage ingests the foreign substance and digests it. This provides the stage for T-cell and B-cell interactions when portions of the antigen move out through the cell membrane and become attached to receptors on the cell surface.

Immune Responses

The immune response is a highly complicated and regulated system. It is categorized into two major components: the humoral immune system and the cellular immune system.

Humoral Immunity

Antigens introduced into tissue through a wound or by injection are carried to a regional lymph node. Orally ingested antigens go to gut-associated lymphoid tissue.

Antigens in the bloodstream arrive at the spleen. In these tissues the antigen stimulates proliferation of specifically committed lymphocytes of the B-cell type. If the antigen has not previously been encountered, lymphocytes in a mass of proliferating cells synthesize a specific IgM against the antigen and release it into the plasma. With a single dose of antigen, there is no stimulus for continued production of lymphocytes; proliferation ceases, and the plasma level of IgM decreases. Some lymphocytes become the memory cells that remain in peripheral lymphoid tissues. A second dose of the same antigen evokes a rapid and greater response from the now large population of memory cells capable of responding. Proliferation yields a high proportion of plasma cell and antibody with IgG rising rapidly in the plasma. The magnitude of an antibody response depends on the nature of the antigen, the frequency of exposure, and duration of each exposure.

Immunoglobulins

Five known glycoproteins are designated as immunoglobulins (Ig); IgG, IgM, IgA, IgE, and IgD.

IgG IgG is the most common. It makes up about eighty percent of total Igs in plasma. It is also found in saliva, tears, and cerebrospinal fluid. It is the smallest Ig and can cross the placental membrane. Small amounts are produced after first exposure; large amounts are produced and released after second and subsequent exposures to most bacteria, bacterial toxins, viruses, and fungi. They serve as a main defense against pyrogenic (fever-producing) bacteria.

IgM IgM has the highest molecular weight, making up about ten percent of the total Igs in plasma. The numbers are increased in chronic infection and particularly in viral infections. IgM is formed predominantly in the presence of gram-negative bacteria. It makes up the ABO system of antigens on red blood cells. If transfusion errors are made, agglutination in the blood can cause blockage of small vessels and result in organ damage.

IgA IgA is synthesized by plasma cells associated with mucous membranes, especially of the respiratory and alimentary tracts. It aids in transport across mucosal epithelium. It is the main Ig in salivary and bronchial secretions, bile, and tears. It is also found in breast milk and colostrum, where it transfers immunity to a child.

IgE IgE occurs in low concentrations. It is bound to the membrane of basophils and mast cells in tissues. A reaction with antigens leads to disruption of these cells causing release of the contents of their granules. IgE causes certain hypersensitivity reactions. It is present in increased amounts in patients with allergic rhinitis and allergic asthma.

IgD IgD's function is unknown; it may affect B-cell maturation.

Cellular Immunity

Cellular (cell-mediated) immunity is a specific response to antigens mediated primarily by lymphocytes and macrophages. It is responsible for functions such as organ transplant rejection, killing of tumor or virus-infected cells, and hypersensitivity reactions. Certain antigens (i.e., tubercle bacillus and foreign cell membranes) induce proliferation of committed small lymphocytes of the T-cell types. Little antibody is released. Antigens being associated with particulate matter are carried to lymphoid tissue after phagocytosis by reticuloendothelial cells. With continued exposure to the antigen or with a second exposure, large numbers of lymphocytes derived by proliferation of the original specifically committed group are released into circulation and accumulate in the vicinity of the source of the antigen in the tissues (killer cells). Combining these cells with antigen results in the release of a number of factors, including a substance that is lethal to the antigenic cells (lymphotoxin), a substance that induces lymphocyte division, and substances that mediate and cause the inflammatory reaction.

Cellular immunity provides the main-line defense against invasion by pathogenic viruses, acid-fast bacilli, fungi, and parasites. It is also responsible for rejection of incompatible tissue grafts and the elimination of neoplastic cells. A lack of humoral immunity, as in inherited disorders, is due to deficiency or absence of B cells, which increases susceptibility to bacterial infections, but not to viral infections or neoplastic disease. Conversely, attenuation of cellular immunity without a corresponding reduction in the reactive capacity of B cells increases susceptibility to viral infection and neoplasm, but not to bacterial infection. If all antigenic sites are combined with humoral antibody, then the antigen becomes masked from the T cells (which are more devastating in attacks on the antigen). The humoral antibody is then described as the blocking antibody. This may be how a neoplasm becomes established.

Lymphocytes

Antibody-antigen reaction is an interaction that involves weak reversible bonds. Action results from an arrangement of amino acids providing binding sites complementary to those in the antigen. Most antigenic proteins usually contain a number of antigen sites. Substances with low molecular weight do not normally elicit antibody production. They can be coupled to proteins, and then they are capable of stimulating antibody production. The low molecular weight constituent is known as a hapten. These combinations have only one antigen site and do not cause a precipitation reaction. A complement is a complex of lipoprotein and globulins in plasma, playing a secondary role after the formation of antigen-antibody (IgG and IgM) complex. One part binds to the antibody molecule after the antigen-antibody reaction, resulting in cell lysis with opsonization of cellular debris (making it more susceptible to phagocytosis).

Lymphoid tissue becomes colonized with mesodermal stem cells. In the thymus, the stem cells differentiate into lymphocytes called thymocytes. Toward the end of intrauterine development, lymphocyte stem cells leave the thymus and take up stations with red cells of the bone marrow. Some stem cells remain in the thymus and proliferate and mature. Mitosis of lymphocytes in the thymus goes on without antigen stimulation as required in peripheral lymphoid tissue. Lymphocytes formed in the bone marrow first pass to the thymus, divide, mature, and acquire the ability to recognize and respond to specific antigens. Figure 17.4 shows the components and flow of the lymphatic system. Cells that leave the thymus and establish in peripheral tissues are T-cell lymphocytes. Lymphocytes formed from stem cells in bone marrow are B cells.

The connective tissue capsule of lymph nodes turns in to form lobe-like portions. Adjacent to the connective tissues is a meshwork of sinuses and sinusoids. Lymph passes through these sinusoids and percolates into interstitial tissue, where it encounters macrophages and scattered lymphocytes. If the lymph contains antigens, they can stimulate lymphocyte division for the committed lymphocytes, which leave the node.

The capsule and trabeculae of the spleen consist of fibrous tissue and bundles of smooth muscle cells. Masses of lymphocytes and macrophages make up the white pulp. Nodules of white pulp are scattered through vascular loose connective-tissue

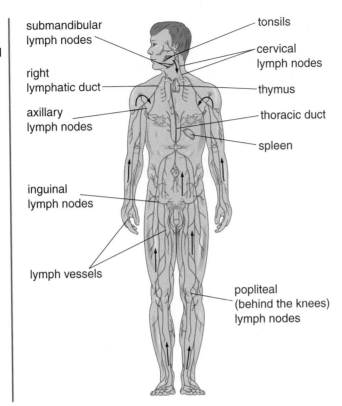

Figure 17.4

Components and Flow of the Lymphatic System

submandibular lymph nodes

tonsils

cervical lymph nodes

right lymphatic duct

thymus

axillary lymph nodes

thoracic duct

spleen

inguinal lymph nodes

lymph vessels

popliteal (behind the knees) lymph nodes

matrix termed red pulp. Walls of the sinusoids and the red pulp contain many macrophages and degenerating erythrocytes and leukocytes. Capillaries and venous sinuses allow the passage of blood cells between the vessels and the pulp.

The reticuloendothelial system comprises several types of cells.

- Histocytes are found in loose connective tissue.
- Kupffer cells are found in blood sinusoids in the liver; similar cells are in the blood sinuses of the bone marrow.
- Monocytes are found in the blood.
- Microglia are found in the central nervous system (CNS).

With the exception of the microglia, reticuloendothelial cells are interconvertible and have the capacity to transform and differentiate into other types of cells derived from mesoderm. The reticuloendothelial cell's primary function is the phagocytosis of bacterial and cellular debris.

Opsonization is the enhancing of phagocytosis of bacteria. Opsonization is a combination of bacterial antigen with specific antibody followed by fixation with complement. It is thought that these phagocytic cells act to control metastasis. Reticuloendothelial cells work with lymphocytes in developing the immune response to bacteria and other antigenic particles. After phagocytosis, such antigens do not reach the lymphocyte directly, but information about the antigen is passed to the lymphocyte, possibly by cell-to-cell contact, by liberating RNA that contains a message to lymphocytes about the antigen taken up. Nonmetabolizable substances remain in reticuloendothelial cells. Drugs affecting lymphoid and reticuloendothelial tissue, such as corticosteroids with glucocorticoid activity, produce involution of lymphoid tissue. These drugs cause the breakdown of large numbers of lymphocytes in the thymus, lymph nodes, and spleen, and inhibit division of the remaining

Table 17.2	Most-Commonly Used Antirejection Drugs		
Generic Name	**Brand Name**	**Dosage Form**	
azathioprine	Imuran	tablet, IV	
basiliximab	Simulect	IV	
cyclosporine	Sandimmune	capsule, oral solution, IV	
daclizumab	Zenapax	injection	
muromonab-CD3	Orthoclone OKT3	IV	
mycophenolate	CellCept	capsule	
sirolimus	Rapamune	solution	
tacrolimus	Prograf	capsule, IV	

lymphocytes. The numbers of circulating lymphocytes fall, reticular connective tissue degenerates, and the lymphoid organs become smaller. Ameboid and phagocytic activity of reticuloendothelial cells is suppressed.

Monoclonal Antibody Antirejection Drugs

Table 17.2 presents the most-commonly used antirejection drugs.

Monoclonal antibody names all end in "mab," which is the abbreviation for monoclonal antibody. The one or two letters before "mab" describe the antibody's source ("u" is human, "o" is mouse, and "xi" is combination). An internal syllable identifies the antibody's target (sometimes the third consonant is left off of this syllable), and the first syllable gives the antibody a distinctive name. For example, the syllables in the term "abciximab" signify the following.

- ⬥ abc the antibody's distinctive name
- ⬥ ci circulatory
- ⬥ xi combination source
- ⬥ mab monoclonal antibody

Orthoclone OKT3 (muromonab-CD3) is for treating acute allograft rejection in renal transplant patients; it is effective in reversing acute hepatic, cardiac, and bone marrow transplant rejection episodes resistant to conventional treatment. It binds T cells and interferes with their function. The first dose can cause severe pulmonary edema. The patient should be monitored carefully for forty-eight hours after the first dose. It is strongly recommended that a corticosteroid precede the first dose. It is also recommended that acetaminophen and antihistamines be given concomitantly. The edema is markedly reduced with subsequent administration of this drug.

Simulect (basiliximab) is indicated for prophylaxis of acute organ rejection in renal transplantation. It is a chimeric monoclonal antibody which blocks the alpha chain of the interleukin-2 receptor complex. This receptor is expressed in activated T lymphocytes and is a critical pathway for activating cell-mediated allograft rejection. Intact vials should be stored under refrigeration. The drug should be reconstituted with sterile water for injection and shaken gently to dissolve. It is then further diluted with normal saline or 5% dextrose. The bag should be inverted gently to avoid foaming.

Zenapax (daclizumab) is part of a regimen that includes cyclosporine and corticosteriods for prophylaxis of acute organ rejection in patients receiving renal transplants. It inhibits the binding of interleukin-2 to the high-affinity receptor, thus suppressing T-cell activity against allografts. Its active ingredient is a humanized monoclonal antibody. The syllables in daclizumab signify the following:

- ◇ dac   distinctive name
- ◇ liz   interleukin
- ◇ u   human
- ◇ mab   monoclonal antibody

Zenepax should be kept refrigerated and protected from light. It should be diluted only in normal saline and used within twenty-four hours of admixture if refrigerated and within four hours if not refrigerated.

Other Antirejection Drugs

Imuran (azathioprine) is used with other agents in preventing rejection of solid organ transplants. It is also used in rheumatoid arthritis. The patient should check with the physician if persistent sore throat, unusual bleeding, bruising, or fatigue occur.

Sandimmune (cyclosporine) is an immunosuppressant that may be used with azathioprine and/or corticosteroids to prolong organ and patient survival in kidney, liver, heart, or bone marrow transplant. It inhibits production and release of interleukin-2. In preparing the dose, the patient should use only glass droppers and glass containers and rinse the dropper to get the full dose. It may be mixed with milk, chocolate milk, or orange juice, preferably at room temperature. The patient should stir it well and drink it all at once. The dose should be taken at the same time each day.

CellCept (mycophenolate) inhibits guanosine nucleotide synthesis on which both T cells and B cells are highly dependent. It suppresses antibody formation by B cells. It is used to prevent kidney rejection in organ transplantation. The side effects are diarrhea, leukopenia, sepsis, and vomiting.

Prograf (tacrolimus) is a potent immunosuppressive agent used for recipients of liver, kidney, heart, lung, or small-bowel transplant. It suppresses humoral immunity by inhibiting T-lymphocyte activation. It should not be taken within two hours of an antacid.

Rapamune (sirolimus) is indicated to prevent renal organ rejection. It inhibits T-lymphocyte activation and proliferation in response to antigenic stimulation. Its mechanism of action differs from other immunosuppressants. It should not be administered with grapefruit juice and should be taken consistently either with or without food. In other words, always take it with food or always take it on an empty stomach. This is to minimize variability.

Hypersensitivity

Anaphylaxsis is an exaggerated reaction of an organism to a foreign substance, resulting from the release of histamine, serotonin, and other vasoactive substances. It can be partly antagonized by large doses of antihistamines. Anaphylactic shock is rapid in onset. For full shock effect to be exhibited, the antigen must enter the bloodstream and build up rapidly to a fully effective concentration. Anaphylactic shock is countered by sympathomimetic amines with pressor and bronchodilator activity and antihistamines as adjunctive therapy.

TYPE I REACTIONS Type I (anaphylactic) reactions are produced when the antigen has stimulated the production of antibody, which then becomes fixed to basophils and mast cells in the tissues. What follows is a disruption of the cytoplasmic granules and release of histamine, leukotrienes, and heparin. There may also be activation of enzymes forming kinins and prostaglandins.

TYPE II REACTIONS Type II (cytolytic) reactions are due to reactions of circulating antibodies of the IgG, IgM, or IgA class with an antigen associated with a cell membrane. Formation of the antibody-antigen complex is followed by complement fixation and lysis of the cell. Transfusion of incompatible blood leads to a type II reaction. Drug reactions are of the type II kind. The drug combines as a hapten with a constituent of the cell membrane. The hapten-complex elicits antibody production. On subsequent exposure to the drugs it combines with the cell membrane, destroys the cell, and may result in marked depletions of the cell type or damage to basement membrane (as in kidneys).

TYPE III REACTIONS Type III (toxin-precipitin) reactions occur when the precipitin complex, which is normally formed by reaction of free circulating antibodies with soluble antigens, such as bacterial toxins, is removed from the bloodstream by reticuloendothelial cells in the spleen. There are no deleterious consequences. If the toxin is present in great excess, the complex is deposited in the endothelial lining of small blood vessels, producing damage that results in an inflammatory reaction with the formation of local thromboses and infiltration of monocytes and lymphocytes into surrounding tissue. Deposition in the connective tissue of the joints produces a disorder resembling rheumatoid arthritis.

Serum sickness is an example of a type III reaction. It is caused by serum proteins of animals, such as in sera used for passive immunization. Symptoms include urticarial skin rash, swelling of the joints with stiffness and pain, albuminuria, and a rise in body temperature. Symptoms may last a few days.

TYPE IV REACTIONS Type IV (cell-mediated hypersensitivity) reactions (T-cell dependent) depend on the presence of T-cell (killer) lymphocytes that combine with the antigen. These are termed delayed hypersensitivity reactions because the response comes after a lapse of twelve to seventy-two hours. The injection site has characteristic erythema and induration (abnormally hard spot), formation of vesicles (blistering), scaling of the skin (exfoliation), and a weeping exudative fluid. The reaction of T cells with antigenic cells results in death of those cells, and this initiates an inflammatory response. In addition to release of preformed histamine, the histamine-forming capacity is increased above normal in tissue.

The best-known examples are produced by the tuberculin test; others are produced from the organisms that cause leprosy and various fungal, protozoal, and parasitic diseases. Sensitization occurs after these diseases have been in course for some time and remains after eradication of the disease.

Contact dermatitis is a type IV-delayed reaction that can result from chemical substances from several plant species (poison ivy), many industrial chemicals, and occasionally drugs and household chemicals.

Summary of Body Defenses

The human body presents three lines of defense against invasion by pathogens:

1. The body surfaces of intact skin and mucous membranes; infection-fighting chemicals in saliva, tears, and other body fluids; the normally harmless bacteria inhabiting body surfaces that resist pathogen invasion; and the flushing effect of tears, urination, diarrhea, sneezing, and coughing.
2. A nonspecific defense: inflammation and increase in the numbers of white blood cells, macrophages, complement proteins, blood clotting proteins, and other infection-fighting chemicals.

3. The immune response: T cells and B cells produce communicating and antigen-fighting substances.

The immune system has two features: 1) specificity, to attack a certain antigen and 2) memory, to remember the antigen for future invasion. Cells that recognize the antigen and enter the fight are effector cells, while those that enter a resting phase are memory cells.

The immune system has the ability to identify not only infecting agents, tumor cells, dying and dead cells, but also the products of cellular degeneration. Antigens are any substances that immune cells view as "foreign" to the body. As T cells recognize a "foreign" substance, cytokines are released that are involved in inflammation. Macrophages then release interleukin-1 and tumor necrosis factor, both of which are involved in inflammation, fever, and cellular destruction.

T cells form in bone marrow, travel to the thymus gland for differentiation into helper T cells and cytotoxic T cells, acquiring T-cell receptors (TCRs) that recognize complexes of antigen and major histocompatability complex (MHC). These cells take up residence in the lymph nodes and spleen. They ignore MHC or "self" molecules that are unbound to an antigen.

As a macrophage binds to, ingests, and fragments an antigen, the fragments form a complex with MHC molecules on the cell surface. Helper T cells bind to the MHC-antigen complex. The macrophages and helper T cells secrete interleukins that bring about rapid cell division of the cytotoxic T cells and memory cells. The cytotoxic T cells kill the pathogens or pathogen-containing body cells by contact, secreting protein molecules called perforins that cause pores to form in the target cell membrane; cytoplasm is expelled, organelles are disrupted, DNA becomes fragmented, and the cell dies.

B cells also arise from bone marrow but do not enter the thymus and differentiate; instead they start producing an antibody molecule that protrudes from the surface of the cell membrane. Antibodies are shaped like a Y, formed from four polypeptide chains with identical antigen binding sites on each arm. The tail becomes embedded in the cell membrane lipid layer with the arms sticking out. When a B cell contacts an antigen, it binds to the antibody. The antigen is taken into the cell and processed with fragments complexing with surface MHC molecules. Helper T cells bind to the complex, secrete interleukin that stimulates B cell division and massive antibody production. Free circulating antibody molecules bind to antigen, labeling or identifying it for destruction.

NEOPLASTIC DISEASE (CANCER)

Mitosis is one of the most vital characteristics of living organisms, providing growth, cell division, and repair. Neoplastic disease occurs when normal cellular growth control mechanisms become altered. It is a disease of uncontrolled cellular growth that involves developing and reproducing abnormal cells. Cancer is a leading cause of death in the United States.

Consistent findings in the cells regardless of the type of cancer:

- Structural alteration with loss of function occurs regardless of the cell type (e.g., epithelium, muscle, bone).
- Uncontrolled cellular reproduction resulting in production of groups of cells with no useful function and may increase in number at a rate faster than that of normal body cells.

Malignancy is characterized by the following.

◇ Abnormal, uncontrolled growth threatens normal body functions and can lead to death.
◇ DNA and RNA synthesis is increased.
◇ Metabolism is altered, so that as the tumor grows, it robs the body of the nutrients necessary for body cells, producing loss in weight and vitality.
◇ Cells lose their contact inhibition. Normal cells have a property that prevents division if the cells become crowded together in a tissue or organ; cancer cells continue to divide even when the pressure of surrounding cell masses is considerable.

Types of cancer are:

◇ **Primary Site** Cancer occurs at the original location.
◇ **Secondary Site** Detached and relocated cells form tumors in other body areas (metastasis).
◇ **Solid Tumors** These can be palpated when they become significantly large or accessible.
◇ **Diffuse Tumors** These are not restricted to one location but are scattered, as in leukemia and Hodgkin's disease.

Agents for Chemotherapy

Several modalities are available and are often used in combination when treating cancer. Surgery is used for solid tumors that are surgically accessible; it is followed by radiation in several treatments. Radiation is most often used after surgery or chemotherapy. Chemotherapy is used for diffuse tumors to kill cancer cells remaining after surgery or radiation. Table 17.3 lists the most-commonly used agents for chemotherapy.

Table 17.3	Most-Commonly Used Agents for Chemotherapy		
Generic Name	**Brand Name**	**Dosage Form**
Alkylating Agents		
busulfan	Myleran	tablet
carboplatin	Paraplatin	IV
carmustine	BiCNU	IV
cisplatin	Platinol	IV
cyclophosphamide	Cytoxan	tablet, injection
dacarbazine	DTIC-Dome	IV
ifosfamide	Ifex	IV
lomustine, CCNU	CeeNU	capsule
streptozocin	Zanosar	IV
temozolamide	Temodar	capsule
Antibiotics		
bleomycin	Blenoxane	IM, IV, SC
dactinomycin	Cosmegen	IM, IV, SC
daunorubicin	Cerubidine	IV
doxorubicin	Adriamycin	IV
epirubicin	Ellence	IV
idarubicin	Idamycin	IV
mitomycin C	Mutamycin	IV
plicamycin	Mithracin	IV
valrubicin	Valstar	injection (into bladder)

continues

Warning
Cisplatin and carboplatin can be misread.

| Table 17.3 | **Most-Commonly Used Agents for Chemotherapy (Continued)** |

Generic Name	Brand Name	Dosage Form
Antimetabolites		
capecitabine	Xeloda	tablet
cytarabine	Cytosar-U	IM, IV, SC
floxuridine	FUDR	IV
fludarabine	Fludara	IV
fluorouracil (5-FU)	Efudex	cream, topical solution, IV
hydroxyurea	Hydrea	capsule
mercaptopurine	Purinethol	tablet
methotrexate	Rheumatrex, Folex	IM, IV
thioguanine	6-TG	tablet
Hormones		
aminoglutethimide	Cytadren	tablet
bicalutamide	Casodex	tablet
flutamide	Eulexin	capsule
goserelin	Zoladex	implant, SC
leuprolide	Lupron Depot	SC
megestrol	Megace	suspension, tablet
mitotane	Lysodren	tablet
tamoxifen	Nolvadex	tablet
Nitrogen Mustards		
chlorambucil	Leukeran	tablet
estramustine	Emcyt	capsule
mechlorethamine	Mustargen	IV
melphalan	Alkeran	IV
thiotepa	Immunex	IV
Plant Alkaloids		
etoposide	VePesid	capsule, IV
vinblastine	Velban	IV
vincristine	Oncovin	IV
Topoisomerase I Inhibitors		
irinotecan	Camptosar	IV
topotecan	Hycamtin	IV
Miscellaneous Agents		
alitretinoin	Panretin	gel
altretamine	Hexalen	capsule
asparaginase	Elspar	IM, IV
levamisole	Ergamisol	tablet
mitoxantrone	Novantrone	IV
paclitaxel	Taxol	IV
procarbazine	Matulane	capsule
Cytoprotective (Rescue) Agents		
amifostine	Ethyol	IV
dexrazoxane	Zinecard	IV
folinic acid, leucovorin	Wellcovorin	tablet, IM, IV, oral solution

Antitumor drugs are most efficient during cancer cell DNA synthesis and rapid cell division. A young tumor has most of its cells making DNA and dividing. As it ages, the growth fraction decreases; growth slows and drug sensitivity is reduced. The curable tumors are discovered when 30% to 100% of cells are in the growth fraction.

Antineoplastic drugs are extremely toxic because they also destroy normal cells, especially those with a normal growth rate close to that of tumor cells, such as those in the bone marrow, the GI tract, and the skin. Therapy usually causes toxicity of these tissues, resulting in bone marrow depression (anemia, leukopenia, and thrombocytopenia), stomatitis, GI tract ulceration, and hair loss (alopecia). Therapy is generally structured to allow for a two- to six-week drug-free period between treatments.

The goal of most chemotherapy is to put the cancer in remission. Remission puts the tumor into an inactive period when there is no active cell division and growth. It does not cure the disease, but extends the patient's life.

Resistance is a lack of responsiveness of the cancer cells to chemotherapy. Cells continue to reproduce even in the presence of the drug. Combinations of agents with different mechanisms of action are used to attack different areas of the cancer cell, providing more efficient therapy.

ALKYLATING AGENTS Alkylating agents bind irreversible cross-links in DNA so that the DNA and cells cannot reproduce.

Temodar (temozolamide) is a prodrug that undergoes rapid nonenzymatic conversion at physiological pH to alkylate DNA. The drug's mechanism is similar to dacarbazine. However, Temodar is taken orally and dacarbazine is given IV. Temodar was FDA approved in 1999 and was the first new drug for the treatment of brain cancer to be approved in more than twenty years. The dose-limited adverse event associated with Temodar is myelosuppression.

ANTIBIOTICS Antibiotics inhibit DNA-dependent RNA synthesis or delay or inhibit mitosis.

Valstar (valrubicin), a semisynthetic analog of doxorubicin is indicated for intravesical therapy of the urinary bladder. The powder has a red color and red-tinged urine is typical for the first twenty-four hours after administration of the drug. Valstar should be stored in the refrigerator. If a waxy form precipitates from the solution, the vial should be warmed until it is clear. Valstar should be prepared and stored in glass. It is diluted with normal saline. A urethral catheter is inserted into the patient's bladder after it is drained and the diluted valrubicin solution is instilled slowly. The patient will then need to retain the drug for two hours.

Ellence (epirubicin) is an anthrycycline cytotoxic agent related to doxorubicin. It is able to penetrate into cells more readily because it is more lipophilic. Ellence is indicated as adjuvant therapy in patients with axillary node tumor following resection of primary breast cancer. Cardiotoxicity is a major risk with this drug.

ANTIMETABOLITES Antimetabolites incorporate into normal cell constituents, making them nonfunctional, or inhibit the normal function of a key enzyme.

Xeloda (capecitabine) is enzymatically converted to 5-fluorouracil. This is a three-step process in which the last step is to catalize the drug by an enzyme that is present in higher concentrations in carcinogenic cells than normal tissue. Because the drug is absorbed and metabolized in a higher concentration for tumor tissue than normal tissue, the risk of systemic toxicity is reduced over standard fluorouracil (5-FU). Xeloda is indicated in cases of breast cancer which have shown resistance to paclitaxel and anthracycline-containing regimens. The most prominent side effects of this drug are nausea and vomiting. When diarrhea occurs, it can usually be controlled with loperamide. Xeloda is given daily with food over a period of two weeks. This period is followed by a one-week rest period. Therapy is given in three-week cycles. The daily dosage is administered in two divided doses, twelve hours apart. It should be taken with food.

HORMONES Hormones inhibit the synthesis of adrenal steroids. Their target neoplasms are

- ◇ **Cytadren (aminoglutethimide)**: breast, prostate
- ◇ **Casodex (bicalutamide)**: prostate
- ◇ **Eulexin (flutamide)**: prostate
- ◇ **Zoladex (goserelin)**: prostate, endometriosis, metastatic breast cancer in premenopausal women. It acts by suppressing estrogen production to postmenopausal levels to reduce growth of estrogen-responsive tumors
- ◇ **Lupron Depot (leuprolide)**: prostate carcinoma, endometriosis, central precocious puberty
- ◇ **Megace (megestrol)**: breast, endometrial
- ◇ **Lysodren (mitotane)**: adrenal cortex
- ◇ **Nolvadex (tamoxifen)**: breast. The National Cancer Institute is now alerting oncologists to limit tamoxifen use to five years. A five-year course of this agent after lumpectomy or mastectomy significantly reduces the risk of recurrence and improves survival. New evidence says that longer use does not further survival and might even be detrimental by increasing risk of uterine cancer.

NITROGEN MUSTARDS Nitrogen mustards bind irreversible cross-links in cellular DNA and RNA, disrupting normal nucleic acid function so it cannot reproduce.

PLANT ALKALOIDS Plant alkaloids inhibit formation of spindle fibers, arresting the metaphase of cell division.

TOPOISOMERASE I INHIBITORS Topoisomerase I inhibitors lead to DNA damage when cells replicate. The target neoplasms are

- ◇ **Camptosar (irinotecan)**: colorectal cancer. A second-line drug, it can cause severe diarrhea.
- ◇ **Hycamtin (topotecan)**: ovarian (second-line after Taxol)

MISCELLANEOUS AGENTS Miscellaneous agents have different mechanisms of action to destroy malignant cells.

Taxol (paclitaxel) is indicated for metastatic ovarian cancer after failure of first-line or subsequent chemotherapy and for breast carcinoma after failure of combination chemotherapy. Patients should be warned to avoid pregnancy because of harm to the fetus and should be told that alopecia occurs in almost all patients. A patient should alert the physician if tingling, burning, or numbness occurs in the extremities, as the dosage may need to be reduced if these symptoms occur.

Warning
Paclitaxel and paroxetine can look alike.

Matulane (procarbazine) has side effects of bone marrow depression, leukopenia, thrombocytopenia, ulceration of skin and GI tract, hair loss, nausea, vomiting, nephrotoxicity, and teratogenicity. It is used to treat Hodgkin's disease.

Panretin (alitretinoin) is related to vitamin A. It is indicated for the treatment of cutaneous lesions in patients with AIDS-related Kaposi sarcoma (KS). Panretin inhibits the growth of KS cells in vitro. The adverse events associated with Panretin occur almost exclusively at the site of application. Most reactions are mild to moderate in severity. Lesions should be covered with a generous coating of the gel. It should be allowed to dry for three to five minutes before covering the treated areas. Application of the drug to normal skin should be avoided. Patients who are being treated with Panretin should be advised to minimize exposure of treated areas to sunlight and sunlamps. Following topical application, little Panretin is absorbed systemically.

CYTOPROTECTIVE (RESCUE) AGENTS Cytoprotective agents are administered to reduce the side effects and toxicity of the chemotherapy agents. Timing is critical when this is done. The chemotherapy agent must be active in the body long enough to kill the malignant cells, then the antidote or "rescue agent" is administered to prevent destruction of the healthy cells.

Ethyol (amifostine) is a prodrug that is converted primarily in tumor tissue to an active form. It may also tie up free radicals in healthy cells. When used with cisplatin, it reduces kidney toxicity. Side effects are reduced blood pressure, nausea, vomiting, flushing, feeling of warmth, chills, dizziness, somnolence, hiccups, and sneezing. It is adjunctive therapy for use with chemotherapeutic agents.

Zinecard (dexrazoxane) interferes with the iron radical thought to be responsible for cardiomyopathy. It is used to reduce the incidence and severity of cardiomyopathy associated with Adriamycin administration in women with metastatic breast cancer. The side effects include alopecia, nausea, vomiting, fatigue, stomatitis, fever, diarrhea, pain of injection, and kidney toxicity.

Wellcovorin (folinic acid, leucovorin) reduces toxicity of agents that antagonize folic acid (WBCs) in methotrexate administration and enhances toxicity of 5-fluorouracil when given together.

Warning

Folinic acid and folic acid mix-ups are common errors.

Biologic-Response Modifiers

Biologic-response modifiers are substances that can alter the host immune response in ways that promote destruction of human malignancies. Five are discussed: interferon, interleukin-2, tumor-necrosis factor, colony-stimulating factors, monoclonal antibodies.

INTERFERON Interferon inhibits viral replication. Small proteins are produced by cells in response to viral infection or other biologic inducers. All are similar in structure.

- **alpha** produced by leukocytes
- **beta** produced by connective tissue cells
- **gamma** produced by T lymphocytes

Interferons bind to specific cell receptors, causing intracellular changes that induce antitumor enzymes. They also stimulate macrophages and make tumor cells more susceptible to immune responses. They are produced by recombinant DNA in *E. coli*. Roferon (alfa-2a) differs from Intron (alfa-2b) in only one amino acid. Interferons are approved for use in hairy cell leukemia. Additional studies are being done with melanoma, non-Hodgkin's lymphoma, other leukemias, and tumors; however, results are not as good. Side effects include flu-like symptoms, such as fever, chills, fatigue, myalgias, confusion, and hypotension. Symptoms are dose-related and diminish with continued use.

INTERLEUKIN-2 Interleukin-2 is secreted by T cells. Increased doses activate lymphocytes and enhance their ability to lyse a broad variety of tumor cells. Extremely high doses are given for several days, followed by removal of activated lymphocytes, which are incubated for three to four days, then reinfused along with additional high doses. Treatment is highly toxic. Response occurs in twenty-five percent of patients with renal cell carcinoma or melanoma, with lesser percentages for other common malignancies. The side effects are hypotension, fluid retention, arthralgia, dyspnea, malignant hyperthermia, MI, delirium, and coma.

TUMOR-NECROSIS FACTOR Tumor-necrosis factor is secreted by macrophages in response to endotoxin. It directly causes lysis of susceptible tumor cells.

COLONY-STIMULATING FACTORS Colony-stimulating factors increase the host's ability to produce blood cells. Selectively enhanced production of granulocytes, monocytes, or red blood cells is now possible and could be used widely as adjunctive therapy to reverse chemotherapeutic-induced bone marrow suppression. These agents are well tolerated. They are used in hematopoietic malignancies, testicular cancer, ovarian cancer, and small-cell carcinoma of the lung. They allow higher doses of chemotherapy, which increases the likelihood of effectiveness, while reducing danger from white and red blood cell platelet levels.

MONOCLONAL ANTIBODIES Monoclonal antibodies are used to direct attacks against specific objectives. Antibodies to a specific tumor or tissue are developed by stimulating lymphocytes to specific antigens. They are used to deliver toxic payloads to malignant cells, to target malignant cell deposits, and to deplete the immune system of cells that prevent tissue rejection of a transplant, such as kidney or bone marrow. Currently MAbs (monoclonal antibodies) are used in diagnostic assays, localization of proteins in histochemical investigations, and cell labeling as well as for drug targeting.

Pain

Cancer pain often is not adequately controlled, which causes needless suffering. It also weakens the patient's appetite, reduces sleep, and increases fear and anxiety. There is little need to worry about a cancer patient's becoming addicted to pain medication. Studies indicate that where there is real pain, a lesser risk of addictions exists. Treatment should deal with the immediate problem of controlling the pain. If the patient survives and the need for pain medication is eliminated, the issue of physical dependence can be dealt with at that time. Demerol is not a good choice for chronic pain, as it is too short-acting and has a toxic metabolite that can accumulate and lead to seizures.

Oral Complications

Oral complications are common manifestations of toxicity and tissue injury associated with the administration of certain anticancer drugs and radiation. The most common of these oral complications are mucositis and concomitant ulceration and infection. Similar problems are encountered with irradiation to the head and neck.

Oral mucositis and ulceration, with the accompanying pain and discomfort, can interfere with the patient's ability to eat, necessitate use of potent analgesics, and create favorable conditions for a local infection that can lead to septicemia and compromise the entire treatment protocol and prognosis. Although oral mucositis and ulceration cannot be prevented, proper management can minimize the duration, discomfort, and potential for infection. Table 17.4 lists the most-commonly used agents for mucositis.

Table 17.4   Most-Commonly Used Agents for Mucositis

Generic Name	Brand Name	Dosage Form
dyclonine	Dyclone	solution
hydrogen peroxide	Peridex, Peroxyl	solution
lidocaine-diphenhydramine-Maalox	Magic Swizzle	solution
phenol sodium borate-sodium bicarbonate-glycerin	Ulcer Ease	solution
pilocarpine	Salagen	tablet

Dyclone (dyclonine) provides effective anesthesia in two to ten minutes, which lasts much longer than that induced by other topical agents. It is best to use the most dilute solution that affords relief. The patient should be warned of a side effect of numbness of the tongue or buccal mucosa, which increases the danger of biting trauma. Topical anesthesia can also impair swallowing and enhance the danger of aspiration; the patient should be cautioned not to eat when the mouth is profoundly numb. Use of this agent should be strictly controlled to limit systemic toxicity.

Hydrogen peroxide has some antibacterial effects, but its primary benefit is the nonmechanical cleansing action produced by the nascent oxygen. It should never be used full-strength for oral lavage of irritated tissues, but should be diluted with water or saline, preferably in a ratio of one part hydrogen peroxide to one or more parts diluent. **Peroxyl** is a ready-to-use form and should be used at the recommended strength of 1.5%. This pleasant, mint-flavored, aqueous solution is well accepted. Twice-daily brushing and a thirty-second rinsing are recommended.

Magic Swizzle (lidocaine-diphenhydramine-Maalox) is often made by the pharmacy technician by combining the three agents in equal parts. The patient holds the solution in the mouth, swishes it around, and then expectorates. It gives some relief. This formula has many names ("Pink Magic" for one). It does not need to be refrigerated and may be made with an antacid other than Maalox.

Ulcer Ease (phenol sodium borate-sodium bicarbonate-glycerin) provides topical desensitization and some antimicrobial effect. It contains 0.6% phenol. It may be used as the primary rinse of an oral care regimen to reduce the discomfort of the other cleansing measures.

Salagen (pilocarpine), artifical saliva, stimulates the salivary glands, alleviating chronic dry mouth, which is painful and makes it hard to eat or speak. It can lead to tearing, sweating, and runny nose. The patient should be told to drink plenty of fluids when taking this medication.

Extravasation of Chemotherapeutic Agents

Extravasation is an escape of the IV fluids into the surrounding tissue. When chemotherapeutic agents are infused without a central line there is a high probability that the drug will "leak" into the tissue surrounding the injection site. When this happens, often the affected tissue must be debrided. Certain drugs are used to stop or slow the spread of the "leaked" drug. The pharmacy technician will need to be familiar with these agents.

Tinver (sodium thiosulfate) is used for Cisplatin. Tinver is mixed with 4 mL of 10% drug with 6 mL of sterile water. Then, 4 mL of the solution is injected into the IV line while 2 mL is injected directly in the damaged tissue.

Wydase (hyaluronidase) modifies the permeability of connective tissue through hydrolysis. The vial of 150 units is reconstituted with normal saline. It should be diluted to a concentration of 15 units per mL. Then, 2/10 mL is injected into the damaged tissue. It complexes with Cisplatin to form a compound that is nontoxic to both normal and cancerous cells.

Chapter Summary

Recombinant DNA

◇ Biotechnology is the method of applying biologic systems and organisms to industrial and technical use.

◇ Protein extraction from plasma or tissue has a number of disadvantages: limited sources, small quantities, and high risk of contamination.

◇ Manufacturing protein consists of two major enzyme activities: (1) cutting DNA into fragments and (2) rejoining the DNA fragments.

◇ The desired gene may be introduced into a bacterial, fungal, or mammalian cell.

◇ Plasmids are small circular rings of DNA found in bacteria. They replicate themselves and move freely between bacterial cells. Plasmids can carry genes resistant to antibiotics.

◇ Cloning produces identical copies of the gene of interest.

◇ The environment of the host cell is critical for the proper folding of the protein.

◇ Studies are showing that the expense saved by curtailing hospital stays, shortening the duration of illnesses, and decreasing the incidence of disease more than pays for these products, even though the cost is extremely high.

◇ The positive clinical implications of the colony-stimulating factors (CSFs) include: decreasing the period of severe neutropenia after cytotoxic chemotherapy or marrow transplantation, treatment of aplastic anemia, and treatment of other immunodeficiency states associated with cytopenia.

◇ Epoetin (erythropoietin) increases RBCs; filgrastim increases WBCs.

◇ Colony-stimulating factors are Neupogen, Prokine, Epogen, and Procrit.

◇ Biologic response modifiers reduce cytokines and increase T-suppressor cell activity. They reduce the frequency of clinical exacerbations in ambulatory patients with relapsing multiple sclerosis. They are Betaseron and Avonex.

◇ Human growth hormone is used for the long-term treatment of growth failure from lack of adequate endogenous growth hormone secretion. It may be given SC every day or three times a week at twice the usual daily dose.

◇ Activase is a tissue plasminogen activator that catalyzes the conversion of tissue plasminogen to plasmin in the presence of fibrin.

◇ Pulmozyme reduces sputum thickness in cystic fibrosis.

◇ Factor VIII is used in hemophilia.

Immune System

◇ There are several types of immunoglobulins. IgG is the smallest and most common. IgM has the highest molecular weight. IgA is the main Ig in salivary and bronchial secretions, bile, and tears; it is also found in milk and colostrum. IgE is responsible for hypersensitivity reactions and is present in increased amounts in patients with allergic rhinitis and allergic asthma; IgD has unknown functions.

◇ Opsonization is the enhancing of phagocytosis of bacteria.

◇ The magnitude of an antibody response depends on the nature of the antigen, the frequency of exposure, and duration of each exposure.

◇ A lack of humoral immunity, as in inherited disorders, is due to a deficiency or absence of β cells, which increase susceptibility to bacterial infections, but not viral infections or neoplastic disease. Conversely, attenuation of cellular immunity without a corresponding reduction in the reactive capacity of β cells increase susceptibility to viral infection and neoplasm, but not to bacterial infection.

◇ CellCept, Imuran, Prograf, Sandimmune, and Orthoclone OKT are antirejection drugs.

◇ Hypersensitivity reactions are characterized as anaphylactic, cytolytic, toxin precipitin (serum sickness), and cell-mediated (contact dermatitis).

◇ The body presents three lines of defense: 1) surfaces of intact skin and mucous membranes, 2) nonspecific, and 3) immune response.

◇ The immune response has two features, specificity to attack a specific antigen and memory to remember the antigen for future invasion.

Neoplastic Disease (Cancer)

◇ Neoplastic disease occurs when cells become resistant to normal growth controls.

◇ Generally the side effects of chemotherapy are bone marrow depression, leukopenia, thrombocytopenia, ulceration of skin, ulceration of GI tract, hair loss, nausea, vomiting, nephrotoxicity, and teratogenicity.

◇ Remission puts the tumor into an inactive period when there is no active cell division and growth. It does not cure the disease, but extends the patient's life.

◇ Alkylating agents prevent cell division by cross-linking DNA strands, which leads to death within the cell.

◇ Antibiotics inhibit DNA-dependent RNA synthesis or delay or inhibit mitosis.

◇ Antimetabolites incorporate into normal cell constituents, which are then nonfunctional, or by inhibiting the normal function of a key enzyme.

◇ Hormones inhibit the synthesis of adrenal steroids.

◇ Nitrogen mustards bind irreversible cross-links in cellular DNA, and thus DNA and RNA cannot reproduce.

◇ Plant alkaloids inhibit formation of spindle fibers, arresting the metaphase of cell division.

◇ Topoisomerase I inhibitors lead to DNA damage when cells replicate. Other agents work by producing toxic metabolites and inhibiting RNA and protein synthesis.

◇ Cytoprotective or rescue agents are Zinecard, Ethyol, and Wellcovorin.

◇ Interferon inhibits viral replication.

◇ Tumor necrosis factor is secreted by macrophages in response to endotoxin.

◇ Colony-stimulating factors increase the host's ability to produce blood cells, which enhances production of granulocytes, monocytes, or RBCs.

◇ Monoclonal antibodies are used to direct attacks against specific objectives.

◇ Most cancer patients do not get adequate pain relief. Demerol is not a good choice for chronic pain because of the short half-life. Agents commonly used are Duragesic Patch, morphine, Dilaudid, Percocet, and Percodan. These were discussed in Chapter 7.

◇ Oral complications are common manifestations associated with chemotherapy. Treatments include Dyclone, Magic Swizzle, Peridex, Peroxyl, Salagen, and Ulcer Ease.

Drug Summary

Most of the drugs listed here are rarely referred to by generic name; the few that are have been listed in other chapters. Asterisks have been omitted.

Recombinant DNA Agents
Colony-Stimulating Factors
erythropoietin, epoetin alpha (Epogen, Procrit)
filgrastim (Neupogen)
sargramostim (Prokine, Leukine)

Biological-Response Modifiers
aldesleukin (Proleukin, Interleukin-2)
erythropoietin beta (Marogen)
interferon alfa-2a (Roferon)
interferon alfa-2b (Intron)
interferon alfa-n1 (Wellferon)
interferon beta-1a (Avonex)
interferon beta-1b (Betaseron)

Human Growth Hormones
somatrem (Protropin)
somatropin (Humatrope, Nutropin)

Fibrinolytic Agent
alteplase (Activase)

Secretion-Thinning Agent
dornase (Pulmozyme)

Hematologic Agent
antihemophilic factor, factor VIII (Hemofil)

Fusion Protein
denileukin (Ontak)

Antirejection Drugs
azathioprine (Imuran)
basiliximab (Simulect)
cyclosporine (Sandimmune)
daclizumab (Zenapax)
muromonab-CD3 (Orthoclone OKT3)
mycophenolate (CellCept)
sirolimus (Rapamune)
tacrolimus (Prograf)

Agents for Chemotherapy
Alkylating Agents

busulfan (Myleran)
carboplatin (Paraplatin)
carmustine (BiCNU)
cisplatin (Platinol)
cyclophosphamide (Cytoxan)
dacarbazine (DTIC-Dome)
ifosfamide (Ifex)
lomustine, CCNU (CeeNU)
streptozocin (Zanosar)
temozolamide (Temodar)

Antibiotics
bleomycin (Blenoxane)
dactinomycin (Cosmegen)
daunorubicin (Cerubidine)
doxorubicin (Adriamycin)
epirubicin (Ellence)
idarubicin (Idamycin)
mitomycin C (Mutamycin)
plicamycin (Mithracin)
valrubicin (Valstar)

Antimetabolites
capecitabine (Xeloda)
cytarabine (Cytosar-U)
floxuridine (FUDR)
fludarabine (Fludara)
fluorouracil, 5-FU (Efudex)
hydroxyurea (Hydrea)
mercaptopurine (Purinethol)
methotrexate (Rheumatrex, Folex)
thioguanine (Tabloid)

Hormones
aminoglutethimide (Cytadren)
bicalutamide (Casodex)
flutamide (Eulexin)
goserelin (Zoladex)
leuprolide (Lupron Depot)
megestrol (Megace)
mitotane (Lysodren)
tamoxifen (Nolvadex)

Nitrogen Mustards
chlorambucil (Leukeran)

estramustine (Emcyt)
mechlorethamine (Mustargen)
melphalan (Alkeran)
thiotepa (Immunex)

Plant Alkaloids
etoposide (VePesid)
vinblastine (Velban)
vincristine (Oncovin)

Topoisomerase I Inhibitors
irinotecan (Camptosar)
topotecan (Hycamtin)

Miscellaneous Agents
alitretinoin (Panretin)
altretamine (Hexalen)
asparaginase (Elspar)
levamisole (Ergamisol)
mitoxantrone (Novantrone)

paclitaxel (Taxol)
procarbazine (Matulane)

Cytoprotective (Rescue) Agents
amifostine (Ethyol)
dexrazoxane (Zinecard)
folinic acid, leucovorin (Wellcovorin)

Agents for Mucositis
dyclonine (Dyclone)
hydrogen peroxide (Peridex, Peroxyl)
lidocaine-diphenhydramine-Maalox
 (Magic Swizzle)
phenol sodium borate-sodium bicarbonate-glycerin (Ulcer Ease)
pilocarpine (Salagen)

Extravasation Agents
sodium thiosulfate (Tinver)
hyaluronidase (Wydase)

Chapter Review

Pharmaceuticals and Body Functions

Select the best answer from the choices given.

1. Betaseron is used to treat
    a. infections.
    b. multiple sclerosis.
    c. Kaposi's sarcoma.
    d. chronic hepatitis.

2. T cells respond directly to antigens to form
    a. B cells.
    b. plasma cells.
    c. clones.
    d. IgG.

3. The most common antibody is
    a. IgG.
    b. IgM.
    c. IgE.
    d. IgD.

4. The Ig with the highest molecular weight is
    a. IgG.
    b. IgM.
    c. IgE.
    d. IgD.

5. The main Ig in salivary and bronchial secretions, bile, and tears and also found in milk and colostrum, where it transfers immunity to a child, is
    a. IgG.
    b. IgM.
    c. IgE.
    d. IgA.

6. A delayed hypersensitive reaction occurs after
    a. twelve to seventy-two hours.
    b. two to three hours.
    c. one to two hours.
    d. ten to eleven hours.

7. Cells that recognize the antigen and enter the fight are
    a. effector cells.
    b. memory cells.
    c. T cells.
    d. killer cells.

8. Cells that enter a resting phase are
   a. effector cells.
   b. memory cells.
   c. T cells.
   d. killer cells.

9. Mitosis gives
   a. growth.
   b. cell division.
   c. repair.
   d. All of the above

10. Remission
    a. puts tumor into an inactive period.
    b. cures the disease.
    c. gives the patient less time.
    d. results in active cell division.

The following statements are true or false. If the answer is false, rewrite the statement so it is true.

_____ 1. The side effects of chemotherapy are bone marrow depression, leukopenia, nausea, and vomiting.

_____ 2. Prokine must be mixed in D_5W (5% dextrose).

_____ 3. Somatropin must be shaken well.

_____ 4. Colony-stimulating factors allow higher doses of chemotherapy.

_____ 5. Extravasation is leaking of drug around the injection site, causing tissue damage.

_____ 6. Interferon increases the host's ability to produce blood cells.

_____ 7. Interleukin is secreted by macrophages in response to endotoxin.

_____ 8. Tumor necrosis factor inhibits viral replication.

_____ 9. Alkylating agents inhibit DNA-dependent RNA synthesis or delay or inhibit mitosis.

_____ 10. Antimetabolites are incorporated into normal cell constituents, which are then nonfunctional, or inhibit the normal function of a key enzyme.

Diseases and Drug Therapies

1. List the disadvantages of extracting protein from plasma or tissue.
2. List the three types of cells into which the desired gene can be introduced.
3. List four types of hypersensitive reactions.
4. List the three lines of defense the human body has against invasion by pathogens.
5. Define remission.
6. Define resistance.

Dispensing Medications

1. Mrs. Brown brings in the following prescription. She has been taking the drug for at least 5 years. What should be done?

R_X **MT. HOPE MEDICAL PARK**
ST. PAUL, MN (651) 555-3591

DEA# _____

Pt. name _Sue Brown_ Date _8-7-05_

Address _____

Tamoxifen 10 mg bid   #60

_____ Dispense as written

✓ Fills _12_ times (no refill unless indicated)

J. Bean _____ M.D.

2. Mrs. Green brings in the following prescription for her son. She says he really does hate to get a shot and screams and yells every time she administers it. What suggestion can the technician make to the pharmacist?

R₂

MT. HOPE MEDICAL PARK
ST. PAUL, MN (651) 555-3591

DEA# _____

Pt. name _John Green_ Date _8-7-05_

Address _____

Humatrope 0.08 units/Kg q d
dispense one month's supply

_____ Dispense as written

_____ Fills _____ times (no refill unless indicated)

_____ *J. Bean* _____ M.D.

Patient weight 50 lbs
Humatrope 5 mg = 13 units = 5 mL

Rewrite the prescription as it is going to be dispensed.

Internet Research

Use the Internet to complete the following activities.

1. The antirejection drugs covered in this chapter are an important component of successful organ transplantation. Find data on common organ transplantation procedures. Create a table giving an overview of three procedures. Include the number of transplants done per year, the disease states/conditions which lead to the need for transplantation, the cost of the procedure, and the Internet sites from which you obtained your information.
2. New chemotherapeutics are being developed continuously. Research new chemotherapeutics, focusing on one particular type of cancer (e.g., colorectal, breast, liver, lung). Create a table listing three new agents. If you include drugs that are currently in clinical trials, indicate what phase of testing has been completed. Be sure to include the type of cancer researched in your table. List your Internet sources.

Vitamins, Nutritional Supplements, Natural Supplements, Antidotes, and CODE Blue Emergencies

Chapter 18

Learning Objectives

◇ Understand total parenteral nutrition, its purposes, ingredients, stability, and complications.

◇ Discuss and calculate electrolyte levels.

◇ Recognize herbs, their values, uses, and dangers.

◇ Know the various types of emergencies and the general guidelines for handling them.

◇ Understand the importance of the Blue Alert cart, its supplies, and its maintenance.

Intake of substances other than drugs can have far-reaching effects on the body in health and in sickness. Foods contain vitamins, minerals, and other nutrients that maintain body function and aid in disease prevention and treatment. The electrolytes regulate the body's electrical activity and need to be kept in balance with body fluids. Among plant substances that can affect the body are the herbs, many of which have medicinal applications. Ingestion of some substances can result in poisoning, causing critical states and necessitating use of lavage measures, antidotes, and supportive therapy. Recent improvements have been made in dealing with life-threatening diseases and emergencies. The pharmacy technician plays an important role by understanding a hospital CODE blue emergency system and the use of the Blue Alert cart and its maintenance.

TOTAL PARENTERAL NUTRITION

Total parenteral nutrition (TPN) is important to the survival and well-being of some patients. It provides the patient with all the nutritional requirements through the parenteral route. The system has evolved over more than 300 years, as advances have been made to provide patients with the nourishment they need. Important landmarks in the history of TPN are shown in Table 18.1.

The provision of parenteral nutritional support has become increasingly more complex. Although total parenteral nutrition can be life-saving, careless use caused by inadequate understanding or poor supervision can result in devastating consequences. Water, electrolytes, carbohydrates, and protein are maintained in proportions within a narrow range through a combination of dietary intake, metabolism, and excretion. Imbalances can be produced by disease or injury and determined by blood analysis. It is much easier to maintain body cell mass or restore small deficiencies than to restore a seriously ill patient. However, at times the most compassionate and cost-effective thing to do for a patient is to recognize that nutritional support will only extend suffering, not provide healing.

Table 18.1	Important Landmarks in Total Parenteral Nutrition
1656	Infusion of wine. Sir Christopher Wren, designer of St. Paul's Cathedral in London, was the first to do an IV infusion. He hollowed out a bird quill, inserted it into a vein, and infused a wine solution.
1843	Sugar infusion. This was the first nutrition solution. It was used on animals, but did not do well, probably because of the preparation.
1909	Rectal administration of protein. It was not successful.
1920	First fat emulsion. The patient did not do well. The particles in early fat products were large and did not pass effectively through small vessels.
1936	Protein solution.
1945	First use of 20% dextrose.
1967	Central venous catheter. A large catheter was inserted into the subclavian vein behind the clavicle. This was the start of modern parenteral nutrition. It allowed administration of concentrated nutrition solutions.
1980	Wide use of TPN using crystalline amino acids.

Malnutrition

Moderate to severe malnutrition has been demonstrated in up to twenty percent of all hospitalized patients. There are two types of protein stores, somatic and visceral. Somatic protein stores are skeletal muscle protein. Visceral protein stores are plasma proteins, and they make up 5% of body mass. These consist of albumin, globulin, transferrin (to transport iron), immunoglobulins, clotting factors, white blood cells, red blood cells, and lymphocytes.

A 20% reduction in body mass is considered moderate malnutrition; 40% is considered severe malnutrition. There are two types of protein malnutrition. The first type, marasmus, is a form of protein-calorie malnutrition with growth retardation. The patient appears thin, owing to low caloric intake. The condition develops over months, sometimes up to two years. There is an imbalance between protein and caloric intake. The second type, kwashiorkor, is a protein deficiency. It may be due to a lack of dietary protein or from the stress of infection, burns, traumatic injury, or disease, which consumes the body's intake and reserves.

Malnutrition causes poor wound healing and an increase in the number of infections. Thus the patient is much more prone to serious infection. Malnutrition destroys red blood cells as a source of energy for protein. It causes organ failure of the cardiovascular, renal, and gastrointestinal (GI) systems. Because the lungs require a lot of energy to function correctly, the malnourished patient may experience serious respiratory failure. The body's stores of protein and calories and lean body mass decreases. The body needs a certain percentage of body fat to offset high stresses and help a patient through a crisis, and the malnutrition decreases these fat stores. In addition, malnutrition decreases glycogen stores. In healthy patients, these sugar reserves provide quick energy between meals.

Cell membranes are the primary barriers to the movement of solute in the body. All membranes are permeable to water, which passes freely. Small solutes may diffuse through all membranes at a rate slower than that of water. The size of lipoproteins determine the lipoprotein crossing. Lipid-soluble gases, oxygen, and carbon dioxide, and lipid-soluble urea pass readily. Small hydrophilic ions and glucose use aqueous channels, moving slower than lipid-soluble substances; it is a passive process from higher to lower concentrations. TPN is formulated so as to insure adequate absorption of nutrients from circulation, providing fluids, carbohydrates, and protein while maintaining osmolarity.

Indications for Total Parenteral Nutrition

When oral feeding is not possible, patients may be fed through a tube that leads to the small intestine; this is called enteral nutrition and is preferred over feeding through the veins as in TPN because the lower abdomen continues to function.

These preparations are enteral feedings. Enterals are prepared by the pharmacy technician. A blue dye is added in order to enable the practitioners to differentiate it from other body fluids. If the enteral used is a ready-to-hang (RTH), the dye is in the tubing and the fluid will turn blue as it traverses the tubing.

The indications for TPN are poor wound healing, infections, anemia, and specific GI disease and/or hypermetabolic states. It may also be used when there is a failure to tolerate enteral nutrition.

The following patients may require parenteral nutrition.

⬥ Patients who cannot eat at all because of GI problems, obstruction, or tumor.
⬥ Patients who cannot eat enough because they have abnormal nutrition requirements. Patients with severe burns or short-bowel syndrome need almost three times the normal nutritional allotment.
⬥ Patients who can eat, but refuse to do so because of eating disorders such as anorexia nervosa.
⬥ Patients who can eat, but should not. This includes those with pancreatitis, severe gallbladder disease, inflammatory bowel disease, or severe diarrhea.

Conditions in which TPN may be indicated include

⬥ perioperative support
⬥ short-bowel syndrome
⬥ acute pancreatitis
⬥ enterocutaneous fistulas
⬥ inflammatory bowel disease
⬥ malignant disease
⬥ AIDS
⬥ pregnancy
⬥ severe gastroparesis (paralysis of the stomach)

Complications of Parenteral Nutrition

Some complications of TPN include

⬥ hyperglycemia or hypoglycemia
⬥ dehydration
⬥ liver toxicity
⬥ elevated serum triglycerides
⬥ high serum lipid concentrations
⬥ hypoalbuminemia
⬥ hyperammonemia
⬥ acid-base imbalance
⬥ failure to induce anabolism
⬥ imbalance of electrolytes

Even nondiabetic patients may show increased blood sugar when on TPN; therefore, insulin may be added to the solution even for the nondiabetic. Hypoglycemia is more significant than hyperglycemia. When patients with high sugar intake decrease it too quickly, the glucose level drops rapidly and to such low levels that coma, brain damage, or even death may occur.

Infections can often be a problem. TPN solutions are rich in nutrients and capable of growing all types of bacteria and fungi. Aseptic technique and testing of solution for growth around the line should be performed. The area around the central line often becomes infected, and the line has to be pulled and another put in to clear the infection.

Albuminar (albumin) is a major plasma protein. It is used clinically to reduce edema by osmotic effect, shifting fluid volume from the body into the circulation and increasing serum protein levels in hypoproteinemia (plasma protein lost in the urine). It is also used to increase plasma volume by osmotic effect to diminish red blood cell aggregation and reduce blood viscosity. Antigenic reactions can cause problems. Renal involvement due to high specific gravity may make albumin toxic to the kidney. Antithrombic activity prolongs clotting time and could lead to disseminated intravascular coagulation (DIC).

Preparing Total Parenteral Nutrition Solutions

There are two types of TPN solutions. TPN generally refers to amino acid-dextrose formulas, whereas total nutrient admixture (TNA) refers to the amino acid-dextrose-lipid content of three-in-one formulations. The advantages of the three-in-one formula are

◇ decreased cost of preparation and delivery
◇ reduced nursing time for administration
◇ potentially reduced risk of sepsis with fewer violations (breaks, points of entry) of the administration line

The disadvantage of the three-in-one is that precipitants cannot be seen if they occur and they are not stable as long as TPNs prepared without lipids.

The TPNs without lipids last about twice as long as those with lipids. The TPN with lipids, if stored properly, may have an expiration of up to seven days after mixed. The two-in-one (without lipids) may have up to a twenty-one-day expiration date. The lipid emulsions will oil out or crack with prolonged or incorrect storage. Producing a compatible three-in-one formulation has been challenging, requiring the amino acid products to be buffered to a higher pH. The electrolytes are added to the mixture when it is initially prepared, but the vitamins are always added just before administration. They are stable for twenty-four hours after addition. The TPN may remain at room temperature for twenty-four hours (usually a bag is hung this long). Otherwise it is always stored in the refrigerator.

A three-in-one formula contains protein, glucose, lipids and electrolytes, with vitamins added later. When mixing TPN it is necessary to be cautious regarding the addition of electrolytes. Pooling is controversial. This process in which all the electrolytes except phosphate are put into a small-volume parenteral bag and then transferred into each batch saves considerable time. Cysteine is sometimes added to prevent precipitation of the electrolytes in the TPN. If pooling is used, be sure to separate the phosphates from the calcium and magnesium. The phosphates should be injected into the bag first, and then the amino acids, dextrose, lipids, water, and then pooled electrolytes. When done this way, it is very unlikely that precipitates would occur.

To provide all nutrients intravenously, parenteral nutrition solutions must contain a large number of different components in a relatively small volume of fluid. Table 18.2 lists common additions to the parenteral nutrition mixture. The possibility of component interactions and microprecipitation is quite high and must be considered when mixing each batch. Solutions that do not contain lipid should be inspected during preparation against both black and white backgrounds with proper lighting.

All bags with precipitates should be refiltered or discarded. It is advantageous to look for particulate matter before adding insulin or albumin, since particles can be removed by passage through a filter into another bag, but albumin and insulin cannot pass through microfilters. Since vitamins degrade more rapidly, they should be added as close to the time of patient administration as possible.

Solutions containing lipids should be carefully inspected in the pharmacy and before infusion for cracking or oiling out. Cracking can be demonstrated by adding hydrochloric acid to the TPN. The result is a distinct separation of the oil, easily visible.

Calcium and phosphorus are the electrolytes that cause the most problems with precipitation. The phosphate ion should always be added first into the bag and mixed thoroughly with other ingredients; after the TPN is mixed, add the calcium ion with constant swirling. Calcium chloride should not be used. The sulfate salt is the preferred form for magnesium. The actual concentration of magnesium depends on the amount of calcium, since both are divalent cations and destabilize the lipid emulsion. The only insulin administered by IV infusion is "R." Regular is added to the parenteral nutrition; it is a solution and the others are suspensions. As little as ten units per liter has been found to be clinically effective in lowering mild elevations of blood glucose.

After final inspection, each batch should be clearly labeled with the patient's name, address or ward, solution name, concentration and volume, and additives. Instructions for the additives, such as vitamins, should be given on the label, and there must be an expiration date on any IV product.

Table 18.3 lists the recommended multivitamin additions. These come in one bottle and are added to the TPN just before administration. Tables 18.4 and 18.5 list other additions that may vary according to the product.

Warning

All IV products must contain expiration dates.

Table 18.2   Common Additions to the Total Parenteral Nutrition Mixture

Electrolytes	Daily Adult Dose
chloride	100 to 150 mEq
sodium	100 to 150 mEq
potassium	80 to 100 mEq
calcium	5 to 15 mEq
phosphorus	15 to 45 mEq
magnesium	8 to 30 mEq

Table 18.3   Recommended Multivitamin Additions

Vitamin	Daily Adult Dose
ascorbic acid (C)	60 mg
retinol (A)	800 mg
ergocalciferol (D_2)	200 mg
thiamine (B_1)	1.1 mg
riboflavin (B_2)	1.3 mg
pyridoxine HCl (B_6)	1.6 mg
niacinamide (B_3)	15 mg
tocopherol (E)	12 mg
biotin	150 mcg
folic acid (B_9)	180 mcg
cyanocobalamin (B_{12})	2 mcg

Table 18.4   Recommended Trace Element Additions

Trace Elements	Daily Adult Dose
chromium	10 to 15 mcg
copper	0.5 to 1.5 mg
manganese	0.15 to 0.80 mg
zinc	2.5 to 4.0 mg

Table 18.5   Per Liter Additions

Additive	Amount per Liter
calcium	9 mEq
magnesium	12 mEq
phosphate	21 mEq
potassium	80 mEq
sodium	patient tolerance
chloride	limited by cation
acetate	limited by cation
insulin, regular	30 U (dependent on blood glucose level)

VITAMINS, FLUID LEVELS, AND ELECTROLYTES

Vitamins are essential organic constituents present in many foods and are necessary for normal metabolic functioning. If inadequate dietary intake results in deficiency, the body cannot synthesize the vitamin. Labs should be drawn regularly (usually weekly) on TPN patients, depending on the disease state and patient's nutritional state. It is important to review these labs before mixing the next TPN because changes may need to be made in the formulations.

In humans, deficiencies occur as five major diseases. Most signs and symptoms can be reversed by administering the appropriate vitamin.

- ◇ Keratomalacia is a vitamin A deficiency that causes softening of the cornea.
- ◇ Rickets is a vitamin D deficiency that causes bending of the bones.
- ◇ Beriberi is a vitamin B_1 deficiency that causes polyneuritis, edema, and cardiac pathology.
- ◇ Pellagra is a vitamin B (niacin) deficiency that causes dermatitis and diarrhea.
- ◇ Scurvy is a vitamin C deficiency that causes anemia, spongy gums, hemorrhages, and brawny induration of calf and leg muscles.

Vitamins

Vitamins are classified as fat soluble and water soluble. Fat-soluble vitamins are maintained in large stores by the body, mainly in the liver. Deficiency develops after several months of restricted intake. As excessive amounts collect, toxic signs develop. Water-soluble vitamins, B and C, are present in extracellular fluids, which are readily excreted by the kidney. Deficiency shows quickly in inadequate dietary sources. Overdose is not likely to be as serious as with other substances, since the kidney quickly removes the excess.

FAT-SOLUBLE VITAMINS **Vitamin A (retinol)** is in milk, butter, cheese, liver, fish oils, and other foods. It can be formed in the body from plant pigments and carotene from fruits and vegetables, and is converted in the wall of the small intestine. Impaired ability to absorb lipids affects absorption of vitamin A. The body uses vitamin A for normal growth, bone formation, shedding and repair of epithelial tissue, retinal function, reproductive function (male and female), and stability of cell membranes.

Symptoms of vitamin A deficiency include night blindness, conversion of mucous surfaces to squamous cells, failure of epithelial surfaces to shed superficial layers, and corneas becoming dry. Overdose results in increased irritability, loss of appetite, itching, and hypertrophy of bone in the skull and extremities. More severe symptoms include increased intracranial pressure, sluggishness, headache, vomiting, and peeling of skin.

Vitamin D (D_2, ergocalciferol; D_3, cholecalciferol) is found in butter, milk, cheese, egg yolk, and fish oils. Bile is necessary for absorption; vitamin D is transported in chylomicrons into the lymphatics. It is normally formed by ultraviolet irradiation of the skin, converting precursors into active forms. Calciferol is formed from D_2 and D_3, which is then rapidly absorbed into the bloodstream. The major effects of vitamin D are seen on calcium and phosphate balance. Deficiency in children causes rickets, with distortion of long bones of the legs and bones of the pelvis and spine due to poor mineralization of newly formed bone. Deficiency in adults causes osteomalacia, which is demineralization and weakening of the skeleton. Toxicity is exhibited by calcium deposits in soft tissues (such as the kidneys and blood vessel walls), with symptoms including loss of appetite, GI disturbances, pain in joints, muscular weakness, psychosis, convulsions, and coma. Death is due to renal failure.

Vitamin E is a group of compounds called tocopherols. Sources include soybean oil, wheat germ, rice germ, cottonseed, nuts, corn, butter, eggs, liver, and green leafy vegetables. Vitamin E acts as an antioxidant for unsaturated fatty acids. Requirements increase with increased intake of fatty acid. A deficiency is exhibited by increased irritability, edema, and hemolytic anemia.

Vitamin K (phytonadione) functions in the formation of prothrombin in the liver (blood clotting). The sources are leafy green vegetables, wheat bran, and soybean products.

WATER-SOLUBLE VITAMINS **Vitamin C (ascorbic acid)** is found in green plants, tomatoes, citrus fruits, and potatoes, with smaller amounts in animal tissues. It is the most powerful reducing agent to occur naturally in living tissue; it causes the loss of oxygen from molecules. It acts as a cofactor. Ascorbic acid and oxygen are essential to the formation of hydroxyproline from the amino acid proline; hydroxyproline is found in collagen and epithelial basement membranes. In deficiencies, collagen formation is impaired, resulting in reduced structural integrity of connective tissue, including bone and epithelial basement membranes, which are compromised. Vitamin C is also one factor involved in maintaining normal cell membrane permeability. Adequate levels are necessary for normal production of thymosin, which confers immune ability to T lymphocytes. Vitamin C increases the phagocytic functioning of leukocytes, has anti-inflammatory activity, and promotes wound healing.

The original vitamin B is not a single vitamin, but a group of vitamins. Sources are yeast, meats, whole meal flour, peas, and beans. Most are synthesized by intestinal flora.

B_1, thiamine, acts as a coenzyme in carbohydrate metabolism. Sources include pork, liver, kidney, whole cereal, grains, peas, beans, and yeast. Deficiency results in beriberi. Alcoholics are often deficient of this vitamin and therefore it is often administered to them.

B$_2$, riboflavin, carries out phosphorylation in intestinal mucosa and functions to maintain the integrity of mucous membranes and metabolic energy pathways. Sources are milk, liver, kidney, heart, cereals, green vegetables, and intestinal synthesis.

B$_3$, nicotinic acid (Niacin, Nicobid), is involved in fat synthesis, electron transport, and protein metabolism. It is found in yeast, liver, lean meats, peanuts, peas, beans, whole wheat, rice grains, and in lesser amounts in potatoes and vegetables. The three Ds of deficiency are diarrhea, dementia (depression, memory loss, confusion) and dermatitis, a dark red coloration on all areas of the skin exposed to air and light. The skin becomes dry and fissured, atrophies (decreases in size), and becomes brown. There are also chronic inflamed mucous membranes, fluid and bloody feces, and central nervous system involvement (confusion, hallucinations, and delirium).

B$_5$, pantothenic acid, forms part of the coenzyme system. It is found in most vegetables, cereals, yeast, liver, kidney, and heart. Symptoms of deficiency include fatigue, headache, sleepiness, nausea, GI pain, muscle spasms, and disturbances of coordination.

B$_6$, pyridoxine, is a coenzyme in amino acid and fatty acid metabolism. It is found in practically all foods of plant and animal origin. A deficiency in infants may cause convulsions; adults may experience irritability, depression, nausea, and impaired peripheral nerve function manifested as peripheral neuritis (sharp shooting pains through the extremities). Other effects include skin disorders such as angular stomatitis and cheilosis (thick, smooth, bleeding tongue), and the skin does not heal well. Vitamin B$_6$ is given to alcoholics who have nerve damage. Tuberculosis patients taking isoniazid (INH) have depleted B$_6$. It is also given to patients for peripheral neuropathies caused by hydralazine or INH.

B$_9$, folic acid, is found in liver and fresh green vegetables. Together B$_{12}$ and B$_9$ provide for production of healthy red blood cells. B$_{12}$ deficiency results in nerve damage manifested as degenerative changes in the spinal cord. A diagnosis of B$_{12}$ deficiency requires the presence of two of the three following criteria: weakness, sore tongue (swollen, smooth), and numbness and tingling of extremities. Methotrexate, an antineoplastic, causes acute lymphocytic leukopenia. When Leucovorin, an active metabolite of folic acid is given within an hour of the cancer drug, it saves many of the white blood cells. If the cause of an anemia is unknown, the best treatment is B$_{12}$ and folic acid. This vitamin is also often given to alcoholics.

B$_{12}$, cyanocobalamin, is a cofactor and is only effective given IM. It is the intrinsic factor for the production of red blood cells. It is found in animal tissue, and the deficiency is exhibited as pernicious anemia.

Biotin is a water-soluble vitamin found in yeast, egg yolk, vegetables, nuts, and cereals. A coenzyme, it is formed by intestinal flora in greater amounts than ingested. Deficiency is characterized by dermatitis and anorexia.

Body Fluids

Bread may be the staff of life, but water is the elixir. Total body water varies between men and women. Figure 18.1 shows the average water percentage of body weight for adult men and women. The difference is due to skeletal weight and the inverse relation of water to adipose tissue.

Water is the major constituent of living cells. Body fluids are in equilibrium across the capillary walls and are divided into two compartments: intracellular (inside cells) and extracellular (outside the cells in the interstices, lymph, and plasma).

Fluid levels vary according to conditions (variations in percentage of total body water), weight, sex, and age. Fat holds little water; therefore the proportion of water in fat persons may be as little as 55%, whereas that in lean, well-muscled persons may be 70%. Women have more fat than men; therefore, they have proportionally

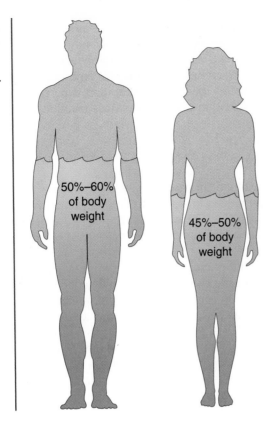

Figure 18.1

Average Water Percentage of Body Weight for Adult Men and Women

50%–60% of body weight

45%–50% of body weight

less body water. The body loses water with aging. Newborns may have up to 75% or more; the elderly have 60% or less.

Water and electrolyte deficits are caused by loss of body fluids as a result of such disorders as vomiting, diarrhea, edema, and excessive sweating from fever.

EXTRACELLULAR VOLUME DEFICIT Death can occur as a result of losing 25% of body water. The causes of water loss are large urine output and acute weight loss (more than 5% of body weight). This can cause dryness of skin and mucous membranes, longitudinal wrinkling of the tongue, hypotension, tachycardia, and lowered body temperature.

EXTRACELLULAR VOLUME EXCESS Retention of water without sodium is usually due to ingestion of excess fluids or infusions of fluids over long surgical procedures. This can cause confusion, bizarre behavior, inability to talk, nausea and vomiting, periods of violence and noisiness, delirium, muscle weakness, drowsiness, and coma.

IV THERAPY The goal of IV therapy is to provide the patient with sufficient water and electrolytes to maintain intracellular and extracellular fluids and excrete the end products of metabolism.

Isotonicity is the relationship of a solution to the body's own fluids and is measured by determining the number of dissolved particles in solution. Hypotonic solution is one with fewer particles than body fluids, so that water enters the body cells and causes them to swell. Hypertonic solution is one with more particles than body fluids, which draws water from the cells, so that they shrink. An isotonic solution is one with the same level of particles, 0.9% sodium chloride, and has the same tonicity as body fluid. It is a solution in which body cells can be bathed without net flow of water across the semipermeable cell membrane. Solvent is water, the liquid that dissolves the substance. Solute is a substance (electrolytes) dissolved in a solvent. Minerals exist as acids, bases, and salts and are dissolved in body fluids.

A common measurement of solution concentration is percent composition of grams of solute per 100 cc of solution. A 5% dextrose solution would contain 5 g of dextrose in 100 cc of water.

Electrolytes

Electrolytes are substances that can carry an electrical charge when in solution. Electrolytes are those compounds that separate into ions (positive and negative charged particles) when dissolved in water. Electrolytes are measured in milliequivalents of an ion in each liter of solution.

SODIUM (Na^+) Sodium is the primary cation ($^+$) of extracellular fluid. The average diet has sufficient sodium to meet the body's requirements. Kidneys are responsible for maintaining normal sodium concentrations in plasma and other body fluids. Sufficient losses of sodium can occur through vomiting and/or diarrhea, which reduce extracellular fluid volume. Fluids then move out of the cells in an effort to maintain blood volume. If water and sodium are not replaced, then blood volume and pressure are reduced and circulatory collapse may occur. Sodium functions to retain fluid in the body, generate and transmit nerve impulses, maintain acid-base balance, regulate enzyme activities, and regulate osmolarity and electroneutrality of cells.

POTASSIUM (K^+) Potassium is the primary cation of intracellular fluid. Potassium depletion produces loss of muscle tone, weakness, and paralysis; an excessive concentration can produce cardiac arrhythmias and heart block. Always use caution with concentrated potassium solution as it can burn out veins and can be lethal. Potassium functions to maintain regular cardiac rhythm, deposit glycogen in liver cells, regulate the enzymes and enzyme systems necessary to produce cell energy, transmit and conduct nerve impulses, and regulate osmolarity and electroneutrality of cells.

CALCIUM (Ca^{++}) Calcium is important in bone formation and dynamics, muscle contraction, and blood coagulation. Deficiency results in hyperexcitability of nerves and muscle fibers (tetany). An excess may cause muscle weakness leading to cardiac and respiratory failure. When a patient has low calcium on a blood test, the albumin levels should be checked. Low calcium may indicate low albumin, as a lot of calcium is bound to albumin.

Warning

Watch out for the calciums.

Various sources of calcium are used for different purposes. There are four primary sources of calcium in use: calcium chloride, calcium carbonate, calcium acetate, and calcium gluconate.

Calcium chloride is three times the strength of calcium gluconate. The chloride salt is the fastest salt to get into the bloodstream so it is the salt primarily used in cardiac emergencies. It moderates nerve and muscle performance through action potential excitation threshold regulation. It should never be mixed or infused in the same IV line as a phosphate because it will precipitate. It is only manufactured as an injection.

Calcium carbonate is usually used as an antacid. It has many brand names. It is also used as a dietary supplement to prevent a negative calcium balance. TUMS is frequently prescribed for this purpose. It is only taken by mouth.

Calcium acetate is used to control hyperphosphatemia in end-stage renal failure. It binds to the phosphorus in the GI tract better than other calcium salts due to its lower solubility and subsequent reduced absorption and increased formation of calcium phosphate. It is also used in parenteral nutrition. It can be administered as a capsule, tablet, or injection.

Calcium gluconate is used to prevent negative calcium balances. It moderates muscle and nerve performance and allows normal cardiac function. It is used in TPN and can be taken by mouth or parenterally.

CHLORIDE (CL⁻) The main effect of a chloride ion excess or deficiency is on acid-base balance. The concentration of chloride ions in parenteral nutrition solutions should usually be adjusted to equal that of sodium ions by adding non-chloride salts of sodium and potassium. Chloride functions to transport carbon dioxide (chloride shift), form hydrochloric acid in the stomach, retain potassium, and maintain osmolarity of the cell.

HYDROGEN IONS (H⁺) These ions determine the acidity or alkalinity of body fluids. Acidosis (blood pH below 7.35) is a metabolic condition due to excessive loss of bicarbonate or sodium as a result of diarrhea, starvation, or diabetic coma. In the respiratory system, the carbon dioxide concentrations increase. Alkalosis (blood pH above 7.45) is a metabolic condition due to excessive loss of potassium or chloride and is most often caused by vomiting or diarrhea. Respiratory system manifestations are hyperventilation and lowered carbon dioxide levels.

NATURAL SUPPLEMENTS

Various terms are used in the literature to describe herbs. The term generally means a plant or plant parts extracted or dried and valued for their savory, aromatic, or other qualities. Most of the information that consumers obtain about herbal products comes from individuals selling them or from books and pamphlets written and sold by them. Many authors have simply copied what they found in older books, so there is similarity in wording. English language herbals are actually copies of copies of copies. Most references can be traced back to one original source, *Gerard's Herbal*, written in the sixteenth century. Pharmacopeias in most Third World countries include herbal materials. The Chinese *Pharmacopeia* of 1979 contained more than 1,000 monographs on herbs. Herbs were the original sources of many important drugs and have served as models for many synthetic agents.

Natural Supplement Safety

Some people think that plants are nontoxic. It is commonly believed that herbs are completely safe, while drugs (nonherbs), including prescription drugs, are highly toxic. Some facts about natural supplements should be considered. Many relatively poisonous plants are excluded from sale because of the poison laws of the Food and Drug Administration (FDA). Many herbs are used in small amounts, in dilute forms, or for short periods so that risk of toxicity is minimal. Herbs are generally less toxic on a weight basis. Also, some persons are confused by the literature on herbs.

It is difficult to evaluate the safety of herbal products because the scientific name of the material in question is not known or the product may contain a mixture of materials. Several different plants may have the same common name. Even if the product is known, it is difficult to find information on toxicity.

Some of the most toxic chemicals are from plants, so herbs may be as toxic as synthetic drugs. People who pick their own herbs should be absolutely certain that the herb they pick is the one they seek. An old saying covers this: "There are old mushroom pickers, there are bold mushroom pickers, but there are no old bold mushroom pickers." The belief that herbs are not toxic, coupled with increasing the dosage, has led to toxicity from herbs that were considered safe in smaller amounts.

When potent herbs are compared with equally potent prescription drugs, the side effects are comparable or more severe. Licorice, for example, contains natural corticoids and has effects similar to equally potent doses of prescription corticoids. The ephedrine herb has greater side effects than phenylpropanolamine. Rauwolfia serpentine has side effects comparable to those of potent antihypertensives and has greater side effects than comparable tranquilizers.

Healthcare professionals are expected to warn patients about side effects of prescription drugs. Herbs, on the other hand, are sold as food without a listing of their side effects on the label or in the promotional literature.

Herbs have many interactions with drugs. For example, feverfew, gingko, garlic, and ginger increase the risk of bleeding in patients taking aspirin or warfarin. Gingseng, ephedra, and yohimbine can all increase blood pressure and decrease the effects of hypertensive drugs. Hawthorn can potentiate digoxin. It can also be difficult to predict how herbals will interact with each other.

Plants, with their natural composition of chemicals, have effects different from the chemicals isolated from them. There are some known differences between herbs and the purified chemicals. The chemical in a drug is more potent by weight. Herb overdose may be difficult because of a bitter or unpleasant taste. Other herbs would require an amount too massive for accidental ingestion.

To date, no study has shown herbs to be more effective than the chemicals purified from them. Prescription drugs that have been compared with herbs have been shown to produce essentially the same actions as quantities of the herb. There have been no demonstrated differences in activity from chemicals taken from plants and concentrated synthetic chemicals.

Most persons survive many illnesses, such as colds and coughs that run their course, without treatment. Infections usually are terminated when the body's defense mechanisms are mobilized; cuts, bruises, and broken bones heal alone. Another fact is that most patients with chronic and debilitating illness (cancer, arthritis) have "good days" and "bad days" since spontaneous periods of regression occur in the normal course of disease. Positive reinforcement and a desire to be cured may account for some positive response, even with a placebo.

There is no widespread cooperation between herbalists and healthcare professionals in the United States. Some herbalists believe that herbs are natural to the body, lack side effects, and are beneficial. Most medical practitioners believe the more desirable drugs are single entities and are proven by FDA standards. These are the most efficient because if there is an adverse event, it is more likely that the causative agent can be isolated.

Federal regulations permit the sale of herbs as foods, so they are labeled as to content, but not as to medical uses, doses, and dangers. No quality control exists, and false claims are numerous. The content of herbal products varies widely. It is not always clear which ingredients within each particular herb cause the desired effect. The need for standardization among herbal products presents a challenge. An herb's composition will vary depending on how the plant is grown, harvested, extracted, and stored. Standardization would require that the manufacturer ensure that each bottle contain the same quantity of active ingredients. However, the variance inherent in herbal farming methods makes standardization from manufacturer to manufacturer nearly impossible.

People consider herbs to be "natural" and "nontoxic." They often do not realize that herbs contain natural ingredients that can cause problems or may interact with other drugs.

There are two major problems with herbs. First, patients may mistake one plant for another which could result in serious effects or an allergic response. Second, the patient may treat with herbs and forgo effective treatment until a disease is too far advanced for help.

Most-Commonly Used Natural Supplements

Table 18.6 presents common herbs used for medicinal reactions. These herbs are considered to be in widespread use. The most-commonly used herbs are St. John's wort for depression, melatonin for sleep, ginseng (gingseng) for energy, gingko to improve memory, feverfew for migraines, saw palmetto for prostate disease, ma-huang as a bronchodilator and stimulant, valerian as a tranquilizer, chromium picolate for weight loss, glucosamine for arthritis, and eleuthera for energy. The last is also called Siberian ginseng.

Ginkgo is indicated for peripheral vascular disease and cerebral insufficiency. A number of well-regarded studies support the use of ginkgo. Twelve symptoms in elderly persons are claimed to be typical of cerebral insufficiency and are said to be relieved by gingko treatment. They are difficulties of concentration, absentmindedness, confusion, lack of energy, tiredness, decreased physical performance, depressive mood, anxiety, dizziness, tinnitus, headache, and memory difficulties.

Melatonin is a hormone produced naturally in the body during the hours of darkness. It helps the body adjust to night and day. This is a function of the circadian rhythm. Young people have much more melatonin in their body than older persons. Some researchers think this may be related to the fact that young people fall asleep so much easier than older people. Travelers are using melatonin as an antidote to jet lag,

Table 18.6	Most-Commonly Used Natural Supplements and Their Uses	
Common Name	**Use**	**Safety/Efficacy**
camomile	anti-inflammatory, antispasmodic, anti-infective	safe and effective; steep 3 g in 250 mL of hot water for 15 minutes; drink three to four times daily
chromium picolate	weight loss, improve insulin metabolism	benefits diabetes by improving insulin metabolism
ephedra (ma-huang)	anorectic, bronchodilator	ineffective as anorectic; effective as bronchodilator; unsafe for those with hypertension, diabetes, or thyroid problems; avoid caffeine
feverfew	migraine prophylaxis	safe and effective; 125 mg of leaves containing not less than 0.2% parthenolide; use one to two times daily
ginger	antiemetic	safe and effective; 1 to 2 g three times daily
ginkgo	circulatory stimulant	safe and effective; 60 mg of standardized extract twice daily
ginseng	energy	safe, but not very efficacious
glucosamine	arthritis	may help osteoarthritis
melatonin	sleep	works for some people; do not exceed recommended dosage
St. John's wort	depression	300 mg three times daily; "Nature's Prozac" works as well as prescription antidepressants for mild depression with fewer side effects

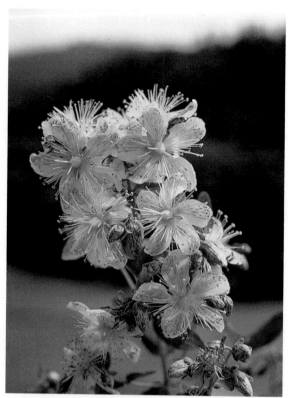

St. John's wort is a popular dietary herbal supplement. However, it has been discovered that it can reduce the effectiveness of some oral contraceptives. Patients should consult with their physician before taking herbal supplements such as St. John's wort.

stress, and insomnia. With traditional sleeping pills one can be groggy the next day, but this is not the case with melatonin. Some stomach discomfort has been the only reported side effect.

St. John's wort is being used for depression and is referred to as Nature's Prozac. It is also used for anxiety and insomnia. Contrary to popular belief, it does not interact with some foods as the MAOIs do. However, one should be very careful to not combine it with an antidepressant. It also causes photosensitivity, and it interacts with some prescription drugs.

Chromium picolate improves glucose tolerance. It is used widely for weight loss, but can have a devastating effect on the heart if taken inappropriately. It has been shown to benefit diabetics by improving the efficiency of their insulin metabolism.

Glucosamine stimulates the biosynthesis of a cartilage-building compound and can thereby help restore damaged tissue through the synthesis of cartilage, tendons, and synovial fluid. This herb may also provide some anti-inflammatory effects. Some research suggests that glucosamine might slow the progression of osteoarthritis. (The agent has no affect in rheumatoid arthritis.) Patients with osteoarthritis who take glucosamine experience less pain and have reduced knee joint deterioration. This supplement seems to work as well as NSAIDs for pain and is better tolerated. It also slows joint damage. The effects of glucosamine may not be felt by the patient until four to six weeks after the initiation of therapy. Glucosamine may increase insulin resistance and exacerbate diabetes. This agent can also cause GI discomfort, but this effect is minimal compared to that of the NSAIDs.

Chondroitin interferes with the enzymes that break down cartilage. This agent, like glucosamine, is widely used as a supplement to treat arthritis. Chondroitin is not as effective as glucosamine.

A reputable study supports the use of **NADH (Enada)**, a co-active enzyme in niacin, as a treatment for chronic fatigue syndrome. This agent reportedly increases energy and mental concentration.

POISONS AND ANTIDOTES

Prevention of accidental poisoning should be a major concern of healthcare professionals. More than two thirds of accidental poisonings occur in children under six years of age and generally by ingesting compounds in household use. It also frequently occurs among older persons who inadvertently receive or give household chemicals mistaken for medication or it happens as a result of occupational exposure to noxious chemicals. Ingestion is the most common route of poisoning.

Once the substance is taken, there are two concerns: 1) eliminating it from the patient's GI tract to prevent absorption, and 2) diminishing the effects of the dose absorbed.

Several drugs cause the most childhood poisonings.

◇ Iron tablets are the leading cause of fatal poisonings in children. Just a few iron or pre-natal tablets can kill a small child.
◇ Tricyclic antidepressants are extremely toxic in children. Small amounts can cause heart arrhythmias, seizures, and shock.
◇ Calcium channel blockers are becoming a big problem; they lead to low blood pressure and heart failure.
◇ Opiates (even Lomotil) can cause respiratory failure.
◇ Aspirin poisoning is down dramatically because of the childproof caps and the increased use of non-aspirin OTC pain relievers. Symptoms include tinnitus; nausea and vomiting occur with doses greater than 150 mg/kg.
◇ Alcohol is often overlooked. Small amounts can cause low blood sugar, coma, and seizures. Some mouthwashes contain enough alcohol to harm a child.

Common Routes of Poisoning

There are several common routes of poisoning. Skin contamination is the most important route of exposure to industrial poisons. When the skin has been exposed to a toxic chemical, the area should be properly irrigated. Chemicals may not only damage the skin, but may also produce systemic toxicity if absorbed through the skin. Inhalation poisoning is damage due to local irritation of the respiratory tract or to systemic absorption. The patient should be immediately carried into fresh air, and breathing support should be provided if necessary. Eye contamination is treated by immediate irrigation of the eye with water or an eye flush solution to diminish the poison's strength.

Supportive Therapy

Supportive therapy consists of establishing the airway and providing cardiopulmonary resuscitation (CPR); maintaining body temperature, nutritional status, and fluid and electrolyte balance; and preventing circulatory collapse, hypoglycemia, uremia, and liver failure. Often supportive measures are the only therapy available. Emptying the stomach, administering an adsorbent (charcoal), and inducing catharsis are potential treatments that should be considered when a sufficient amount of a potentially toxic substance has been ingested within a specific time.

GASTRIC LAVAGE This procedure is indicated for patients in coma, convulsing, or with no gag reflex. The first step in handling ingestion is to eliminate the ingested poison; however, this is usually not fully effective. Next, three steps are taken to diminish the effective dose of the ingested absorbed poison.

Step 1. Pharmacologic antagonists (specific antidotes) are given to counteract the effects of the poison.
Step 2. Forced diuresis by giving large quantities of fluid, orally, rectally, or IV. This is even more effective if the pH can be adjusted appropriately: acid is given for an alkaline chemical, or alkaline for an acid chemical.
Step 3. Dialysis and exchange transfusion are needed if the patient has ingested a very large dose of a water-soluble poison. They are contraindicated if the ingested substance is fat-soluble, protein-bound, or tissue-bound.

The agents for gastric lavage are syrup of ipecac, apomorphine, activated charcoal, and cathartics. **Syrup of ipecac** is the most-commonly used agent, but the drug should only be used as a last resort. It is the drug of choice in the home or hospital setting. It comes from the roots of two plants, *Cephaelis ipecacuanha* and *C. acuminata*. They contain two alkaloids that have CNS effects, stimulating the chemoreceptor trigger zone (CTZ) to cause vomiting. The suggested doses are

◇ younger than one year: 10 mL, followed by 100 mL of water or milk
◇ age one year or older: 15 mL, followed by 200 mL of water or milk
◇ adult: 15 to 30 mL followed by 1 L of fluid

It is very important to keep the patient awake for the next several hours after the ipecac dose. The drug induces drowsiness, and the patient could choke on vomitus. Just because the patient has vomited once does not mean it will not happen again.

Apomorphine is an alternative drug to ipecac. Its onset of action is usually faster than that of ipecac. It depresses respiration and the CNS.

Activated charcoal has become the primary emergency room treatment to prevent absorption of poison from the GI tract. Cathartics are used in conjunction with activated charcoal to further decrease the absorption of the ingested agent. Speeding the travel of gastric contents decreases the likelihood of absorption. Saline cathartics, such as magnesium sulfate and magnesium citrate, or hyperosmotic cathartics such as sorbitol, are the agents of choice.

PHARMACOLOGIC ANTAGONISTS (ANTIDOTES) A variety of drugs serve as antidotes, including chelating agents. An antidote is a drug that reduces a poison's negative effects. Table 18.7 lists the most-commonly used antagonists.

Atropine is used in poisoning from cholinergic agents to treat drug-induced bradycardia.

Cyanide antidote kit contains amyl nitrate inhalers, sodium nitrite ampules for injection, and sodium thiosulfate ampules for injection.

N-Acetylcysteine (mucomyst) is used for acetaminophen overdose.

Ethyl alcohol is a competitive inhibitor for the metabolism of methyl alcohol and ethylene glycol. It prevents biotransformation into formaldehyde and other compounds.

Table 18.7	**Most-Commonly Used Antagonists**	
Antagonist		**Chemical It Binds**
Generic	*Brand*	
N-acetylcysteine	Mucomyst	acetaminophen
atropine		cholinergic agents
calcium disodium	EDTA	lead
deferoxamine	Desferal	iron
dimercaprol	BAL	lead, arsenic, mercury, gold, bismuth, chromium, nickel, copper
fomepizole ethyl alcohol	Antizol	ethylene glycol-methyl alcohol
flumazenil	Romazicon	benzodiazepines
fomepizole	Antizole	ethylene glycol
methylene blue	Urolene Blue	nitrates
naloxone	Narcan	narcotics
nitrites and thiosulfate		cyanide
penicillamine	Cuprimine	copper, zinc, mercury, lead
physostigmine	Antilirium	atropine and other belladonna alkaloids
pralidoxime	Protopam	organophosphates
vitamin K$_1$	AquaMEPHYTON	warfarin

Urolene Blue (methylene blue) is used to treat nitrate and nitrite poisoning.

Narcan (naloxone) reverses narcotic respiratory depression.

Protopam (pralidoxime) is an acetylcholinesterase reactivator used for acetyl-cholinesterase-inhibiting pesticides (organophosphates). It is given after atropine in life-threatening situations.

Physostigmine is a cholinesterase inhibitor used to reverse toxic effects of drugs producing cholinergic crisis (i.e., atropine and other belladonna alkaloids).

Vitamin K promotes formation of clotting factors and is an antagonist for warfarin.

Antizol (fomepizole) is used to reverse ethylene glycol and methanol toxicity. It complexes with and inactivates alcohol dehydrogenase, thus preventing the formation of the toxic metabolites of the alcohols. Antizol is diluted in normal saline and dextrose and is stable for at least forty eight hours when refrigerated. The solution may become solid in the bottle and in this case it should be warmed by rotating it in the hand or running it under warm water.

EDTA (calcium disodium) is an edetate calcium disodium injection that enhances mobilization and excretion of lead from the body.

BAL (British Anti-Lewisite), also called **dimercaprol**, forms a stable chelate with lead, arsenicals, mercurials, gold salts, bismuth, chromium, nickel, and copper. It also reactivates enzymes shut down by these metals.

Desferal (deferoxamine) is a chelator for ferric iron used in acute iron poisoning.

Cuprimine (penicillamine) is a chelator of copper, zinc, mercury, and lead. It promotes the excretion of these metals in the urine.

ANTIVENOMS Snake antivenin is produced by hyperimmunization of a host. The dose required may be large. A high percentage of patients have serum sickness. Antivenin is developed against two species of North American pit vipers (rattlesnakes), but is clinically effective against venoms of pit vipers, whose bites are deadly. The drug must be on hand at the time of the emergency, together with epinephrine 1:1000, IV antihistamine, and hydrocortisone. There is a need to pretest, and if a reaction occurs, the value of giving the antivenin must be weighed against the risk of reaction.

A black widow spider bite is usually survived by most healthy adults with only supportive care. Antivenin is indicated for patients over sixty-five years and under twelve years with medical problems such as hypertension and cardiovascular disease. The venin is prepared from horse immunization. For a brown recluse spider bite, some physicians prescribe **Avlosulfon (dapsone)** in an attempt to preserve the skin around the bite. Dapsone is a sulfone antimicrobial. It causes photosensitivity, and the physician should be notified if persistent sore throat, fever, malaise, or fatigue occurs.

SUPPORTIVE DRUGS Many of these drugs have been discussed in other chapters. They are used in poisoning because of specific beneficial actions.

Cogentin (benztropine) is used to treat extrapyramidal side effects (EPS) caused by phenothiazines.

Benadryl (diphenhydramine) is used to treat EPS reaction to psychotic drugs.

Xylocaine (lidocaine) is used for ventricular arrhythmias.

Dilantin (phenytoin) is used to treat ventricular arrhythmias.

Antilirium (physostigmine) is indicated in seizures, severe hallucinations, hypertension, and anticholinergic-induced arrhythmias.

Inderal (propranolol) blocks excessive heart action (rate and strength).

Clinically Significant Drug-Food Interactions

The drug-food interactions should be avoided unless the physician is making an attempt to exploit an anticipated increase in drug effect. There is a clinically significant increase in absorption and/or effect when ketoconazole (Nizoral), nitrofu-rantoin (Macrodantin), and propafenone (Rythmol) are taken with food and when griseofulvin (Fulvicin) is taken with a fatty meal.

Grapefruit juice has been found to affect a good many drugs—specifically those drugs that are metabolized by cytochrome P450 in the liver and wall of the gut. However, it is important to note that not all drugs metabolized by these isozymes have clinically important interactions with grapefruit juice. Based on current data, the following drugs should not be given concurrently with grapefruit juice.

- all calcium channel blockers
- estrogens
- cyclosporine
- midazolam
- triazolam

The magnitude of the interactions between grapefruit juice and these drugs vary from person to person and from drug to drug. For example, an individual might actually benefit from taking cyclosporine with grapefruit juice. In some cases, the juice's ability to potentiate the drug could allow the desired effect to be achieved with a lower dosage.

The following drugs experience a clinically significant decrease in absorption and/or effect when taken with food or enteral nutrition.

- Achromycin (tetracycline)
- Cipro (ciprofloxacin)
- Didronel (etidronate)
- Dilantin (phenytoin)
- Noroxin (norfloxacin)
- Retrovir (zidovudine)
- Synthroid (levothyroxine)
- Videx (didanosine)

CODE BLUE EMERGENCIES

A CODE is a system to communicate when a patient is in a life-threatening situation, such as when a patient's heart and/or breathing have stopped. In response to a blue alert emergency, hospital personnel respond with appropriate emergency procedures. A patient in cardiac arrest has a flat ECG.

Various terms categorize the causes of death. Sudden cardiac death is death that occurs within twenty-four hours of the onset of illness or injury. Most patients have no symptoms immediately before collapse. The aim of treatment is to prevent ventricular fibrillation or to treat the arrest itself.

Sudden arrhythmic death is the loss of consciousness and pulse without prior circu-latory collapse. It is *not* preceded by circulatory impairment, but is preceded by chronic CHF. Death results from ventricular fibrillation associated with MI, transient myocardial ischemia, and underlying myocardial abnormalities (usually from previous MI).

Myocardial failure is a gradual circulatory failure and collapse before loss of pulse. It is due to hemorrhage, trauma, infarction, stroke, or respiratory failure.

The emergency procedures to deal with the conditions leading to sudden death are to stabilize the patient at the scene and then transport to a site of continuing care. Basic life support involves measures to prevent circulatory or respiratory arrest or provide external support for circulation and respiration if they have failed. Advanced cardiac life support (ACLS) ensures ready access to adjunctive equipment to support ventilation, give IV infusions, administer drugs, and provide cardiac monitoring, defibrillation, arrhythmic control, and postresuscitation care. The objectives are to

- ◇ correct hypoxia
- ◇ reestablish spontaneous circulation
- ◇ optimize cardiac function
- ◇ suppress sustained ventricular arrhythmias
- ◇ correct acidosis
- ◇ relieve pain
- ◇ treat CHF

The American Heart Association (AHA) has recommended guidelines for use of oxygen. The aim is to increase the oxygen level of the blood, thereby raising levels in organs and tissues. Indications include acute chest pain due to suspected or confirmed heart attack, suspected hypoxia of any cause, and cardiopulmonary arrest.

Agents for Cardiac Emergencies

Table 18.8 presents the most-commonly used agents for cardiac emergencies.

CARDIAC STIMULATION Cordarone (amiodarone) is used for first line management of life-threatening recurrent ventricular fibrillation. It is an antiarrhythmic agent which inhibits adrenergic stimulation, prolongs the action potential and refractory period in

| Table 18.8 | Drugs Recommended by ACLS Guidelines for Cardiac Emergencies |

Generic Name	Brand Name	Dosage Form
Cardiac Stimulation		
amiodarone	Cordarone	IV
diltiazem	Cardizem	IV
dobutamine	Dobutrex	IV
epinephrine	Adrenalin	IV
ibutilide	Corvert	IV
isoproterenol	Isuprel	IV
procainamide	Procan, Pronestyl	IV
verapamil	Isoptin	IV
Hypotension		
dopamine	Intropin	IV
Antidote Extravasation		
phentolamine	Regitine	IV
Bradycardia		
atropine	Atropair	IV, SC
Esophageal Bleeding		
ethanolamine	Ethamolin	local injection
vasopressin	Pitressin	IV
Cerebrovascular Accident		
nimodipine	Nimotop	liquid-filled capsule

myocardial tissue, and decreases atrioventricular conduction and sinus node function. During a CODE blue emergency, this drug may be mixed and infused in a plastic container. However, if the patient is put on a drip, it must be mixed in a glass container. It is incompatible with most drugs and must be protected from light.

Adrenalin (epinephrine) is the most-commonly used agent in cardiopulmonary arrest. A strong heart stimulant, it increases contractility and excitability. It is used in any form of cardiopulmonary standstill, and helps to convert fine ventricular fibrillations to a coarser form that is easier to defibrillate. *Precaution:* Use cautiously in liver disease, low cardiac output, and allergy.

Isuprel (isoproterenol) is a beta stimulant that increases heart rate. It is used for rates of 40 or less and for slow rates not responsive to atropine. *Precautions:* Increases oxygen demands on the heart or in arrhythmias or hypotension.

Procan and **Pronestyl (procainamide)** decrease the fibrillation threshold and prevent recurrence; they are used to suppress arrhythmias not responsive to lidocaine or in lidocaine allergy. They are not used in ventricular fibrillation because of slow onset of activity. *Precautions:* Can cause hypotension, ECG changes, and kidney disease.

Isoptin (verapamil) is a calcium channel blocker (slows the movement of calcium ions through slow channels). It slows SA node action, slows AV node conduction, and dilates coronary artery smooth muscle. It is used in atrial fibrillations and/or flutter that results in fast ventricular rates. *Precaution:* May result in hypotension and heart block.

Dobutrex (dobutamine) is a sympathomimetic adrenergic agonist. It increases heart rate with little action on β_2 or alpha receptors. Dobutrex is used to increase cardiac output in the short-term treatment of patients with cardiac decompensation caused by depressed contractility from organic heart disease, cardiac surgical procedures or acute myocardial infarction. It is compatible with dopamine, epinephrine, isoproterenol, and lidocaine. The drug is stable for forty-eight hours after mixing if refrigerated and for six hours if not refrigerated. It may turn a slight pink color, but this color change does not indicate a significant loss of potency.

Corvert (ibutilide) is used for acute termination of atrial fibrillation or flutter. It prolongs the action potential in cardiac tissue. It is stable for twenty-four hours at room temperature and forty-eight hours if refrigerated.

Cardizim (diltiazem) is used for atrial fibrillation or flutter and paroxysmal supraventricular tachycardia. The IV form of this drug, which is the only way it can be used for a code blue emergency, is refrigerated. Therefore it cannot be stored on the Blue Alert cart. It should not be used if the patient has severe hypotension.

Hypotension Intropin (dopamine) increases blood pressure by causing constriction of peripheral vessels while maintaining blood flow to internal organs and kidneys. It is used to support blood pressure and decrease cardiac and kidney function. *Precautions:* May result in arrhythmias, blood pressure control problems, nausea, vomiting, or IV extravasation (leaking of drug around the injection site) causing tissue death. It is also used as adjunctive treatment of left ventricular failure secondary to acute myocardial infarction, adjunct treatment of males with impotence, and in hypertensive crisis from sympathomimetic amines.

Antidote Extravasation Regitine (phentolamine) is used when there is extravasation from an injection. This drug can cause hypotension and skeletal weakness, tachycardia, and GI upset. It is also used as an antidote to the extravasation of dobutamine. The drug is diluted with normal saline and injected into the extravasated tissue. It will immediately reverse the blanching.

Bradycardia **Atropair (Atropine)** blocks vagus stimulation, which slows the heart, allowing the sympathetic system to speed the rate. It is most useful in bradycardia for rates less than 60 bpm and in asystole. However, it increases oxygen demands on the heart in arrhythmias or hypotension.

Esophageal Bleeding **Ethamolin (ethanolamine)** is a fatty acid compound for injection into dilated veins of the esophageal wall. *Precaution:* It is a chemical cauterizing agent that causes sclerosis or scarring.

Pitressin (vasopressin) is an antidiuretic hormone (ADH) injected into the superior mesenteric artery. It is used as an adjunct with an esophageal inflation device to control bleeding.

Cerebrovascular Accident **Nimotop (nimodipine)** is a calcium channel blocker with a greater effect on blood vessels of the brain than on heart cells. It is used to treat blood vessel spasm after subarachnoid hemorrhage in patients in good neurologic condition. Between days 4 and 14 after hemorrhage, cerebral arterial spasm is common, with frequent severe ischemic neurologic deficits or death. *Precautions:* Adverse effects are headache, nausea, bradycardia, flushing, and fluid retention.

Miscellaneous Agent **Betapace (sotalol)** is a beta blocker used to treat sustained ventricular arrhythmias and to maintain normal sinus rhythm in patients with symptomatic atrial fibrillation and flutter. When taken in a non-emergency situation it should be taken on an empty stomach.

The Blue Alert Cart

Blue Alert carts are stocked with the following drugs listed in Table 18.9. In hospitals, it is the pharmacy technician's responsibility to keep all these drugs stocked and up to date.

The technician must remove any expired drugs and any that will expire in the next one to two months. Expiration dates must be checked at least twice. Blue Alert carts must be checked regularly by the pharmacist. Always make sure the pharmacist has checked the cart before it is returned to the hospital floor. When a cart has been returned to the pharmacy, the drugs must be restocked and the expiration dates checked.

Dextrose 50% is included for diabetic coma. Naloxone is to reverse narcotic overdose. Flumazenil is for benzodiazepine overdoses.

Warning

In an emergency situation it would be very easy to confuse dobutamine and dopamine. Be sure they are not stored together on the Blue Alert cart.

Table 18.9	**Blue Alert Cart Drugs**

◇ adenosine	◇ isoproterenol
◇ aminophylline	◇ lidocaine
◇ amiodarone	◇ magnesium sulfate
◇ atropine sulfate	◇ naloxone
◇ calcium chloride	◇ procainamide
◇ dextrose 50%	◇ phenytoin
◇ diazepam	◇ sodium bicarbonate
◇ dobutamine	◇ sodium chloride
◇ dopamine	◇ sotalol
◇ epinephrine	◇ vasopressin
◇ flumazenil	◇ verapamil

Chapter Summary

Total Parenteral Nutrition

- It is much easier to maintain body cell mass or restore small deficiencies than to restore a seriously ill patient.
- The results of malnutrition are poor wound healing, infections, anemia, organ system failure, and decreased body stores of protein and calories.
- Enterals which are fed through a tube directly into the small intestine are preferred over TPN because the lower abdomen continues to function. A blue dye is added in order to differentiate the enteral from other body fluids.
- The advantages of three-in-one formulations are decreased costs of preparation and delivery, reduced nursing time for administration, and potentially reduced risk of sepsis with fewer violations of the administration line.
- The disadvantages of three-in-ones are the short stability and the inability to see precipitants if they have occurred.

Vitamins, Fluid Levels, and Electrolytes

- Vitamins are classified as water-soluble and fat-soluble. B and C are water-soluble; the rest are fat-soluble.
- Water is the major constituent of living cells. Body fluids are divided into two compartments, intracellular and extracellular.
- Water and electrolyte deficits are caused by loss of body fluids as a result of such things as vomiting, diarrhea, edema, and excessive sweating from fever.
- Death can occur as a result of losing 25% of body water. Causes of water loss are large urine output and acute weight loss, more than 5% of body weight. This can cause dryness of skin and mucous membranes, longitudinal wrinkling of tongue, hypotension, tachycardia, and lowered body temperature.
- "Isotonic" implies the same level of particles as the body fluids, 0.9% sodium chloride.
- Sodium is the primary cation of extracellular fluid.
- If there is a loss of water and sodium in the body, blood volume is reduced, blood pressure is reduced, and circulatory collapse may occur.
- Potassium is the primary cation of intracellular fluid.
- Calcium is associated with bone formation and dynamics, muscle contraction, and blood coagulation.
- Each calcium salt has a specific use.
- Hydrogen ions regulate the acidity or alkalinity of body fluids.

Natural Supplements

- Herbs were the original source of many important drugs and have served as models for many synthetic drugs.
- Licorice contains natural corticoids and has similar effects to equally potent doses of prescription corticoids.
- Herbs have many drug interactions.
- Two major problems with herbs are mistaken identity and allergy and forgoing professional treatment.

Poisons and Antidotes

◇ Once a poison is ingested there are two concerns: 1) eliminating it and 2) diminishing the effects.

◇ The drugs that cause the most childhood poisonings are iron tablets, tricyclic antidepressants, calcium channel blockers, opiates, aspirin, and alcohol.

◇ Syrup of ipecac is most commonly used to induce vomiting. Never induce vomiting of a caustic agent. Attempt to neutralize it. It may do more damage as it comes back out. This drug should be reserved for serious situations.

◇ Activated charcoal has become the primary treatment to prevent absorption from the GI tract in emergency room patients.

◇ The following drugs have a much better absorption if given with food: Plendil, Procardia, Fulvicin, Nizoral, Mevacor, Macrodantin, and Rythmol.

◇ The following drugs have a clinically significant decrease in absorption if taken with food: Cipro, Videx, Didronel, tetracycline, AZT, Noroxin, Dilantin, and Synthroid.

◇ Drug-food interactions should be avoided unless making an attempt to exploit an anticipated increase in effect, or decrease dosages in others.

CODE Blue Emergencies

◇ The pharmacy technician is the individual responsible for keeping the Blue Alert carts stocked. All medications must be kept up to date. An out-of-date medication could cost someone his or her life.

Drug Summary

Because of the nature of this chapter, brands and generics have not been asterisked. Those that would need the asterisk have already been covered in other chapters.

Vitamins
biotin
vitamin A, retinol
vitamin B
    B_1, thiamine
    B_2, riboflavin
    B_3, nicotinic acid (Niacin, Nicobid)
    B_5, pantothenic acid
    B_6, pyridoxine
    B_9, folic acid
    B_{12}, cyanocobalamin
vitamin C
vitamin D
    D_2, ergocalciferol
    D_3, cholecalciferol
vitamin E
vitamin K

Electrolytes
sodium, Na^+
potassium, K^+
calcium, Ca^{++}
    calcium acetate
    calcium carbonate
    calcium chloride
    calcium gluconate
chloride, Cl^-
hydrogen ions, H^+

Natural Supplements
camomile
chondroitin
chromium picolate
ephedra (ma-huang)
feverfew
ginger
ginkgo
ginseng
glucosamine
melatonin
NADH (Enada)
St. John's wort

Agents for Gastric Lavage
activated charcoal
apomorphine
atropine
calcium disodium (EDTA)
cyanide antidote kit
deferoxamine (Desferal)
dimercaprol (BAL: British Anti-Lewisite)
fomepizole ethyl alcohol (Antizol)
flumazenil (Romazicon)
fomepizole (Antizole)
methylene blue (Urolene Blue)
N-aylcysteine (mucomyst)
naloxone (Narcan)
penicillamine (Cuprimine)
physostigmine (Antilirium)
pralidoxime (Protopam)
syrup of ipecac
vitamin K_1 (AquaMEPHYTON)

Supportive Drugs
benztropine (Cogentin)
dapsone (Avlosulfon)
diphenhydramine (Benadryl)
lidocaine (Xylocaine)
phenytoin (Dilantin)
physotigmine (Antilirium)
propranolol (Inderal)

CODE Blue Emergencies
Cardiac Stimulation
amiodarone (Cordarone)
diltiazem (Cardizem)
epinephrine (Adrenalin)
ibutelide (Corvert)
isoproterenol (Isuprel)
procainamide (Procan, Pronestyl)
verapamil (Isoptin)

Hypotension
dopamine (Intropin)

Antidote Extravasation
phentolamine (Regitine)

8. Which vitamin is used in treating and preventing colds?
   a. A
   b. B
   c. C
   d. D

9. Which vitamin helps calcium move into the bone?
   a. A
   b. B
   c. C
   d. D

10. Which vitamin is usually purchased as a complex of vitamins?
    a. A
    b. B
    c. C
    d. D

The following statements are true or false. If the answer is false, rewrite the statement so it is true.

_____ 1. The leading cause of childhood poisoning is iron tablets.

_____ 2. Some indications for TPN are poor wound healing, infections, and anemia.

_____ 3. Causes of water loss are large weight loss, lowered body temperature, and large urine output.

_____ 4. An isotonic solution has fewer particles than body fluids.

_____ 5. Ginkgo is recommended as an antiemetic.

_____ 6. Melatonin is a hormone produced naturally in our bodies.

_____ 7. Feverfew is an anti-inflammatory, antispasmodic, and anti-infective.

_____ 8. Ginseng is recommended for increasing circulation.

_____ 9. There are no major problems with herbs.

_____ 10. Opiates can cause respiratory failure.

Diseases and Drug Therapies

1. List three specific gastrointestinal diseases and/or hypermetabolic states that could be an indication for TPN.
2. List ten complications of TPN.
3. What is the phone number of the poison prevention center in your area?
4. List twelve symptoms that may be helped by ginkgo.
5. List the symptoms of extracellular volume excess.

Dispensing Medications

1. A mother runs into the pharmacy to get ipecac. She is upset. What instructions should she be given on the label for dosing it and what precautions should be taken?
2. What drugs must be in the emergency room before administering snake antivenin? The technician must get these together.

Internet Research

Use the Internet to complete the following activities.

1. Create a table listing tips for adults on preventing accidental poisonings in the home and instructions for dealing with a case of suspected poisoning. In a third column include a list of useful resources for parents concerned about the potential for accidental poisoning (e.g., phone numbers, Web sites). List your Internet sources.
2. Herbal medicines have become increasingly popular. Use the Internet to research two of the herbal remedies covered in this chapter. List two or three medicinal benefits as well as precautions of use for each. List your Internet sources.

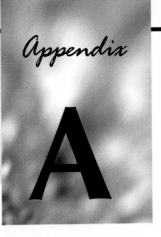

Equivalent Measures and Conversions

Appendix

A

Equivalent Measures

Metric	Volume	1 liter	= 1,000 milliliters
		1 milliliter	= 1 cubic centimeter
	Weight	1 gram	= 1,000 milligrams
		1 milligram	= 1,000 micrograms
Apothecary	Volume	1 fluid ounce	= 6 drams
		1 fluid dram	= 60 minims
Household	Volume	1 gallon	= 4 quarts
		1 quart	= 2 pints
		1 pint	= 16 fluid ounces
		1 ounce	= 6 teaspoonsful
		1 cup	= 8 ounces
		1 tablespoonful	= 3 teaspoonsful
		1 teaspoonful	= 100 drops
	Weight	1 pound	= 16 ounces
	Length	1 yard	= 3 feet
		1 foot	= 12 inches
Other		1 unit	= 1,000 milliunits

Measurement Conversions

	Household	Apothecary	Metric
Volume	1 quart	32 fluid ounces	1 liter
	1 pint	16 fluid ounces	473 milliliters
	1 cup	8 fluid ounces	240 milliliters
	2 tablespoonsful	1 fluid ounce	30 milliliters
	1 tablespoonful	3 fluid drams	15 milliliters
	1 teaspoonful	1 fluid dram	5 milliliters
	60 drops	1 fluid dram	5 milliliters
	1 drop	1 minim	
Weight	2.2 pounds	1 kilogram	
	1 pound	0.45 kilogram	
Length	1 inch	2.5 centimeters	

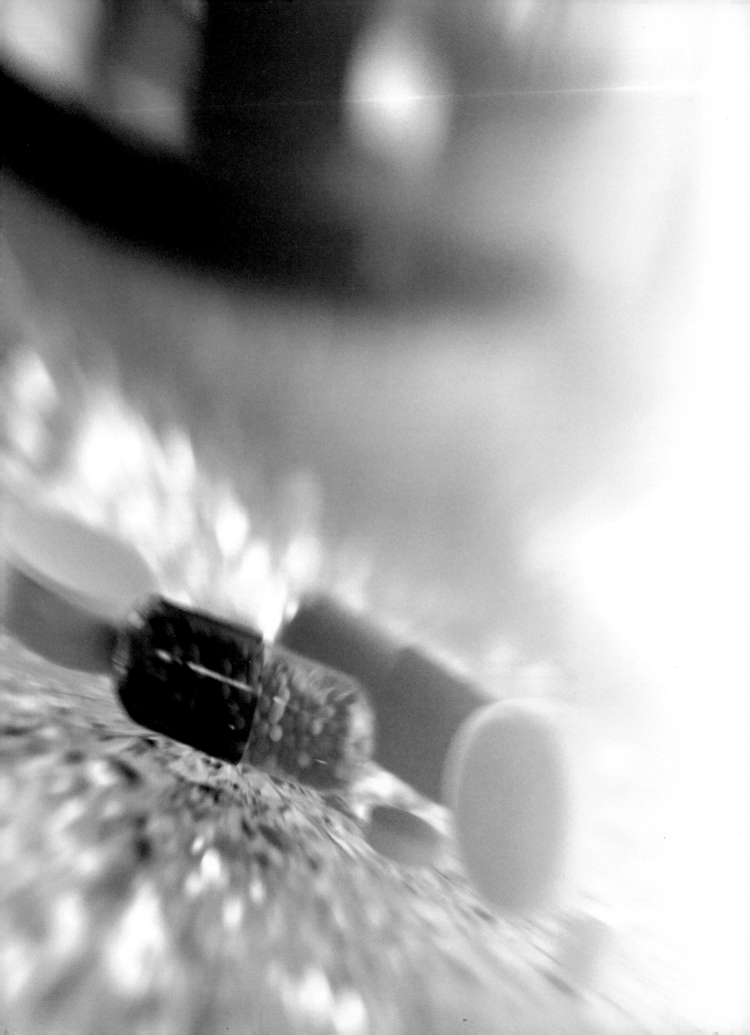

Abbreviations

ACE	angiotensin-converting enzyme
ACh	acetylcholine
ACLS	advanced cardiac life support
ACTH	adrenocorticotrophic hormone
ADA	American Dental Association
ADD	attention-deficit disorder
ADH	antidiuretic hormone
ADHD	attention-deficit hyperactivity disorder
ADP	adenosine diphosphate
ADR	adverse drug reaction
AHA	American Heart Association
AIDS	acquired immune deficiency syndrome
ALS	amyotrophic lateral sclerosis
AMA	American Medical Association
ANS	autonomic nervous system
APhA	American Pharmaceutical Association
ATP	adenosine triphosphate
AV	atrioventricular
BP	blood pressure
BPH	benign prostatic hypertrophy
BUN	blood urea nitrogen
cAMP	cyclic adenosine monophosphate
CBC	complete blood count; complete blood [cell] count
CCU	coronary care unit
CDC	Centers for Disease Control
cDNA	complementary DNA
CF	cystic fibrosis
CHF	congestive heart failure
CMV	cytomegalovirus
CNS	central nervous system
CO	cardiac output
COMT	catechol-o-methyl transferase
COPD	chronic obstructive pulmonary disease
CPR	cardiopulmonary resuscitation
CRF	corticotrophin-releasing factor
CSF	colony-stimulating factors
CTCL	cutaneous T-cell lymphoma
CTZ	chemotrigger zone
CV	cardiovascular
CVA	cardiovascular accident

DEA	Drug Enforcement Administration
DIC	disseminated intravascular coagulation
DMARD	disease-modifying antirheumatic drug
DNA	deoxyribonucleic acid
DOC	drug of choice
DT	delirium tremens
DVT	deep vein thrombosis
ECG	electrocardiographic
ECT	electroconvulsive therapy
EEG	electroencephalographic
EPS	extrapyramidal symptoms
EPSE	extrapyramidal side effect
ERT	estrogen replacement therapy
ESR	erythrocyte sedimentation rate
ESRD	end-stage renal disease
FDA	Food and Drug Administration
FSH	follicle-stimulating hormone
GABA	gamma-aminobutyric acid
G-CSF	granulocyte colony-stimulating factor
GERD	gastroesophageal reflux disease
GH	growth hormone
GHRF	growth hormone releasing factor
GI	gastrointestinal
GM-CSF	granulocyte-macrophage colony-stimulating factor
GMP	good manufacturing practice
GRF	gonadotrophic-releasing factor
HCG	human chorionic gonadotropin
HDL	high-density lipoprotein
HIV	human immunodeficiency virus

HPA	hypothalamus/pituitary/ adrenal [axis]		PEP	post-exposure prophylaxis
HRT	hormone replacement therapy		PG	prostaglandin
			pH	acid-base balance
			PI	protease inhibitor
IBS	irritable bowel syndrome		PID	pelvic inflammatory disease
IBW	ideal body weight		PMDD	premenstrual dysphoric disorder
ICU	intensive care unit			
IgE	immunoglobulin E		PMS	premenstrual syndrome
IgG	immunoglobulin G		PNS	peripheral nervous system
IL-2	interleukin-2		PPD	purified protein derivative
INH	isoniazid		PT	prothrombin time
ISA	intrinsic sympathomimetic activity		PTCB	Pharmacy Technician Certification Board
			PTT	partial thromboplastin time
KS	Kaposi's sarcoma		PTU	propylthoiuracil
			PUD	peptic ulcer disease
LAK	lyphokine-activated killer		PVC	premature ventricular contraction
LDL	low-density lipoprotein			
LH	luteinizing hormone			
LSD	lysergic acid diethylamide		RBC	red blood cell; red blood [cell] count
MAbs	monoclonal antibodies		RDA	recommended daily allowance
MAOI	monoamine oxidase inhibitor			
MCA	monoclonal antibody		RDS	respiratory distress syndrome
mcg	microgram		REM	rapid eye movement
MDI	metered dose inhaler		RF	rheumatoid factor
MHC	major histocompatability complex		RIND	reversible ischemic neurologic deficit
MI	myocardial infarction		RNA	ribonucleic acid
MS	multiple sclerosis		RSV	respiratory syncytial virus
MVI	multiple vitamin complex		RTH	ready-to-hang
NDA	new drug application		SA	sinoatrial
NGU	nongonococcal urethritis		SNS	sympathetic nervous system
NK	natural killer		SR	sustained release
NNRTI	non-nucleoside reverse transcriptase inhibitor		SSRI	serotonin-selective uptake inhibitor
NREM	nonrapid eye movement		STD	sexually transmitted disease
NRTI	nucleoside reverse transcriptase inhibitor		$T_{1/2}$	half-life
NSAID	nonsteroidal anti-inflammatory drug		TB	tuberculosis
			TCA	tricyclic antidepressant
			TCR	T-cell receptor
OC	oral contraceptive		TIA	transient ischemia attack
OR	operating room		TNA	total nutrient admixture
OTC	over-the-counter		TNF	tumor necrosis factor
			TPA	tissue plasminogen activator
PABA	para-aminobenzoic acid		TPN	total parenteral nutrition
PAF	prostatic antibacterial factor		TPR	total peripheral resistance
PCA	patient-controlled analgesia		TSH	thyroid stimulating hormone
PCBs	polychlorinated biphenyls			
PE	pulmonary embolism		WBC	white blood cell; white blood [cell] count
PEFR	peak expiratory flow rate			

Lab Values

These are just a few of the reference lab values for adults that the technician may have to look up for the pharmacist. These normal ranges are for reference only. The laboratory doing the tests will provide normal ranges for the results provided.

Serum Plasma
    Albumin 3.2–5 g/dL
    Bicarbonate 19–25 mEq/L
    Calcium 8.6–10.3 mg/dL
    Chloride 98–108 mg/L
    Creatinine 0.5–1.4 mg/dL
    Glucose 60–140 mg/dL
    Hemoglobin, glycosylated 4–8%
    Magnesium 1.6–2.5 mg/dL
    Potassium 3.5–5.2 mEq/L
    Sodium 134–149 mEq/L
    Urea Nitrogen (BUN) 7–20 mg/dL

Cholesterol
    Total < 220 mg/dL
    LDL 65–170 mg/dL
    HDL 40–60 mg/dL
    Triglycerides 45–150 mg/dL

Liver Enzymes
    GGT
        Male 11–63 IU/L
        Female 8–35 IU/L
    SGOT (AST) < 35 IU/L (20–48)
    SGPT (ALT) (10–35) < 35 IU/L

CBC
    Hgb (hemoglobin)
        Male 13.5–16.5
        Female 12.0–15.0
    Hct (hematocrit or "crit")
        Male 41–50
        Female 36–44
    WBC with differential 4.5–11.0 (×10 to the third power over mm cubed)

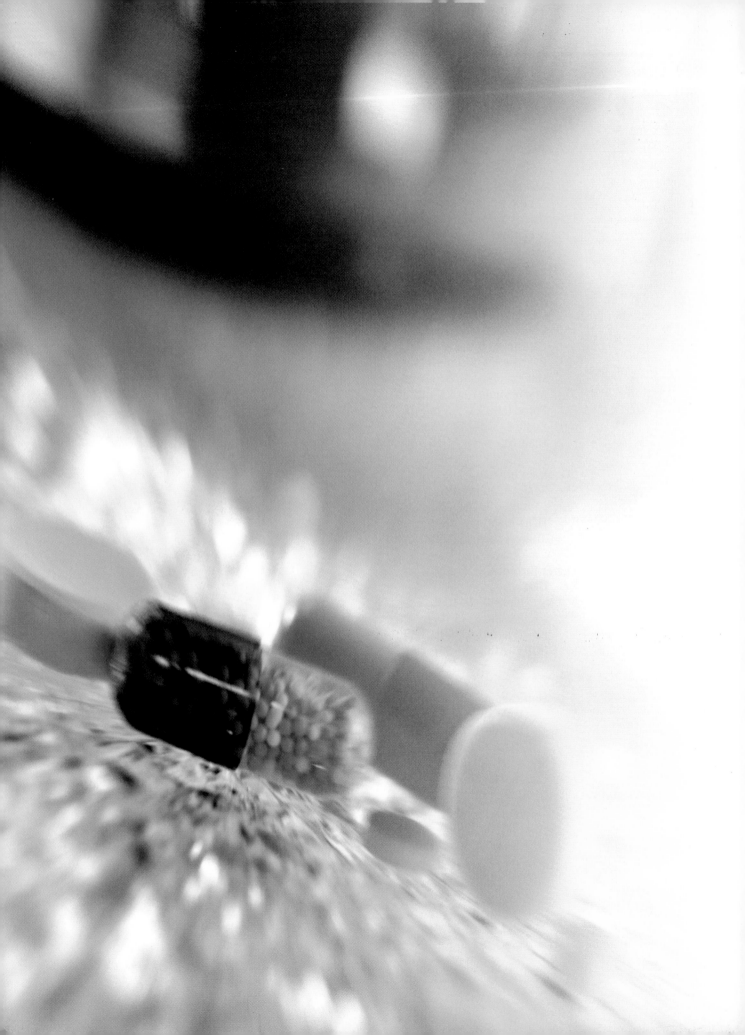

Index

Italicized page locators refer to figures; *t* denotes table.

and cimetidine, 223
enzymes, 27
protease inhibitors metabolized through, 91, 92
system, 90
cytochrome P-450 3A4, 69
cytokine-activated macrophages, 317
cytolytic reactions, 412, 422
cytomegalovirus (CMV) retinitis, 97
antivirals for, 86, 87, 88
Cytomel (liothyronine, T$_3$), 335, 361
cytoprotective (rescue) agents, 417-418, 422
Cytosar, 87
Cytotec (misoprostol), 224, 315
cytotoxic agents/drugs, 250, 327
Cytovene (ganciclovir), 87
Cytoxan (cyclophosphamide), 182, 322

D

daclizumab, 410
dairy products
and quinolones, 68
and tetracycline, 66
dalfopristin, 69
Dalmane, 162
dalteparin, 289
dandruff, 375, 390
Dantrium (dantrolene), 122, 137, 312
dantrolene, 122, 137, 312
dapsone, 445
DEA. See Drug Enforcement Administration
deafness, 70
death, 446
and water loss, 437, 450
Decadron (dexamethasone), 200
decongestants, 105-107, 110, 119
drug summary for, 111
most-commonly used, 106t
side effects and dispensing issues with, 106-107
side effects of, 107t
therapeutic uses of, 106
decosanol, 377
deep-vein thrombosis, 293
and estrogens, 341
risk factors for, 287
definitive host, 236, 237
D$_5$W (5% dextrose), 69
dehydration
and constipation, 229
from diarrhea, 226
from vomiting, 231
delavirdine, 90
Delsym, 109
Deltasone (prednisone), 200
de Materia Medica, 4, 16
dementia, 153, 184, 186
Demerol, 419, 422
denileukin, 405
dental work
and amoxicillin, 74
and cephalosporins, 65
and clindamycin, 71
and quinolones, 69
deoxyribonucleic acid: in viruses, 83, 84
Depakene (valproic acid and its derivatives), 151, 173
Depakote (divalproex), 151, 162, 173
dependence, 130
alcohol, 159
depolarizing agents, 312
depression, 145
with Alzheimer's disease, 184
menopause-related, 340
most-commonly used MAOIs in, 148t
most-commonly used SSRIs in, 146t
most-commonly used TCAs in, 147t
dermatitis, 385
dermatologic system
and antipsychotics, 152
and lithium, 150
dermis, 371
Desferal (deferoxamine), 445

desflurane, 122
desipramine, 183
Desoxyn (methamphetamine), 235
Desyrel (trazodone), 149
Detrol (tolterodine), 252, 259
dexamethasone, 200, 350
dexatroamphetamine, 235
Dexedrine (dexatroamphetamine), 235
dexrazoxane, 418
dextromethorphan, 110
dextrose 50%, 449
dextrose flushes, 403
DiaBeta, 357
diabetes, 352
early treatment of, 6
and heart attacks, 277
and heart disease, 268
and lack of insulin, 353-354
symptoms of, 353
treating, 354-355
types of, 353, 363
diabetic coma: dextrose 50% for, 449
diabetic patients
and cephalosporins, 65
and estrogen, 340
diabetic ulcers, 355
dialysis, 250
dialysis patients: and Vancocin, 70
Diamox (acetazolamide), 388
diaper rash, 381
diarrhea
with protease inhibitors, 91
and quinolones, 69
tetracycline for, 66
traveler's, 237
treatment for, 226-227, 240
diastolic reading: blood pressure, 281
diazepam, 123, 312, 325
and status epilepticus, 171
DIC. See disseminated intravascular coagulation
diclofenac, 320
Dicumarol (warfarin), 289
dicyclomine, 109
didanosine, 88, 89, 446
Didronel (etidronate), 345, 446, 451
diet
and diabetes treatment, 354, 355
and FDA health claims, 13
and heart health, 268, 277
and hypertension, 281
weight-loss, 234
dietary fiber, 227, 240
diet drugs, 242
diethylpropion, 235
difenoxin, 226
Differin (adapalene), 376, 390
diffuse tumors, 414
diflorasone diacetate, 382
Diflucan (fluconazole), 94, 98, 124, 349
digestion, 118
digital clubbing: with cystic fibrosis, 203
digitalis toxicity ("dig toxicity"), 276, 299
digoxin, 8, 274, 275, 299, 440
dihydroergotamine, 136
Dilacor XR, 280
Dilantin (phenytoin), 146, 174, 273, 299, 445, 446, 451
and status epilepticus, 171
Dilatrate-SR (isosorbide dinitrate), 280
Dilaudid, 422
diltiazem, 448
dimenhydrinate, 153
dimercaprol, 445
Dioscrides, 4, 16
Diovan (valsartan), 277
Dipentum (olsalazine), 225, 239
diphenhydramine, 105, 109, 110, 113, 153, 156, 159, 233
diphenoxylate-atropine, 226
diphtheria, 44
diplopia, 181
Diprivan (propofol), 123, 124
dipyridamole, 293, 294
dirithromycin, 68
disease condition: and drug effects, 39

disease-modifying antirheumatic drugs, 322-323, 327
drug summary of, 328
most-commonly used, 322t
diseases
allergic, 47-48
and drug therapies, 80-81
fungal, 93
infectious, 57
theories of, 3-4
disinfectants, 60, 371, 378-380
actions of, 378t
drug summary for, 392
most-used, 379t
diskhalers, 87
disopyramide, 272
Dispensatorium, 5
dispensing issues
with antibiotics, 59-60
with antihistamines, 104-105
with antitussives, 108
with cephalosporins, 65
with decongestants, 106-107
with macrolides, 67
with MAOIs, 148-149
with penicillin, 63
with quinolones, 69
with sulfonamides, 61-62
with tetracyclines, 66-67
for TIA and stroke prevention agents, 293-294
disseminated intravascular coagulation, 432
dissolution, 21
distribution, 20, 22, 25, 28
age-related changes in, 41-42
dosage forms, routes of administration and, 36
and pediatric patients, 43
disulfiram (Antabuse), 75, 160, 163
Ditropan (oxybutynin), 252, 259
diuretics, 41, 250, 255-258, 259, 301, 327
and cholesterol levels, 296
in congestive heart failure treatment, 274
drug summary for, 260
for hypertension, 283
most-commonly used, 257t
and secondary diabetes, 353
and Zyloprim, 324
divalproex, 151, 162, 173
diverticula: portion of colon with, 228
diverticular disease, 228-229
DMARDs. See disease-modifying antirheumatic drugs
DNA. See deoxyribonucleic acid
DNA enzyme, 405
DNA formation: antibiotics and interference with, 59
DNA mutation: by bacteria, 60
DNA sequence, 400
dobutamine, 449
Dobutrex (dobutamine), 448
Domagk, Gerhardt, 6
donepezil, 185
dopamine, 117, 118, 119, 137, 333, 449
and Parkinson's disease, 177, 186
receptors, 180
and seizures, 170
dopaminergic neurons, 177
Dopar, 179
Doral, 162
dornase, 405
dornase alfa, 203, 204
Doryx (doxycycline), 348
dorzolamide, 388
dosage forms, 50
common, 37t
for corticosteroids, 351
routes, 37t
and routes of administration, 36-39
dosages, 23
antiretroviral regimens, 92t
and five "rights" for correct drug administration, 35
with narcotics, 132
and pediatric patients, 43

prescription drugs/over-the-counter drugs, 114
tuberculosis statistics, 216
interstitial cystitis, 252
intestinal flukes, 237
intestinal infections: and metronidazole, 71
intestinal tapeworms, 237
intestinal transit time, 217
intra-abdominal infections
and clindamycin, 71
tetracycline for, 66
intra-arterial route of drug administration, 21
intracellular body fluids, 436, 450
intracerebral hemorrhage, 292
intracranial hemorrhage, 291
intradermal injections, 38
intragastric balloon, 235
intramuscular injections, 38
intramuscular route of drug administration, 21
intraoccular pressure, 387, 388
intrarenal events: and renal failure, 248, 249
intravenous injections, 38, 50
intravenous route of drug administration, 21
Intron (interferon alfa-2b), 404, 418
Intropin (dopamine), 449
invasive aspergillosis: and Cancidus, 96, 98
Invirase, 92
involuntary skeletal muscle contraction, 311
iodine deficiency: and hypothyroidism, 334
ions, 438
Iopidine (apraclonidine), 387
ipecac syrup: vomiting induced by, 232
ipratropium, 197
ipratropium bromide, 199, 202, 211
irinotecan, 417
iron deficiency, 250
iron tablets: and childhood poisonings, 443
irritable bowel syndrome, 229
irritant receptors: and cough reflex, 107
ischemia: causes of, 249
islets of Langerhans, 352
Ismelin (guanethidine), 286
isoetharine, 199, 210
isoflurane, 122
isometheptene-dichloralphenazone-acetaminophen, 136
isoniazid, 206
isoproterenol, 199, 210, 274
Isoptin (verapamil), 448
Isopto Atropine (atropine), 274, 299
isosorbide dinitrate, 280
isotonic, 450
isotonicity, 437
Isuprel (isoproterenol), 199, 274, 448
itching, 373, 390
itraconazole, 95, 96
IV infusions, 430t
of narcotics, 133
IV local anesthetics, 125
IV products: expiration dates for, 433
IV therapy, 437-438

Ketalar (ketamine), 123
ketoconazole, 95, 349, 446
ketones, 354
ketorolac, 321
ketotifen, 388
kidneys, 247
and congestive heart failure, 274
diabetes and damage to, 353
disease of, 247
functions of, 247-248, 255
mixed analgesics and failure of, 316
as site of elimination, 23, 28
and sodium concentration, 438
Kinerase (furfuryladenine), 376
King, Dr. Emil, 6
klebsiella, 60
Klonopin (clonazepam), 176, 183
Koch, Heinrich Hermann Robert, 378
KS. See Kaposi's sarcoma
kwashiorkor, 430
Kwell, 384
Kytril (granisetron), 233

Levulan (aminolevulinic acid), 377
Lewy bodies: and Parkinson's disease, 177
Leydig cells, 337
LH. See luteinizing hormone
libido, 337
lice, 382-384, 391
most-commonly used agents for, 383t
licorice, 440, 450
lidocaine, 125, 273, 445
lidocaine-diphenhydramine-Maalox, 420
lifestyle modifications: and heart health, 268
life-threatening infections: and aminoglycosides, 69
life-threatening situations: and CODE, 446
ligases, 400, 401
limbic system, 128
lindane, 384
Lioresal (baclofen), 184, 186, 313, 325
liothyronine, T$_3$, 335
liotrix, 335
lipase inhibitors, 235-236
lipids, 22
lipid solubility, 20
lipid-soluble molecules, 22
Lipitor (atorvastatin), 297, 302
lipoproteins, 294, 295
liquid dosage forms: for pediatric and geriatric populations, 36
lisinopril, 276
lispro, 356, 357
Lister, Joseph, 6, 378
lithium, 162
lithium compounds: for bipolar mood disorders, 149, 150
lithobid, 150
lithonate, 150
lithotabs, 150
liver, 353
and cholesterol processing, 294
cirrhosis of, 159
as site of elimination, 23, 28
liver enzymes: lab values for, 461
liver toxicity: with antifungals, 96
loading doses, 24, 28, 351
local anesthetics, 125-127, 137
drug summary for, 139
most-commonly used, 127t
local effect, 26
local viral infection, 85
locus ceruleus, 155, 156
Lodine (etodolac), 129, 320
lollipops: anesthetic, 137
Lomotil (diphenoxylate-atropine), 176, 226, 239
long-acting β$_2$ agonists, 197
long-acting insulin, 355
Loniten, 286
loop diuretics, 256, 258, 259, 296, 301
loop of Henle, 256, 257
loperamide, 226, 239, 416
Lopid (gemfibrozil), 298
lopinavir-ritonavir, 91
Loprox, 95
Lorabid (loracarbef), 66, 131
loracarbef, 66, 131
lorazepam, 123, 154
Lortab, 131, 320
losartan, 277
Lotemax (loteprednol), 388
Lotensin (benazepril), 276
loteprednol, 388
lotions, 50
Lotrimin (clotrimazole), 95, 375, 377, 390
Lou Gehrig's disease, 183, 186
Lovenox (enoxaparin), 289
low-density lipoproteins, 228, 236, 294, 295, 296, 301
low molecular weight heparins: drug summary for, 304
Lozol (indapamide), 258
Ludiomil (maprotiline), 147
Luminal (phenobarbital), 175
Lunelle (estradiol cypionate-medroxyprogesterone), 343, 362
lung diseases
cystic fibrosis, 203-204

salicylates, 314-315, 325, 326, 327, 328
salicylic acid, 375
salicylism, 315
salmeterol, 199, 210
salmonella: Chloromycetin for, 71
salt intake: and heart health, 268
Salvarsan, 6
Sandimmune (cyclosporine), 411, 422
SA node. *See* sinoatrial node
saquinavir, 92
Sarafem, 146
sargramostim, 403
saturated fats, 296
saw palmetto, 441
Scabera (lindane), 384
scabicides, 382-385
scabies, 382, *384*
    site of infestation of, on body, *385*
SC doses. *See* subcutaneous doses
Schedule I drugs, 9, 10*t*
Schedule II drugs, 10*t*
Schedule III drugs, 10*t*
Schedule IV drugs, 10*t*
Schedule V drugs, 10*t*
schistosoma, 237
schistosome infections, 236
schistosomiasis, 237
schizophrenia, 151
Schmiedeberg, Oswald, 6
Schwann cells, 126
scurvy, 434
sebaceous glands: disorders of, 372-373
seborrhea, 372
secobarbital, C-II, 158
Seconal (secobarbital, C-II), 158
secondary diabetes, 353, 363
secondary glaucoma, 321
secondary site cancer, 414
secondary-stage infection: with syphilis, 348
second-generation cephalosporins, 65, 74
second-generation sulfonylureas, 357
second-hand smoking: effects from, 207
secretion-thinning enzymes, 405
Sectral (acebutolol), 285
sedation
    with antihistamines, 104, 105
    with narcotics, 129
sedatives, 162
seizures, 169-171, 232
    anticonvulsants for partial and general-
      ized, 172*t*
    causes of, 170
    generalized, 170-171, 186
    partial, 170, 186
    therapeutic regimens for, 173*t*
selective alpha$_1$ adrenergic antagonists, 254
selective estrogen receptor modulator, 346
selective 5-HT receptor agonists: for migraine
    headaches, 135-136
selective serotonin reuptake inhibitors, 146-147
    most-commonly used, in depression, 146*t*
    drug summary for, 164
selegiline, 148, 179
selenium sulfide, 375
Selsun Blue (selenium sulfide), 375
Semmelweis, Ignaz Philip, 6
sense organs, 117, 118
sepsis, 69, 249
Septra (sulfamethoxazole-trimethoprim), 127,
    253
Serax (oxazepam), 154
Serevent (salmeterol), 197, 199, 211
serotonin, 20, 117, 119, 137, 146, 411
    and migraine headaches, 134
    and seizures, 170
serotonin receptors: 5-HT$_1$ and 5-HT$_2$, 134
serotonin-specific reuptake inhibitors, 162
sertraline, 147, 179
serum plasma: lab values for, 461
serum sickness, 104, 412, 422, 445
Serzone (nefazodone), 149
sevelamer, 250
sexually transmitted diseases
    agents for, 349-350, 364
    drugs for, 346-350, 362

most-commonly used agents for, 349*t*
    and quinolones, 69
sexual potency, 337
"shake well before using" sticker, 388
shampoos: summary of, 393
shingles, 374
    antivirals for, 86, 97
    famciclovir for, 87
short-acting β$_2$ agonists, 197
short-acting insulin, 355, 356
Siberian ginseng, 441
sibutramine, 235, 236
side effects, 26, 30, 44
    with ACE inhibitors, 277, 285
    with androgens, 337
    with angiotensin II receptors, 285
    with antiarrhythmic agents, 272-274
    with antibiotics, 59-60
    with anticholinergic drugs, 119
    with anticoagulants, 288-289
    with antihistamines, 104-105
    with anti-Parkinson agents, 178
    with antiplatelet agents, 290
    with antipsychotics, 152
    with antitussives, 108
    with aspirin, 294, 315
    with benzodiazepines, 154
    with beta blockers, 281, 285-286
    with birth control pills, 342
    with cephalosporins, 65
    with chemotherapy, 422
    with cholesterol-lowering agents, 296-298
    with CNS agents, 286
    with combination drugs for hypertension,
      287
    with corticosteroids, 200, 350-351
    with COX-2 inhibitors, 321
    with decongestants, 106-107
    with disease-modifying antirheumatic
      drugs, 322-323
    with drugs for gouty arthritis, 324
    with enzyme inhibitors, 358
    with epinephrine, 197
    with estrogen, 340
    with G-CSFs, 403
    with herbs, 440
    with hypnotic medications, 157-158
    with insulin, 356
    with macrolides, 67
    with muscle relaxants, 312, 325
    with narcotics, 131
    with nitroglycerin, 279-280
    with nonnarcotic analgesics, 314
    with nonsteroidal anti-inflammatory
      drugs, 318, 319, 326
    with oral contraceptives, 339, 341-342
    with penicillin, 63
    with peripheral acting agents, 286
    with prescriptions, 35
    with protease inhibitors, 91
    with quinolones, 69
    with salicylates, 315
    with sulfonamides, 61-62
    with tetracyclines, 66-67
    with TIA and stroke prevention agents,
      293-294
    with tricyclic antidepressants, 147
    with vasodilators, 286-287
    with weight reduction stimulants, 235
signa (sig): on prescription, 33
signs of renal disease, 249
sildenafil, 338
Silvadene (silver sulfadiazine), 380
silver nitrate, 8, 347, 379
silver sulfadiazine, 380
simethicone, 231, 240
Simulect (basiliximab), 410
simvastatin, 297, 302
Sinemet (levodopa-carbidopa), 179, 186
Singulair (montelukast), 200, 211
sinoatrial node, 269
sinus infections: and cephalosporins, 65
sinusitis: relieving, 106
sirolimus, 411
site antagonism, 20, 30

Skelaxin (metaxalone), 313
skeletal muscle relaxants, 139
skeletal muscles, 118, 311
skeletal muscular system: and anesthesia, 120
skin
    anatomy of, *372*
    disorders of, and agents for treatment of,
      372-385, 390-391
    most commonly used agents for treating
      disorders of, 376*t*
    structure and function of, 371-372, 390
    summary of miscellaneous treatments
      for, 393
skin cancer, 373, 375, 377
skin contamination: and poisonings, 443
skin infections
    cephalosporins for, 65
    tetracycline for, 66
sleep disorders, 145, 156-159
    most-commonly used agents for, 158*t*
sleep stages, 156-157
Slo-Phyllin, 199
slow viral infection, 84
small intestine, 22, 217
smallpox, 44
smoking
    and asthma, 195
    and emphysema/chronic bronchitis, 201
    and estrogen replacement therapy, 340
    and GERD, 220
    health endangered by, 207
    and heart disease, 268, 277
    and hypertension, 281
    and strokes, 291
smoking cessation, 207-209, 211
    antidepressants for, 149
    drugs for, 209, 212
    most-commonly used agents for, 209*t*
    personal benefits to, 207*t*
    planning, 193, 208-209
smooth muscle, 20, 118
snake antivenoms, 445
snuff, 207
sodium (Na$^+$), 438, 450
sodium bicarbonate, 8, 373
sodium hypochlorite, 379
sodium phosphate, 230
sodium thiosulfate, 420
soft tissue infections: tetracycline for, 66
Solage (mequinol-tretinoin), 377-378
solid tumors, 414
solubility of drug, 21
soluble fiber, 227
soluble lipoproteins: classes of, 295-296
Solu-Cortef (hydrocortisone), 200
Solu-Medrol (methylprednisolone), 200
solutes, 438
solvents, 438
Soma (carisoprodol), 312, 325
somatic nervous system, 118
somatic pain, 313, 325
somatic protein stores, 430
somatrem, 405
somatropin, 359, 363, 404, 405
Sonata (zaleplon), 158, 162
sotalol, 273, 290, 449
soy protein: labeling of, 13
spacers, 210
Sparine, 151
specificity, 19, 413
Spectinomycin, 347
sperm production, 337
spider bites, 445
spinal column: injections into, 38
spinal cord, 117, 128
spinal cord injuries, 122, 312
spinal local anesthetics, 126
Sporanox (itraconazole), 95, 96, 98
squamous cell carcinoma, 373
SSRIs. *See* selective serotonin reuptake
    inhibitors
St. John's wort, 91, 441, *442*
St. Mary's Hospital (London), 6
stable angina, 278
Stadol (butorphanol), 136

Stadol NS, 136
staph infections: and Vancocin, 70
staphylococcal penicillinases, 63
Staphylococcus, 380, 381
Staphylococcus aureus, 60, 75
status asthmaticus, 195, 199
status epilepticus, 171, 172
stavudine, 89
STDs. *See* sexually transmitted diseases
Stelazine (trifluoperazone), 153
sterility: and gonorrhea, 347
steroid production, *350*
steroids, 23
   topical, 392
   withdrawal from, 352
Stevens-Johnson syndrome, 61
stickers
   "shake well before using," 388
   "take with food," *67, 75, 76,* 321. *See also*
     labels/labeling
sticky ends, 400
stillbirths: and congenital syphilis, 348
stimulants: for weight reduction, 235, 240
stomach, 217, 218
stool-bulking capacity: of fiber, 227
strength of drug: and five "rights" for correct
   drug administration, 35, 50
strepomycin, 206
Streptase (streptokinase), 290
strep throat, 57, 79
streptococcal infections: and penicillin, 73
Streptococcus, 380, 381
Streptococcus pneumoniae, 61
streptogrammins, 69, 75, 78
streptokinase, 290
stress, 333
   and histidine, 45
   and psoriasis, 375
stress ulcers, 219, 239
stretch receptors: and cough reflex, 107, 109,
   113
stroke, 122, 267, 291-294, 301
   causes of, 291
   most-commonly used agents for TIAs and,
     292*t*
   and muscle relaxants, 312
   and oral contraceptives, 341-342
   prevention and management of, 292-294
   risk factors for, 292*t*
   and smoking, 207, 268
   types of, 291-292
strongyloides, 238
subacute bacterial endocarditis: penicillin
   for, 62
subcutaneous doses, 133
subcutaneous injections, 38
subcutaneous route of drug administration, 21
Sublimaze (fetanyl), 137
Sublimaze IV, 124
sublingual route of drug administration, 21, 38
successful aging, 40
succinylcholine, 124
sucralfate, 224
sudden arrhythmic death, 446
sudden cardiac death, 446
sugar infusion, 430*t*
sugarless over-the-counter products, 355*t*
sulfa allergies: and amprenavir, 91
sulfa drugs, 14, 196
sulfamethoxazole-trimethoprim, 253
Sulfamylon (mafenide acetate), 380
sulfasalazine, 225, 239
sulfate salt: in total parenteral nutrition
   mixtures, 433
sulfinpyrazone, 293, 294, 315, 324, 327
sulfonamides (sulfa drugs), 8, 57, 59, 73, 77,
   127
   commonly used, 61*t*
   and photosensitivity, 372
   side effects and dispensing issues with,
     61-62
sulfonylureas: and photosensitivity, 372
sulindac, 321
Sultrin, 349
sumatriptan, 135, 136, 138

sunburn, 47, 373
sunscreens, 373, 376
superinfections, 60, 73
superpotent topical steroid classes, 382*t*
supportive drugs, 445, 452
suppositories, 38, 50
suppuration, 378
Suprane (desflurane), 122
Suprax (cefixime), 65
surfactants, 212
surgery: history of, 119-120
surgical treatment: and obesity, 235
Survanta (beractant), 204
suspension dosage forms of otics: and
   ruptured ear drums, 389, 391
Sustiva (efavirenz), 90
swallowing of medications, 44
sweat glands, 371, 372
sweating, 118
syllables: in spelling of monoclonal antibody
   antirejection drugs, 410, 411
Symmetrel (amantadine), 87, 97, 179
sympathetic nervous system, 106, 118
Synercid (quinupristin-dalfopristin), 69
synergism, 27*t*
synthetic drugs, 8
synthetic organic chemistry, 6
synthetic vaccines, 43
Synthroid (levothyroxine), 335, 361, 451, 446
syphilis, 57, 347-348
   penicillin for, 62
   treatment of, 6, 349
syrup of ipecac, 443, 444, 451
syrups, 36, 50
systemic agents
   antifungal, 94
   antiviral, 87-88
   corticosteroids, 197
   drug summary of, 99
systemic effect, 26
systolic reading: blood pressure, 281

T

tablets, 36, 50
tachycardia, 271
tachypnea, 201
tacrine, 185
tacrolimus, 411
Tagamet, 23
Tagamet (cimetidine), 23, 46, 223
"Take with food" labels/stickers, *67, 75, 76,*
   321
Tambocor (flecainide), 273
Tamiflu (oseltamivir), 87
tamoxifen, 417
tamsulosin, 254, 259
Tapazole (methimazole), 336, 361
tapeworms, 236, 237-238
tardive dyskinesia
   and antianxiety agents, 155
   with antipsychotics, 153
target, 333, 361
target cells, 19
Tasmar (tolcapone), 180
Tavist (clemastine), 105, 110
Taxol (paclitaxel), 417
TB. *See* tuberculosis
TCAs. *See* tricyclic antidepressants
T-cell lymphocytes, 408
T-cell receptors, 413
T cells, 47, 406
TCRs. *See* T-cell receptors
Tegretol (carbamazepine), 151, 162, 175
Temodar (temozolamide), 416
temozolamide, 416
temperature regulation, 371
Tenex (guanfacine), 286
Tensilon (edrophonium), 181
Tenuate (diethylpropion), 235
teratogenic effects: with lithium, 151
Terazol (terconazole), 95
terazosin, 254, 286
terbinafine, 95, 375, 377

terbutaline, 196, 199, 210
terconazole, 95
terminator controls, *401*
tertiary-stage infection: with syphilis, 348
Tessalon Perles (benzonatate), 109
Testoderm, 337
testosterone, 337, 361
tetanus, 44
tetracaine, 127
tetracyclines, 59, 74, 77, 221, 237, 240, 347,
   349, 381, 446, 451
   for acne, 373
   commonly used, 66*t*
   side effects and dispensing issues with,
     66-67
   therapeutic uses of, 66
thalamus, 128, 177
Theo-dur, 199
theophylline, 197, 199, 200, 210
   and cystic fibrosis, 203
   and macrolides, 75
   and quinolones, 69
therapeutic effect, 26
therapeutic range, *24*
thiabendazole, 238
thiamine (B$_1$), 159, 435
thiazide diuretics, 256, 259, 301
   and cholesterol levels, 296
   and photosensitivity, 372
thiopental, 123, 137
thioridazine, 151, 162
third-generation cephalosporins, 74
thoracic stroke, 293
Thorazine (chlorpromazine), 136
three-dimensional (3-D) shape: of protein, 399
three-in-one formulations, 432, 450
thrombi: preventing, 287, 288-289
thrombocytopenia: with chemotherapy, 416
thrombolytic agents, 293
thromboxane A$_2$, 313
thromboxane formation, 293
thrush, 375
thymocytes, 408
thymus cells (T cells), 85
thyroglobulin, 333
thyroid, 333
thyroid cancer, 334
thyroid drugs, 8
thyroidectomy, 336
thyroid hormones, 333-336, 361
thyroiditis, 334
thyroid preparations: drug summary for, 364
thyroid replacement therapy, 334
thyroid stimulating hormone, 333
thyroid storm, 335
Thyrolar (liotrix), 335, 361
thyrotoxicosis, 335
thyroxine (T$_4$), 333
TIAs. *See* transient ischemic attacks
ticarcillin-clavulanate, 63
Ticlid (ticlopidine), 293
ticlopidine, 293
Tigan (trimethobenzamide), 233
time: and five "rights" for correct drug
   administration, 35-36, 50
Timentin (ticarcillin-clavulanate), 63
Tinactin (tolnaftate), 377
Tinver (sodium thiosulfate), 420
tinzaparin, 289, 301
tirofiban, 290
tissue injury: pain pathway in, *314*
tissue plasminogen activator, 290, 405
Titralac (calcium), 346
tizanidine, 184
TNA. *See* total nutrient admixture
TNF. *See* tumor necrosis factor
tocainide, 273
tocixity: and quinolones, 68
tocopherols, 435
Tofranil (imipramine), 156, 183
tolcapone, 180
tolnaftate, 377
tolterodine, 252, 259
tonic-clonic (Grand Mal) seizures, 170, 171
Tonocard (tocainide), 273

Photo Credits

cover Artville; **4** (top) Archivo Iconografico, S.A./CORBIS; **4** (bottom) CORBIS; **5** Bettmann/CORBIS; **6** Minnesota Historical Society/CORBIS; **7** Janeart/Image Bank; **36** McNeil Pharmaceutical, McNeilab, Inc.; **58** (bottom) Copyright Biodisc, Inc.; **84** SuperStock; **93** Lester V. Bergman/CORBIS; **108** Edward Gallucci/Doctor Stock; **109** Custom Medical Stock Photos; **114** Courtesy of Pfizer Inc., New York, NY; **130** Michael English/Custom Medical Stock Photos; **195** Custom Medical Stock Photos; **197** Custom Medical Stock Photos; **203** Courtesy of Dr. Kenneth Nowak; **263** Courtesy of Hoechst Marion Roussel Inc., Kansas City, MO; **264** Courtesy of Proctor & Gamble; **295** (left) Custom Medical Stock Photos; **295** (right) Custom Medical Stock Photos; **307** Reproduced with permission of Glaxo Wellcome Inc.; **383** (left) SPL/Custom Medical Stock Photos; **383** (right) J.L. Carlson/Custom Medical Stock Photos; **384** Custom Medical Stock Photos; **442** Hans Reinhard/OKAPIAPhoto Researchers, Inc.